Stuttering

Meets Stereotype,

Stigma,

and Discrimination

STUTTERING
MEETS STEREOTYPE, STIGMA, and DISCRIMINATION

An Overview
of Attitude Research

Kenneth O. St. Louis

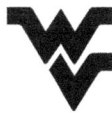

WEST VIRGINIA UNIVERSITY
MORGANTOWN 2015

Published by West Virginia University Press for West Virginia University
Copyright © 2015 West Virginia University Press
All rights reserved
First edition published 2015 by West Virginia University Press
Printed in the United States of America

22 21 20 19 18 17 16 15   1 2 3 4 5 6 7 8 9
ISBN:

cloth   978-1-940425-36-8
paper   978-1-940425-39-9
epub   978-1-940425-37-5
pdf   978-1-940425-38-2

Cataloging-in-Publication Data is available from the Library of Congress

Book and cover design by Than Saffel

Contents

PART III: RESEARCH: ATTITUDES OF PROFESSIONALS

Foreword

Glen Tellis

When Dr. Kenneth O. St. Louis invited me to serve as Chair of the Program Committee for the inaugural Stuttering Attitudes Research Symposium at West Virginia University, I was very pleased to accept his offer. I believed that it was important to have a forum where world-class researchers could present stuttering attitude research. This four-day conference in September 2013—the first conference specifically focused on fluency attitudinal research—was the brainchild of Dr. St. Louis. He and his team worked tirelessly to offer a high-caliber conference with leaders in the field. In response to a circulated invitation, I coordinated peer review by at least three experts in stuttering attitude research of all author submissions for research presentations. From this process, many outstanding proposals were accepted. These proposals were presented as posters— and also as short papers—to complement five invited papers by primary speakers at the symposium. In my judgment, the entire symposium was well organized and efficiently run. The tight-knit group of attendees came from all over the world to discuss research and strategize about future collaborations (St. Louis, Weidner, Gabel, Hughes, & Coleman, 2014).

After a careful review, the West Virginia University Press agreed to publish this volume of selected proceedings from the Stuttering Attitudes Research Symposium. Subsequent to follow-up invitations to authors, manuscripts were prepared for each original presentation. These further peer-reviewed manuscripts include considerations of epidemiology of public attitudes toward stuttering; stigma and stuttering; bullying experienced by those who stutter; Native American cultural perspectives about stuttering; and attitudes about stuttering from several countries, including the United States, Canada, Sudan, Poland, Sri Lanka, Iran, and Kuwait. Other topics covered in these proceedings include job discrimination associated with stuttering, workplace implications for those who stutter, helping professions, and coursework that specifically pertains to stuttering. This book also has chapters that discuss positive aspects of stuttering as perceived by the general public, changing attitudes toward stuttering, and interdisciplinary training programs in stuttering to raise awareness and change attitudes. A chapter on a new clinical tool to measure stuttering attitudes in a client's environment is also included. Finally, an annotated bibliography serves as a good reference list of attitudinal studies.

Chapters by Kenneth St. Louis, Michael Boyle, and Gordon Blood cover variables associated with stuttering, stigma, and coping mechanisms for those who stutter. In the chapter on epidemiology, Kenneth St. Louis thoroughly describes public attitudes toward stuttering, using his *Public Opinion Survey of Human Attributes–Stuttering* (*POSHA–S*) to discuss variables associated with stuttering and those that could potentially predict future changes in stuttering attitudes. Michael Boyle and Gordon Blood provide many models of stigma and summarize coping mechanisms used by people who stutter to deal with stigma associated with stuttering. The authors describe the multidimensional nature of stuttering and offer suggestions to reduce stigma experienced by those who stutter.

In recent years, bullying has surfaced as a major area of concern, especially as it relates to stuttering. Marilyn Langevin, Susanne Cook, and Peter Howell provide information about specific issues that relate to bullying and stuttering. They also suggest several intervention strategies to reduce stuttering-related bullying. In her chapter, Marilyn Langevin outlines peer rejection and coping styles of children who stutter and who are victims of bullying. Susanne Cook and Peter Howell describe the psychosocial impact of bullying and the differences in perspectives between children and their parents with regard to the impact of stuttering and bullying. The authors indicate that in some instances, parents perceive the psychosocial impact and the experience of bullying as more severe than their children. The authors recommend group counseling with parents and children who stutter to discuss education-related concerns and the use of specific strategies to address bullying.

Several researchers from around the world—including Ann Beste-Guldborg, Nichole Campanale, Kenneth St. Louis, Yomna Elsiddig, Charles Haynes, Julie Atwood, Katarzyna Węsierska, Marta Węsierska, Saminda Kuruppu, Chantha Jayawardena, Staci LeMasters, Ahmad Poormohammad, Fauzia Abdalla, Megan Burgess, and Chelsea Kuhn—provide cultural perspectives about stuttering. The common theme that emerges from these papers is that negative attitudes toward stuttering are still pervasive. Results of many of these studies indicate that negative personality stereotypes associated with stuttering still exist; however, moderately positive or neutral reactions to the disorder seem to be emerging.

Ann Beste-Guldborg, Kenneth St. Louis, and Nichole Campanale, in their chapter on helping professions, indicate that the negative stereotype associated with stuttering exists in the workplace. The authors examined the perceptions of professionals in mental health, education, health care, and law enforcement and noted the presence of the stuttering stereotype and anxiety related to communicating with people who stutter. The authors found that the presence of the stuttering stereotype exists in all groups. By and large, these groups were uneasy when interacting with those who stutter. These groups expressed uncertainty about the cause of stuttering and were not aware of where they could receive accurate information about stuttering.

In his chapter on job discrimination associated with stuttering, Rodney Gabel explained theories relating to role entrapment, marginalization, paternalism, and stigma. He indicates that people who stutter may experience discrimination related to employment and provides suggestions for reducing discrimination, including attending speech-language therapy and acknowledgment of stuttering during job interviews. Jill Douglass and John Tetnowski conducted a qualitative study to determine the impact covert stuttering has on workplace performance. In their chapter, the authors describe the professional penalties experienced by people who stutter and suggest reasons they choose to hide their stuttering in the workplace. The major themes that emerged from this research include participants' justification for maintaining their covert status to save face and maintain their professional reputation. Another theme that emerged, however, was the realization that hiding their stuttering professionally was unproductive because of professional penalties associated with keeping quiet instead of speaking up during meetings.

Not every chapter in this book relates to negative stereotypes associated with stuttering. Some authors have argued that it is possible to change attitudes toward stuttering. Lejla Junuzović-Žunić, Mary Weidner, Isabella Reichel, Susanne Cook, Kenneth St. Louis, and Mercedes Ware reviewed the impact on speech-language pathology students' stuttering attitudes of fluency disorders coursework. The authors mention that to potentially change attitudes of a certain group toward stuttering, universities should include sensitivity training during academic coursework. Results of their study indicate that students' attitudes improved after completing fluency disorders coursework. Similarly, Stephanie Hughes and Edward Strugalla provided a chapter on what the general public perceives as positive aspects of stuttering. The authors note that fluent speakers assign the positive traits of compassion, motivation, and perseverance to people who stutter. Two other chapters address changing attitudes toward stuttering. Marilyn Langevin indicated in her qualitative research chapter that school-age children are interested in learning about stuttering. Marilyn noted that children who stutter who are in environments where peers have learned about stuttering may be less vulnerable to bullying and are more likely to be accepted by peers. In Fauzia Abdalla's chapter, she mentions that educating and instructing people on issues related to stigma associated with stuttering may result in more positive attitudes toward people who stutter. Exploring various strategies used to change attitudes, she points out that specially constructed videos have been shown to be beneficial.

Complementing other chapters in the book, Stephanie Hughes, Rodney Gabel, Christopher Roseman, and Derek Daniels propose an interdisciplinary training program in stuttering designed to raise awareness and change attitudes in speech-language pathology students and counseling students. The authors suggested collaborations between students training to be school counselors and speech-language pathology graduate students. After participating in an eight-day intensive stuttering clinic for children who stutter, the students training to be school counselors and speech-language pathology graduate students learned factual information about stuttering, recognized the socio-emotional needs of children who stutter, and began to consider how they could work together to provide optimal services to children who stutter.

This book also introduces a new clinical tool (*Appraisal of the Stuttering Environment*) to measure stuttering attitudes in a client's environment. This tool, developed by Kenneth St. Louis, Chelsea Kuhn, and Lindsey Lytwak, measures the extent to which stuttering attitudes of adults who stutter diverge from those of their family members and close friends, and how these attitudes are different from those of the general public. In the last chapter in this book, Stephanie Hughes provides a comprehensive annotated bibliography. It includes summaries of 76 published studies about attitudes toward stuttering and covers several decades of attitude research. Though every peer-reviewed attitude study could not be covered in this annotated bibliography, Stephanie attempted to provide references to seminal studies, recent research articles, and papers that suggest new avenues for research.

I hope you enjoy and benefit from this compilation of chapters from the inaugural Stuttering Attitudes Research Symposium. I believe that this publication will serve as a wonderful reference for students, researchers, clinicians, and others who are interested in stuttering attitudinal research.

Preface

More than a century of research has sought to identify the causes of stuttering, describe its nature, and enhance its clinical treatment. Those continued efforts have borne real fruit in such areas as understanding genetic factors in stuttering's cause, identifying brain differences in individuals who stutter, generating models that can explain stuttering symptoms, documenting numerous conditions that often coexist with stuttering, and developing more effective strategies to reduce stuttering. By contrast, the environment within which stuttering occurs has not enjoyed such a long history of research interest; studies directly focused upon public and professional attitudes toward stuttering began in the 1970s. From the beginning, this research has identified stereotypes and negative attitudes toward stuttering. Literally hundreds of studies have replicated these findings in numerous ways and in myriad population samples. Recent years have also seen a flurry of comparison studies around the world that have documented the universality of negative public attitudes. Finally, recent efforts have taken this research to new levels, including the development of standard measures; comparing work in stuttering to that in other areas such as mental illness; addressing the widely reported phenomena of teasing, bullying, and discrimination against people who stutter; and attempting to change public opinion toward stuttering to more accepting and sensitive levels.

As editor and author, my personal stake in this area comes from my own stuttering from childhood into adulthood. Although mostly recovered, I still stutter and experience the reactions to that stuttering from those around me. Societal attitudes toward stuttering did affect me negatively as a child and adolescent. Fortunately, most of the reactions are now generally neutral, or even positive. Additionally, my research in this area was motivated as well by a long-held desire to carry out collaborative, international research.

Stuttering Meets Stereotype, Stigma, and Discrimination: An Overview of Attitude Research is the culmination of the first meeting devoted exclusively to research on public attitudes toward stuttering and their ramifications. In September 2013, experts in this area convened in Morgantown, West Virginia, for the inaugural Stuttering Attitudes Research Symposium with presentations representing North America, Europe, the Middle East, Asia, Africa, and New Zealand. The meeting's overarching purposes were to take stock of what has been learned so far in stuttering attitude research and to identify areas where further research would be most fruitful. The hope is that this book will not only become a valuable resource that makes sense of this burgeoning area of research, but also be a catalyst for designing additional high-impact short- or long-term studies. Among the latter would be future research that can inform policy makers, speech-language pathologists, people who stutter, parents of children who stutter, and indeed the public about how best to cope with and mitigate negative public attitudes toward those who stutter.

As the title implies, stuttering is typically met with stereotypes (some negative and a few positive), stigma, and even discrimination. The book is organized in such a way as to lead the reader through a maze of research efforts, emerging with a clear understanding of the important issues involved and ideas of where to go next. It will be immediately clear to any reader that assertions are not simply expert opinion; they are supported by empirical evidence. The annotated bibliography of the review and research chapters is extensive, containing 76 entries. Importantly, the evidence base for stuttering attitude research extends beyond research in this fluency disorder to such areas as mental illness, obesity, and race. Thus, although of interest primarily to those who work, interact, or otherwise deal with stuttering, the book has potential for understanding, ameliorating, or informing research in any of a host of "unwanted" human attributes.

Who, specifically, would be likely to find *Stuttering Meets Stereotype, Stigma, and Discrimination: An Overview of Attitude Research* useful or helpful? Researchers or those interested in research that deals with better understanding public attitudes toward stuttering will find the book a "must read" if they wish to locate the important, current information in one place. It will especially help them distinguish between areas of inquiry that have already been satisfactorily investigated and those that are either in need of further understanding or have not yet been addressed. And just as the research in stuttering has drawn from a larger body of research on other stigmatized conditions such as mental illness, obesity, HIV/AIDS, epilepsy, and so on, researchers in those areas will find information in this book that can inform their own future studies.

People who stutter, and their relatives (especially parents) and friends, will find a wealth of information in this book that they can use to better understand their own attitudes juxtaposed against those of the public. For example, anyone who deals with unsettling public attitudes—ranging from misinformation all the way to illegal discrimination—will discover evidence they can use to cope with, confront, or even fight these situations. Those stutterers and others who are or intend to be advocates in the self-help movement for stuttering will encounter strategies that have been shown to help improve public attitudes and those that are ineffective.

For clinical speech-language pathologists, the book includes existing and new instruments that can be used with stuttering clients and their families. Additionally, in spite of good intentions, speech-language pathologists as well as psychologists, counselors, teachers, health care workers, and other professionals will no doubt be both surprised and dismayed upon reading that professional attitudes toward stuttering no doubt contribute to the stereotypes, stigma, and discrimination that many stutterers experience. Accordingly, this book will be a valuable addition to the library of anyone who is in the business of helping people.

Faculty in the fields of communication sciences and disorders, social psychology, sociology, education, counseling, nursing, and related fields will find relevant information in this book, sufficient to either require all or parts of it in advanced classes or as suggested resources. A considerable amount of the extant research in public attitudes toward stuttering has been carried out by students at both undergraduate and graduate levels. Accordingly, faculty members who advise or direct student research would find the book an especially useful resource.

Since *Stuttering Meets Stereotype, Stigma, and Discrimination: An Overview of Attitude Research* is the only reference work to date devoted entirely to the topic of stuttering attitudes, it will be useful to anyone else who might be interested in any of the topics covered. As such, community, school, and university librarians will find the book to be an important acquisition for policy makers in areas relating to citizen well-being, journalists seeking background for stories about stuttering, lawyers who might be involved in cases of stuttering-related bullying or discrimination, high school students seeking term-paper topics, and anyone from the public seeking an overview or specific information on the topics of stereotype, stigma, and discrimination.

Acknowledgments

Without the help of many people, this book would never have been published. Foremost among those to whom I am most grateful is my wife and best friend, Rae Jean Sielen. Her steady patience was the anchor I required as I conceptualized and brought this project to reality. She willingly permitted me to work far too many extra hours at my office on nights and weekends as the two-year process of planning, organizing, corresponding, writing, editing, and finalizing of this volume progressed. Likewise, I am not sure how I could have completed the project without the willing, able, and valuable assistance of Mary Weidner. She entered our PhD program at West Virginia University just two weeks before the international research symposium took place. That symposium was the genesis of this book. Mary's talent, incredibly hard work, tact, organization, and communication skills were an integral part of every single aspect of the initiative from start to finish.

Of course, I am indebted to all the authors and coauthors for the excellent chapters they wrote, as well as for their willingness to deal with my often picayune editorial suggestions for their chapters. Most of these individuals played critical roles in the peer-review process of other authors' chapters as well, and a few also had volunteered to participate in the original peer review of the symposium presentations. Others who did not contribute chapters to the book were important peer reviewers and reviewers of the book proposal as well. All of them should be acknowledged, not only because it is the right thing to do, but to focus attention on the broad spectrum of expertise that undergirds the content of this book. Listed alphabetically, they are: Fauzia Abdalla, Hayley Arnold, Ann Beste-Guldborg, Paul Blanchet, Michael Boyle, Craig Coleman, Susanne Cook, Joe Donaher, Jill Douglass, Rodney Gabel, Sheryl Gottwald, Jacqueline Guendouzi, Peter Howell, Stephanie Hughes, Farzan Irani, Harsha Kathard, Joe Klein, Mary Ellen Koay, Marilyn Langevin, Margaret Leahy, Norimune Kawai, Sertan Özdemir, Bob Quesal, Jean Sawyer, Lynne Shields, Hilda Sønsterud, Ed Strugalla, Glen Tellis, John Tetnowski, Ying-Chiao Tsao, Mary Weidner, Katarzyna Węsierska, and Scott Yaruss.

Finally, I am indebted to the faculty and staff at West Virginia University's Communication Sciences & Disorders Department in the College of Education & Human Services and to the capable people at WVU Press at West Virginia University for their solid support in making this book a reality. While overjoyed that the book is finished, I have again learned that when people come together for a worthwhile common purpose, extraordinary things happen.

Ken St. Louis, Editor

Introduction

One might imagine that this book constitutes the proceedings for the 2013 symposium. In many ways, it is. Yet, it is *not* titled *Proceedings of the 1st Stuttering Attitudes Research Symposium* for two important reasons. The primary reason is that it includes far more than the information presented at the symposium. Authors of the review chapters in the first half of the book had been invited to make keynote presentations on five main topics at the symposium and then to develop them into chapters. In every case, the review chapters were extensively reorganized, augmented with new material, and carefully edited. Subsequent to the symposium, most—but not all—authors and coauthors whose submitted research proposals had been peer-reviewed and accepted for posters and short oral presentations were invited to develop them into chapters for this book. Another important reason that the book is not a typical proceedings collection is that all the invited chapters, both from the keynote speakers and the research authors, were sent out for further peer review. Upon receiving comments and evaluation of the reviewers, as editor, I carried out an extensive edit myself of each contribution, based on the reviewers' comments and evaluation and my own careful reading. Not every chapter was accepted in its invited form, and most of them—including my own—underwent minor to extensive editorial changes. I subsequently carried out another equally careful review of each revised chapter and, where deemed necessary, requested further clarifications from the authors. In this second review, editorial changes were made or suggested that, unlike a typical collection of papers in a special edition of a journal, would enhance the book's reader friendliness, cohesiveness, and format consistency.

Stuttering Meets Stereotype, Stigma, and Discrimination: An Overview of Attitude Research is organized first into review chapters and research chapters. In order, the review chapters provide extensive reviews on five key subareas relating to the research on stuttering attitudes: (1) *epidemiology* of stuttering attitudes; (2) *stigma* and *self-stigma* resulting from stuttering; (3) *bullying* (and its closely related topic of teasing) in stuttering children; (4) employment *discrimination* and related issues faced by stutterers; (5) and *changing* or *improving* stuttering attitudes.

Following are 15 research chapters, which are brief reports related to specific current studies of stuttering attitudes. The first five describe studies that sought attitudes of members of the *non-stuttering* public at large. The next five relate to investigations of the attitudes of *professionals* who would be likely to interact with individuals who stutter, either children or adults. The final five studies sample the attitudes of children and adults *who stutter themselves*, and in some cases, attitudes of *their family or friends*. Within each category, quantitative research studies are presented first, followed (if present) by mixed-method studies, and then by qualitative studies. Research participants represented in the research chapters are diverse. They represent diversity of nationality (Canadians, Americans, Poles, Bosnian-Herzegovinians, Iranians, Kuwaitis, and Sudanese), ethnic group (e.g., Native Americans), religion (e.g., primarily Christian, Muslim, and Jewish samples), sex (i.e., females versus males), type of stuttering (i.e., covert versus overt), and age (children and adults).

The last contribution is an invited annotated bibliography that contains important previous and recent research studies. This important chapter provides both historical and topical coverage of seminal research studies in stuttering attitudes through brief descriptions of key investigations through the years, placing the review and research chapters into a meaningful perspective.

At the end of the book, a list of references of all the sources cited is included. Additionally, the book contains an author index listing the works of individual authors in each chapter.

A few comments are in order regarding the style of the book. Authors were asked to follow the current version of American Psychological Association (APA) guidelines in their manuscripts. Some would argue that the APA convention of placing the authors' names and dates in all citations renders text harder to read than would be the case with some version of footnotes. That may be true, but since (1) the evidence base for the material in this book is important and (2) most stuttering attitudes investigators are extremely familiar with the author/date citation system, it was maintained. Two departures from recommended APA guidelines do appear in the book. The guidelines currently dictate that any reference with more than six authors be cited as "first author + et al.," even the first time it occurs. In this book, all the authors are listed in the first citation of a multi-authored work. Also, APA guidelines mandate the use of "person-first" language rather than direct labeling, i.e., "person/child/adult who stutters" versus "stutterer." Based on research showing that this distinction makes virtually no difference in judgments of hypothetical people who stutter (e.g., see St. Louis, 1999), the term "stutterer" does appear in some chapters when the authors determined that it was less awkward than using a person-first equivalent. More important, whereupon in the stuttering literature, "person who stutters" and similar nomenclature have been typically replaced by acronyms, e.g., "PWS," "CWS," "PWNS," or "PWDNS," such acronyms do not appear in this book except occasionally in tables or figures. Instead, person-first language is written out in order to foster readability for those unfamiliar with the acronyms and also to avoid the possibility that the acronyms themselves defeat the intended benefit of using person-first language.

Stuttering Meets Stereotype, Stigma, and Discrimination: An Overview of Attitude Research was truly a team effort. Individually and together, the contributors to this book share the goal of one day improving the daily lives of people who stutter.

Part One

REVIEW

Chapter 1

Epidemiology of Public Attitudes Toward Stuttering

Kenneth O. St. Louis

ABSTRACT

Epidemiology of public attitudes toward stuttering concerns comparisons among different populations regarding public attitudes, as well as variables that are associated with or could potentially predict future changes in such attitudes. This chapter reviews the rationale for studying public attitudes and a small sample of the literature that has done so. It focuses primarily on a standard measure of public attitudes that has been translated to other languages and used worldwide, the *Public Opinion Survey of Human Attributes–Stuttering* (*POSHA–S*) (St. Louis, 2011a). The chapter summarizes investigations that have used the *POSHA–S* with different populations, the public at large, teachers, speech-language pathologists (SLPs) or SLP students, people who stutter, and so on. Consideration is given to variables that have been associated with more versus less positive attitudes, such as video or live presentations about stuttering to individuals that have typically resulted in improved ratings on the *POSHA–S*. Future research recommendations are grounded in preliminary investigations that have shown certain variables, such as SLP training, to be associated with—and potential predictors of—more positive attitudes.

Relevance of Epidemiology to the Study of Public Attitudes

A voluminous literature exists on public attitudes toward stuttering. The chapters by Abdalla (Chapter 5), Boyle and Blood (Chapter 2), Gabel (Chapter 4),

Hughes (Chapter 21), and Langevin (Chapter 3) review relevant past research contributions to that literature and important new contributions. New research contributions in this volume are valuable additions to the literature as well. This chapter addresses a relatively new subset of such research, the epidemiology of stuttering attitudes. This is not the common use of the term "epidemiology," which derives from "epidemic" and most often deals with the distribution of diseases. More appropriately, this chapter's content could be considered part of "social epidemiology" (Krieger, 2000), which among many other areas, deals with discrimination. Indeed, as shown clearly by Boyle and Blood (Chapter 2), Gabel (Chapter 4), as well as others, public attitudes toward stuttering can be considered directly harmful to others. In this way, epidemiological research is unlike, for example, surveys of political views of various populations around the world by such organizations as Gallup Politics (2014). A more important distinction as contributions to the literature relating to stuttering is that epidemiology typically seeks to make inferences about populations, unlike most stuttering research, which seeks to infer about individuals or isolated groups. Overlap exists between these two approaches, but epidemiological measures are often designed not to consider individual differences but population trends.

Why Study Public Attitudes Toward Stuttering?

It is widely accepted that most cases of stuttering are due to genetically based, sex-linked physiological differences that affect the coordination and timing of neuromotor aspects of speaking (Bloodstein & Bernstein Ratner, 2008; Howell, 2010). Nearly all of the thousands of research studies devoted to stuttering have addressed why stuttering occurs, how it develops, what its correlates are, and what its effects are on those who have the disorder. Very little, by comparison, has dealt with what those who do not stutter bring to the problem.

The rationale for studying public attitudes toward stuttering and other stigmatizing conditions seems obvious and has been the impetus for most studies. Since the public often holds negative and stigmatizing beliefs, feelings, and thoughts about stuttering or those who stutter, and since people who stutter grow up surrounded by such views, then much of the social penalty experienced by people who stutter derives from these views. Calls for accurate information about stuttering to be disseminated to the public have been widespread, and initiatives to do just that have been carried out at local, regional, national, and even international levels (e.g., Gabel, Brackenbury, & Irani, 2010; International Stuttering Association, 2014; National Stuttering Association, 2014b; The Stuttering Foundation, 2014b). The assumption is that providing better information to the public will result in better attitudes, which will in turn result in less social penalty for those who stutter. Hopefully, they would feel better about themselves (even with the stuttering); would be expected to talk about it more openly; would experience less teasing, bullying, or discrimination; and would be able to function better at home, school, and work.

These are "armchair" deductions that may well be true, but actually little evidence exists to support the underlying assumptions. Until recently, with few exceptions (e.g., de Britto Pereira, Rossi, & Van Borsel, 2008; Van Borsel, Verniers, & Bouvry, 1999; Xing Ming, Jing, Yi Wen, & Van Borsel, 2001), it was not possible to compare public attitudes accurately from one population to another since most investigations used different measures. Neither was it possible to determine if strategies designed to improve public attitudes were more effective than placebo or no treatments or, more specifically, which strategies might be most effective. The lack of such evidence underlies the research summarized in this chapter. It was motivated by the perceived need to develop a *standard measure* of public attitudes toward stuttering such that (1) populations around the world could be compared on the same measure and (2) the effectiveness of various strategies to change stuttering could be compared. If such a measure could be developed, then questions, such as the following, could be answered: (1) When most people interact with a person who stutters, what do they do, what do they feel, and what do they think? (2) What difference do their actions, feelings, thoughts, and knowledge make to people who stutter? (3) Can their beliefs and reactions be changed? (4) If so, how would they be changed, and how long will it take? (5) Would those changes be short term or permanent? (6) Finally, what differences would it make to people who stutter with whom most people interact as their beliefs and reactions were changed?

Development of a Standard Measure of Public Attitudes Toward Stuttering

In several publications, St. Louis and colleagues explicated a new initiative called the International Project on Attitudes Toward Human Attributes (IPATHA) (St. Louis, 2005, 2014, 2012c; St. Louis, Lubker, Yaruss, Adkins, & Pill, 2008). Inaugurated by an invited task force that met in Morgantown, West Virginia, in 1999, the IPATHA initiated development of a prototype of the *Public Opinion Survey of Human Attributes–Stuttering* (*POSHA–S*). It also laid the groundwork for measuring other human attributes, ranging from positive to neutral to negative, against which stuttering could be compared. In the 14 years since its inception, the IPATHA initiative has completed a final version of the *POSHA–S*. Additionally, a parallel version for cluttering has been developed and used (*POSHA–Cl*)

(St. Louis, Filatova, Coşkun, Topbaş, Özdemir, Georgieva, McCaffrey, & George, 2011; St. Louis, Sønsterud, Carlo, Heitmann, & Kvenseth, 2014). Cluttering is a fluency disorder characterized by a rapid rate of speech and attendant sequelae, including any combination of excessive normal disfluencies, abnormally collapsed syllables, and atypical prosody (St Louis & Schulte, 2011). Prototype instruments for mental illness (*POSHA–MI*) (St. Louis & Roberts, 2013) and obesity (*POSHA–Ob*) have been developed as well. Moreover, a Web site has been established, www.stutteringattitudes.com (St. Louis, 2014). The IPATHA vision is "to understand and improve public attitudes toward stuttering and other stigmatizing conditions worldwide through objective measurement." Its mission is "to foster effective use of the *Public Opinion Survey of Human Attributes* (*POSHA*) in comparing public attitudes and reducing stigma related to negative public opinion."

The *POSHA–S* has undergone two major changes since its inception. The first prototype featured a quasi-continuous scale, which, although satisfactory as a measure, was not at all user-friendly for either respondents or those responsible for tallying and reducing the data. The second version used most of the same items but with a 9-point rating scale. It was shown to be equivalent to the first prototype, but required more time to complete than was assumed to be satisfactory for any final version. (The second version was adapted for a clinical instrument called the *Appraisal of the Stuttering Environment* (*ASE*) and described by St. Louis, Kuhn, and Lytwak, [Chapter 16].) The final, much shortened *POSHA–S* was preceded by systematic item analysis (described in St. Louis, 2012c). It is characterized by a simpler rating scale, with 1–5 ratings for demographic and comparisons of stuttering to other attributes and converted 1–3 ratings for most stuttering items. All scaled ratings are converted to values from -100 to +100 with 0 being neutral. In order to avoid response bias, higher ratings do not consistently reflect more positive attitudes. Thus, ratings for some items are inverted in the analysis so that higher scores are consistently associated with more accurate, sensitive, and data-driven responses, and vice versa.

The *POSHA–S* has a demographic section that contains common variables such as age, sex, education, birthplace and current residence, marital and parental status, occupation, race, and religion. It also contains a relative income measure derived from a 1–5 rating of one's income relative to (1) one's family and friends and (2) all the people in one's country in order that incomes can be compared across widely different economies. Additional items ask about physical health, mental health, learning ability, and speaking ability, as well as life priorities that might be related to better versus worse stuttering attitudes, e.g., "being safe and secure," "doing my job or duty," or "having exciting but potentially dangerous experiences." The general section asks respondents to rate three items for each of five human attributes (stuttering, mental illness, obesity, left-handedness, and intelligence), as well as to complete a checklist of those whom they know (including themselves) with each of these attributes. The items relate to "overall impression," "want to be or have [the attribute]," and "amount known about [the attribute]." Finally, a detailed stuttering section asks for ratings on stuttering items, which are categorized as (1) Beliefs about people who stutter that are external to the respondent or (2) Self Reactions to people who stutter that refer to the respondents' own reactions, feelings, and actions when interacting with a person who stutters. Items are combined into components (e.g., Cause or Sympathy and Social Distance), and components are combined into three subscores. Beliefs and Self Reactions subscores are averaged for an Overall Stuttering Score (OSS). In addition the *POSHA–S* has an Obesity/Mental Illness subscore.

The *POSHA–S* is an explicit measure of attitudes using self-report. Attitudes are not inferred (1) implicitly (e.g., Gawronski & Bodenhausen, 2006); (2) from physiological measures (e.g., Guntupalli, Everhart, Kalinowski, Nanjundewaran, & Saltluklaroglu, 2007) or (3) from observation of the behavior of participants (e.g., McDonald & Frick, 1954). Instead, it employs simple, unambiguous, and direct language that enhances accurate translations to other languages. To further enhance reliable translations, it does not include a definition of stuttering, although research has shown that addition of a definition does not change the results (St. Louis et al., 2011; St. Louis et al., 2014). Similarly, the *POSHA–S* does not provide audio or video examples of stuttering for the related reason that they would be extremely difficult to translate to other languages without introducing other variables such as different voices, dialects or accents, faces, races, and so on.

Most of the IPATHA-related research to date has been with the *POSHA–S*, and much of that has related to its development and documentation of sociometric and user-related properties. The *POSHA–S* has been found to demonstrate: (1) satisfactory agreement among the items (internal consistency) (Al-Khaledi, Lincoln, McCabe, Packman, & Alshatti, 2009; St. Louis, 2012c); (2) minimal change in repeated administrations two weeks apart (test-retest reliability) (St. Louis, 2012c; St. Louis, Lubker, Yaruss, & Aliveto, 2009); (3) changes in the expected direction in studies designed to improve attitudes (construct validity) (Abdalla & St. Louis, 2014; Flynn & St. Louis, 2011; St. Louis, Reichel, Yaruss, & Lubker, 2009); and (4) greater differences than similarities with another widely used measure of attitudes, i.e., the Woods and Williams (1976) "bipolar adjective scale" (concurrent or divergent validity) (St. Louis, Reichel, et al., 2009; St. Louis, Williams, Ware, Guendouzi, & Reichel, 2014). The *POSHA–S* has also been shown to manifest: (1) adequate readability and user friendliness (St. Louis et al., 2008); (2) equivalence in two different languages (St. Louis & Roberts, 2010); and (3) equivalence with online versus paper-and-pencil administration (St. Louis, 2012b). The instrument was shown to be (1) amenable for use with probability versus convenience sampling (Abdalla & St. Louis, 2012; Özdemir, St. Louis, & Topbaş, 2011a); (2) robust with respect to small versus large sample sizes (St. Louis, 2008); and (3) comparable from study to study using standard scoring and graphic results carried out by partners or volunteers (e.g., St. Louis, 2012c; Özdemir et al., 2011a; Özdemir, St. Louis, & Topbaş, 2011b; Ip, St. Louis, Myers, & An Xue, 2012; Przepiórka, Błachnio, St. Louis, & Wozniak, 2013).

Arguably, the most important aspect of the IPATHA initiative is the *POSHA–S* database. Interested researchers have been granted permission to translate and/ or use the *POSHA–S* without payment in exchange for sending the author an electronic copy of their raw data to build the database. Circa July 2013, the *POSHA–S* had been translated to 20 different languages and used in 29 countries. These represent 119 different respondent samples from 8,144 respondents. All of these completed the *POSHA–S* only once or more than once. Sixty-nine of these samples involved respondents completing the instrument two or three times. Combining all samples analyzed (first or only time analyzed plus multiple times analyzed) yielded a total of 188 samples, which are listed on the IPATHA Web site.

Standard POSHA–S Graphic Profiles

Figure 1.1 depicts the standard *POSHA–S* radial graph into which individual samples can be placed. Better or more positive attitudes are toward the periphery while worse or less positive attitudes are toward the center. Components listed clockwise after each of the circled subscores—i.e., Beliefs, Obesity/Mental Illness, and Self Reactions—are shown by the dotted and curved arrows. For example, the Beliefs subscore is the mean of the components shown as Traits, [Who Should] Help, Cause, and Potential. Similar components are shown for the Self Reactions subscore and the Obesity/Mental Illness subscore. The lowest and highest sample means for each component and subscore obtained from all the samples analyzed are shown in the graph for first or multiple administrations (e.g., including pre- and post-administrations in studies attempting to change attitudes). Between them is the median of those sample means for the sole or first administration (when multiple administrations occurred). Unlike the lowest and highest values for which extreme values are sought (see below), the median is reported so that extreme mean scores do not affect the average

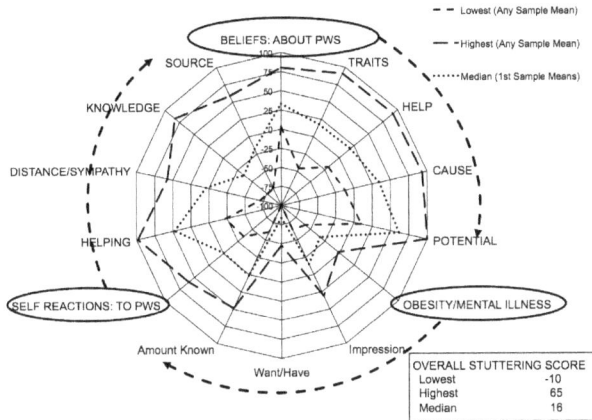

Figure 1.1: *POSHA–S* radial graph showing the lowest, highest, and median database samples for the three subscores and their components, as well as the Overall Stuttering Scores.

as much as would be the case considering the mean of the sample means. The Overall Stuttering Score (OSS) of the sample in question is typically shown in the box at the lower right; however, in Figure 1.1, the OSSs for the lowest, highest, and median values from the 188 means in the *POSHA–S* database are shown, i.e., -10, 65, and 16.

The two highest and two lowest samples obtained to date in the *POSHA–S* database are shown in Figure 1.2. The two highest, based on their OSSs of 65 and 61, respectively, were self-help leaders, most from North America but with a few from Western Europe (St. Louis & George, 2008; St. Louis, Kuhn, & Lytwak, Chapter 16) and SLPs who were fluency specialists in the United States (St. Louis, Tellis, Tuanquin, Wolfenden, & Nicholson, 2004; St. Louis et al., Chapter 16), both administered in English. The two lowest, with OSSs of -10 and -9, respectively, were mid-socioeconomic status (SES) adults from India who responded in Hindi (Kanaka, St. Louis, Usmani, & Rajashekhar, 2012) and mostly professional males from Nepal in English (Knudsen, Kathard, St. Louis, & Shrestha, 2004). The graph shows that the two highest samples comprised or approximated the highest sample means observed to date, with the reverse for the two lowest samples. Large differences characterized the stuttering components and subscores, but much smaller differences were observed for Obesity/Mental Illness ratings.

Not only are the differences visible for the negativity-positivity of the attitudes, the pattern or profile of each of the four tracings is different. A challenge

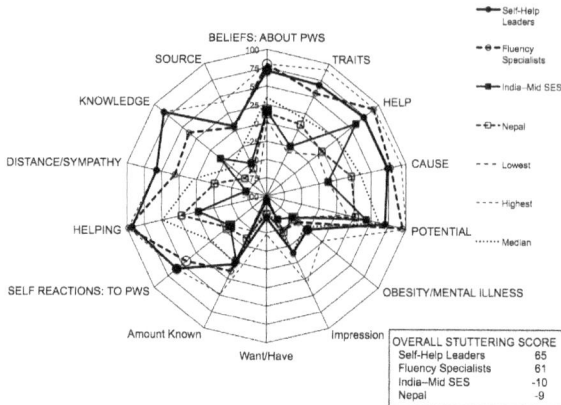

FIGURE 1.2: *POSHA–S* graphs of samples with the two most positive and two least positive attitudes toward stuttering (circa November 2013).

to be faced in future research will be to develop statistical and perhaps other methods to take account of the profile differences among samples, aside from the component, subscore, and OSS values. Until such methods are developed, visual inspection of multiple graphic profiles, such as those seen in Figure 1.2, offers a way to identify both central tendencies and variability across studies.

POSHA–S Graphic Profiles for Different Respondent Categories

The growing *POSHA–S* database provides the raw material with which comparative differences in public attitudes toward stuttering can be achieved. Figures 1.3 to 1.7 are comprised of multiple radial graph profiles, each representing a different study utilizing the final version of the *POSHA–S*, with each figure depicting attitudes of a different category of respondents. Each individual study's design and sample characteristics were different, yet clusters of profiles illustrate the central tendencies and inherent variability mentioned.

Figure 1.3 shows all of the graphic profiles for samples of the *public*, but excluding sample targeting only students, teachers, SLPs or SLP students, or people who stutter. The rationale for sampling attitudes of the public toward stuttering was explained earlier, so it is obvious that most studies have attempted to document attitudes of the non-stuttering majority within the general population. Whereas the 44 profiles included illustrate the considerable variability that characterize the *POSHA–S* samples across the numerous regions, countries, cultures, and languages represented, they also show some striking similarities.

Figures 1.4, 1.5, 1.6, and 1.7 depict samples obtained from the populations excluded from Figure 1.3. Figure 1.4 displays profiles for 14 student samples, 11 for college students but also two samples of sixth-graders and one sample of high school students. One reason for the popularity of college student samples is that academics or students carrying out master's or doctoral research have ready access to them. One criticism that is frequently leveled at such research is that college students may not represent the general population, e.g., Gabel (2006). The profiles show less variability than those for the public (Figure 1.3), quite likely due to the smaller number of samples displayed, sampling from less diverse populations, and containing only three samples with less than high school education. Nevertheless, the central tendency for positivity-negativity of the students tends to mirror those for the public.

Figure 1.5 shows seven profiles for school teachers. Teachers have become popular sample targets for several reasons. Whether correct of not, it is widely assumed that attitudes of children might be changed more easily and effectively than attitudes of adults. In schools, children from wide-ranging backgrounds are provided with information that is regarded to be the best available, yet that information must inevitably be filtered through the personalities and values of individual teachers (Kuruppu & Jayawardena, Chapter 12). Thus, if teachers had negative attitudes toward stuttering, it would follow that teachers' attitudes logically would be those that should be improved. With one exception for the most positive Traits/Personality component for only one sample in all five figures (1.3 to 1.7), the teacher samples in Figure 1.5 appeared not to demonstrate any more positive attitudes than the general public or college students. In fact, in a careful statistical analysis of *POSHA–S* database participants across numerous studies, Arnold and Goltl (2013) reported that attitudes of teachers were *less* positive than those of non-teacher controls.

Profiles of SLPs and students training to become SLPs are shown in Figure 1.6. An often unstated assumption is that SLPs should be on the front line manifesting and fostering the most positive attitudes toward stuttering (c.f., Junuzović-Žunić,-Weidner, Reichel, Cook, St. Louis, & Ware, Chapter 14; Węsierska, Węsierska, St. Louis, & Beste-Guldborg, Chapter 13). The profiles of the 11 samples shown in the Figure 1.6 appear to be somewhat more positive than the profiles for the public, students, and teachers, although neither dramatically nor consistently so.

Figure 1.7 shows the profiles for three samples of adults who stutter. Described in more detail in Chapter 16 by St. Louis et al. (Chapter 16), one of the samples, i.e., leaders in the self-help movement, is featured in Figure 1.2, and it has the most positive attitudes observed to date. The two other samples represent individuals who stutter, or stuttered earlier in their lives who were recruited from

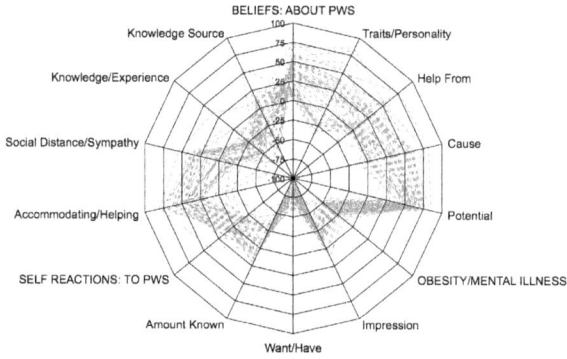

Figure 1.3: *POSHA–S* (final version) profiles of studies that sampled members of the public.

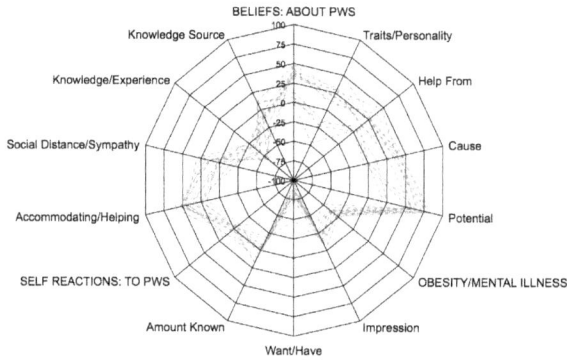

Figure 1.4: *POSHA–S* (final version) profiles of studies that sampled students.

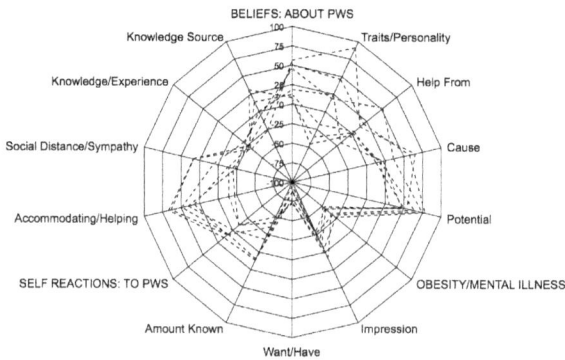

Figure 1.5: *POSHA–S* (final version) profiles of studies that sampled school teachers.

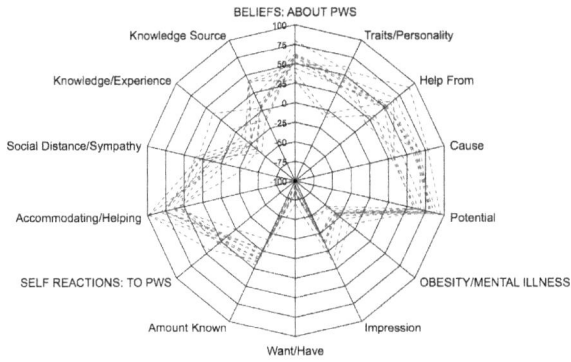

Figure 1.6: *POSHA–S* (final version) profiles of studies that sampled speech-language pathologists (SLPs) or SLP students

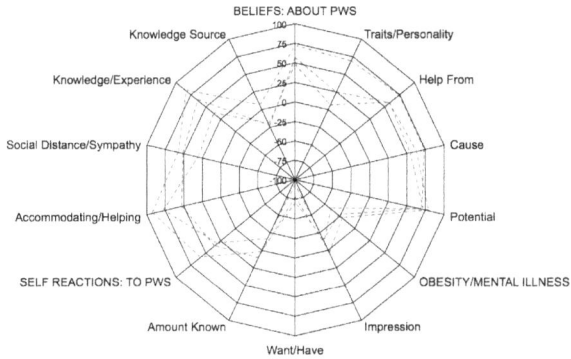

Figure 1.7: *POSHA–S* (final version) profiles of studies that sampled adults who stutter.

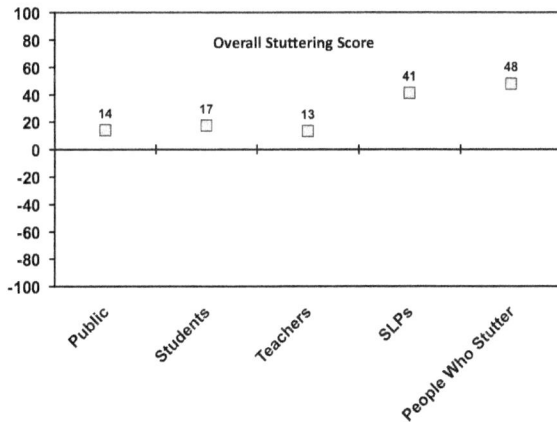

Figure 1.8: Mean Overall Stuttering Scores of samples from the public, students, teachers, SLPs or SLP students, and adults who stutter in the *POSHA–S* database.

(1) clinical and nonclinical populations and (2) individuals who were sampled as members of the public but indicated on the *POSHA–S* general section that they stuttered. These three samples suggest that attitudes of stutterers toward stuttering are the most positive.

Table 1.1 provides the means not only for the OSSs but also the subscores and components for the means of these five categories of respondents. The Beliefs and Self Reactions subscores showed the same general pattern as seen in Figure 1.8, i.e., adults who stutter and SLPs/SLP students having much more positive than average ratings, while the public, student, and teacher ratings having relatively average ratings. A few exceptions occurred. SLPs and SLP students were about the same as the public, students, and teachers for the social distance/sympathy component, but had ratings between the public/students/teachers and the stutterers for the knowledge/experience component. The SLPs and SLP students also rated sources of knowledge overall higher than the other three groups.

In summary, it appears that the same general attitudes emerge on the *POSHA–S* regardless of whether investigators sample students, teachers, or the public, so long as SLPs or SLP students are not included. It currently appears safe to suggest that college students have roughly the same attitudes as convenience samples of older adults on the *POSHA–S*, although more data will be required in the future to draw a firm conclusion. Also, it appears that the attitudes of teachers are no more positive, or even less positive (Arnold & Goltl, 2013), than those of the public.

Effects of Sampling on Public Attitudes

The foregoing suggests that the summary graphs, tabular data for components, subscores, and the OSS, or even the OSS alone, generate roughly the same general conclusions for multiple samples. The question then arises: Is this level of analysis sufficient or satisfactory for comparisons among individual samples? The aforementioned results suggest that individual items of the *POSHA–S* be bypassed in analysis with only the component, subscores, and/or OSS reported, as is the case in most clinical measures of severity (e.g., the *Stuttering Severity Instrument-4* [*SSI-4*]) (Riley, 2009) or self-perceptions, such as the *Overall Assessment of the Speaker's Experience with Stuttering* (*OASES*) (Yaruss & Quesal, 2008). And given the past state of affairs in comparative public attitude research wherein most studies inspected a plethora of different items to draw conclusions about their samples, it would be tempting to recommend the standard *POSHA–S* graph and table such as those shown in Figure 1.2 and Table 1.1. Indeed, that may be what will eventually happen, but evidence exists that this approach will miss important information, as the following example illustrates.

Table 1.1: *POSHA–S* Components, Subscores, and Overall Stuttering Scores for Samples from the Public, Students, Teachers, SLPs or SLP Students, and Adults Who Stutter in the *POSHA–S* Database

POSHA–S Variable	Public	Students	Teachers	SLPs / SLP Students	Adults Who Stutter	POSHA-S Database Median[b]
Number of Samples [a]	44	15	7	9	3	188
OVERALL STUTTERING SCORE	*14*	*19*	*15*	*39*	*48*	*16*
Beliefs about People Who Stutter	*29*	*34*	*28*	*57*	*56*	*33*
Traits	10	17	11	39	31	18
Help From	18	23	10	56	61	19
Cause	29	34	33	56	61	34
Potential	60	63	57	78	71	62
Self Reactions to People Who Stutter	*0*	*3*	*3*	*21*	*40*	*-1*
Accommodating/Helping	39	45	31	76	76	47
Social Distance/Sympathy	5	13	0	12	41	4
Knowledge/Experience	-32	-38	-26	-16	59	-36
Knowledge Source	-14	-11	0	11	-16	-18
Obesity/Mental Illness	*-38*	*-34*	*-38*	*-32*	*-32*	*-34*
Impression	-21	-19	-13	-17	-13	-15
Want/Have	-80	-86	-82	-86	-80	-84
Amount Known	-12	2	-20	6	-4	1

[a]The numbers of samples are slightly different from those in the profiles in figures 1.3 to 1.7 due to different combining of a few samples.
[b]Circa July 2013, the *POSHA–S* database was composed of 8,144 respondents in 29 countries and 20 languages.

The Turkish version of the *POSHA–S* was administered in Turkey to a convenience sample of 106 adults who were recruited in the city of Eskişehir, Turkey, a city of 600,000 inhabitants (Özdemir et al., 2011a). These were compared to a school-based probability sample wherein Census data were used to select a representative region of the city at random, followed by selection of a school at random where the sampling occurred. Sixth-graders were each given four *POSHA–Ss*, one for themselves, one for a parent, one for a grandparent or, if unavailable, another adult relative, and one for an adult neighbor who did not have a child in the same school. Male or female parents and female or male grandparents (or adult relatives) were recommended based on the child's odd

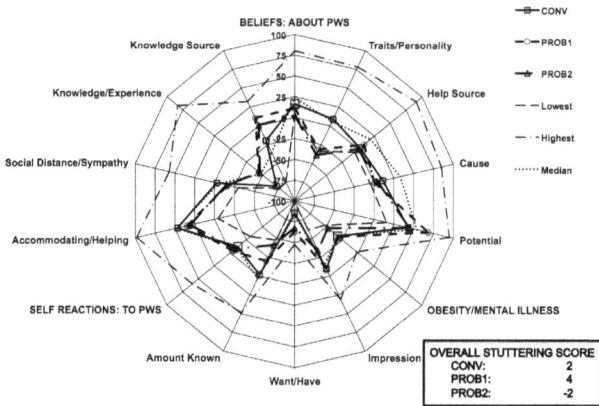

Figure 1.9: *POSHA–S* profiles for one convenience sample of adults (CONV) compared with two probability samples of adults (PROB1 and PROB2) in Turkey (Özdemir et al., 2011a).

or even birthday. This procedure was replicated in another area of the city one year later. Özdemir et al. (2011a) compared the convenience sample of adults with the two neighbor groups in the two school-based probability samples. In this comparison, OSSs differed only by 6 points, with the first probability sample being 2 points below the convenience sample and the second probability sample 4 points above it. These were not significantly different. None of the 15 comparisons for the components, subscores, and OSS were significant between the two probability samples, but 40% (6/15) were significant between the convenience sample and the first probability sample, and 53% (8/15) were significant between the convenience sample and the second probability sample. Adding all the individual *POSHA–S* items to these summary values, none (0%) of the 60 contrasts between the two probability samples were significant compared to 28% between the convenience and first probability sample and 24% between the convenience and second probability sample. Figure 1.9 clearly illustrates the differences in profiles between the convenience sample and the two probability samples. In other words, the profiles of the convenience sample and two probability samples were quite dramatically different even though the OSSs were quite similar.

Two implications emerge. First, it appears to be important to consider the profiles of *POSHA–S* measured attitudes, as well as the OSS and subscores. Second, probability sampling can provide vastly different results from convenience sampling. Accordingly, other studies have used a school-based probability sampling scheme similar to that of Özdemir et al. (2011a) with parents and teachers in Kuwait (Abdalla & St. Louis, 2012, 2014; Al-Khaladi et al., 2009) and the public in Portugal (Valente, Jesus, Leahy, & St. Louis, 2014).

POSHA–S Scoring, Data Conversion, and Sample Comparisons

The *POSHA–S* was designed for users both inside the scientific community, such as clinical researchers and epidemiologists, as well as those outside, such as clinical SLPs, teachers, stakeholders in the self-help movement, or any other group interested in comparing or changing attitudes toward stuttering or other stigmatizing attributes. User-friendliness was an important goal, and with the final version including many "yes," "no," or "not sure" responses, completion time for the *POSHA–S* was reduced to an average of 10 minutes. This was considered the maximum allowable time for widespread public use. With "no" = 1, "not sure" = 2, and "yes" = 3 conversions, the data become a 1/2/3 ratio scale, even though technically these are ordinal scales (Siegel, 1956). As with the data from the first two prototypes, the results are further converted to a -100 to +100 scale for each sample to provide more manageable and intuitive comparisons among and within samples.

Repeated, widespread, and successful use of this procedure has generated a large and growing body of comparisons with the *POSHA–S* that add to its international appeal. Recently, primarily for the scientific community, St. Louis (2012c) reported on studies designed to verify that the possible ordinal-to-ratio scale conversions were justifiable. The same respondents completed both the final version of the *POSHA–S*, i.e., 1–5 (general section) and 1–3 (stuttering section) scales to the 1–9 scale (both sections) two weeks apart, with order counterbalanced. Both paper-and-pencil and online *POSHA–S*s were used (c.f. St. Louis, 2012b). Both scales yielded similar results on the converted -100 to +100 scale, with none of the 60 comparisons being significantly different on pair-wise *t*-tests.

In 16 published *POSHA–S* studies, results were analyzed by independent or dependent *t*-tests as appropriate, and Bonferroni corrections were made for pair-wise comparisons using $p \leq .00417$ (.05/12). Why employ *t*-tests when other more sophisticated statistical analyses could be used? First, *t*-tests are highly robust when some of the underlying assumptions are not met, such as lack of homoscedasticity or skewness (Fagerland, 2012; Stonehouse & Forrester, 1998). Second, a strong case can be made that the *t*-test is the best-understood and most well-known inferential statistic that could render *POSHA–S* results comprehensible and replicable by collaborators or potential users worldwide. Third, and very important to beginning and inexperienced researchers, the *t*-test is easy to calculate, and almost all statistical programs permit unequal frequencies, which is the rule rather than the exception in *POSHA–S* samples. Fourth, the *t*-test can be run on small samples. Numerous samples in the *POSHA–S* database are smaller than 50 respondents (St. Louis, 2014). In a study comparing different types of sampling, St. Louis (2008) found that samples as small as 25 predicted the mean of the "population" of 1,500 respondents in the database as accurately as samples of 50, 100, or 200.

Of course, using multiple pair-wise comparisons increases the likelihood of making a Type I error, or rejecting the null hypothesis and accepting the alternative hypothesis that a significant difference exists when it does not exist. The Bonferroni correction involves dividing the alpha level by the number of comparisons made, which is simple and very effective when 10–20 pair-wise comparisons are made. Yet, with all 60 pair-wise contrasts considering all of the *POSHA–S* attitude ratings, the standard $p \leq .05$ alpha level would become .05/60 = .000833, or extremely conservative. In early publications (e.g., St. Louis et al., 2008), we used for the Bonferroni correction of 12 ($p \leq .05/12 = .00417$) because it reflected the average number of items under each prompt in the *POSHA–E* versions. This provided a conservative approach that required a substantial difference in ratings to manifest a significant difference. Over multiple investigations, this same alpha level has turned out to provide an excellent balance between not making Type I errors (i.e., reporting significant differences when one does not exist), but also, and equally importantly, not making Type II errors (i.e., not reporting differences when they do exist) (e.g., Flynn & St. Louis, 2011; Ip et al., 2012; Özdemir et al., 2011a, 2011b; Przepiórka et al., 2013; St. Louis, 2011a, 2012a, 2012b, 2012c; St. Louis, Lubker et al., 2009; St. Louis, Przepiórka, Beste-Guldborg, Williams, Blachnio, Guendouzi, Reichel, & Ware, 2014; St. Louis, Reichel et al., 2009).

We have also reported Cohen's *d* effect sizes (Cohen, 1988) for statistically significant *t*-test comparisons because *any* consistent difference, no matter how small, will become statistically significant if the sample size is increased sufficiently or if the variance is reduced. Some *POSHA–S* samples are quite large (e.g., Przepiórka et al., 2013); therefore, it is important to temper consideration of statistical power with the magnitude of effect sizes. In recent studies, we have followed significant *t*-tests results with average Cohen's *d* values in order to estimate whether it is the sample size, effect size, or both that should be considered in interpretation of the results. Two examples with modest sample sizes are provided to illustrate this point in Table 1.2. The first is a study comparing male versus female respondents on the *POSHA–S* (St. Louis, 2012a) wherein one male and one female were selected randomly from 50 different samples in the *POSHA–S* database. The table shows the rating pairs for the three subscores and OSS,

Table 1.2: Sample Data from Two Studies Illustrating the Balance Achieved by Using a Bonferroni Corrected Alpha Level of $p \leq .00417$ Followed by Cohen's d Values for Significant Differences

Study and Description	Sample Sizes	Obesity/ Mental Illness Subscores	Belief Subscores	Self Reactions Subscores	Overall Stuttering Scores	Percent Significant at $p \leq .00417$	Percent Significant at $p \leq .05$	Mean Cohen's d Significant ($p \leq .00417$)	Mean Cohen's d Non-significant ($p \leq .00417$)
Representative sample from IPATHA database (St. Louis, 2012a)									
Multi-country Males vs. Females;	50/50	-40/-33	29/27	-12/-7	9/10	0	6.7	n/a	.17
U.S. High School with an oral presentation, video, or both between POSHA-Ss (Flynn & St. Louis, 2011)									
ORAL Pre vs. VIDEO Pre	40/43	-37/-40	38/36	-1/-1	19/18	0	1.9	n/a	.14
ORAL Pre vs. ORAL Post	40/40	-37/-30	38/71	-1/-18	19/44	36.5	48.1	1.0	.48
VIDEO Pre vs. VIDEO Post	43/43	-40/-36	36/53	-1/14	18/33	34.6	42.3	.71	.36
VIDEO Post vs. VIDEO + ORAL	43/43	-36/-40	53/72	-14/14	33/43	13.5	30.8	.80	.24
ORAL Post vs. VIDEO + ORAL	40/43	-30/-40	71/72	18/14	44/43	3.9	15.4	.54	.27

followed by the percentage of significant *t*-test differences using our "conventional" Bonferroni correction (p ≤ .00417), as well as the uncorrected alpha levels (p ≤ .05) for comparison purposes and which generated more significant differences. With the correction, none of the 60 corrected pair-wise differences was significant, meaning essentially no difference between male versus female respondents. Since none were significant, the mean Cohen's *d* is not reported for those significant. As a rather oblique control procedure, I ran Cohen's *d*'s for those contrasts that were not significant (all of them in this case). The mean *d* was 0.17, or "no difference" to "very small," which would be expected. Essentially, when no differences would be expected, as between equal numbers of males and females selected randomly from 50 samples, none of the corrected *t*-tests were significant.

The second example in Table 1.2 involved an attempt to improve high school students' attitudes toward stuttering by listening to a humorous talk by an adult who stuttered, a video presentation featuring this adult (along with others), or both (Flynn & St. Louis, 2011). The study had two groups of students, one who heard the speaker only (ORAL) between pre- and post-*POSHA–S*s, and the other with the video (VIDEO) between pre- and post-*POSHA–S*s followed by a shortened talk (VIDEO + ORAL) and a third *POSHA–S*. Thirty-seven percent of the corrected *POSHA–S* comparisons were significantly improved in the study after the ORAL condition only and 35% after the VIDEO condition. Mean Cohen's *d* values for these differences were 1.00 and 0.71, respectively, or "large" to "very large," with *d*'s of .48 and .36 (or "small" to "moderate") for the non-significant differences. In this case, one could argue that the corrected versions were too conservative. The VIDEO + ORAL condition generated an additional 14% significant differences with "large" effect sizes (mean d = 0.80), but "small" effect sizes for the non-significant differences (mean *d* = .24). To put these into perspective, the first comparison in the table comparing the two groups of students on the two pre-*POSHA–S*s (when no differences would be expected) showed virtually no differences, with non-significant mean *d*'s = 0.17 or "none" to "very small." Comparisons at the end of each condition (i.e., VIDEO + ORAL post-versus ORAL post) yielded 4% of corrected difference significant with a "moderate" effect size (mean *d* = 0.54) but with a "small" effect size (mean *d* = 0.27) for non-significant differences.

These examples illustrate that our "conventional" procedure generates conservative results and provides a good balance between not making either Type I or Type II errors. Inspection of numerous samples analyzed this way, St. Louis (2012c) recommended that >30% of *POSHA–S* pair-wise comparisons indicate large differences between samples. Moderate differences would be indicated by 10–30% of the comparisons, small differences by 5–10% of the comparisons, and no differences by 0–5% of the comparisons. Using these guidelines, the differences between the aforementioned convenience sample and probability samples in Turkey were in the moderate range. It must be emphasized, however, that more sophisticated statistical procedures should be applied to better capture differences in profiles and database predictors. It is possible that such sophisticated analyses could identify factors that could predict attitude changeability.

Predictors and Correlates of Public Attitudes Toward Stuttering

Predictors versus Correlates

One of the goals of much of the epidemiological research on public attitudes toward stuttering has been to identify variables that, given appropriate interventions, might predict better or worse attitudes in the future. In common language, "prediction" refers to estimating that something will happen in the future or be the consequence of something, and in behavioral science, it typically refers to establishing the functional or predictor relationships between variables and outcomes (Reed & Wu, 2013). To be sure that a variable is a predictor and not simply a correlate usually requires statistical modeling, as is often done using regression analysis. Moreover, the predictor and outcome variables must be chosen carefully in order that mathematical prediction is accurate. The *POSHA–S* database is large enough that such prediction research can be carried out; however, research to date has focused on variables that appear to be—or not to be—associated with better or worse stuttering attitudes.

Speech-Language Pathology Profession

Being a person who stutters and having experience in the self-help movement for stuttering are variables associated with some of the most positive attitudes toward stuttering that have been observed (e.g., St. Louis & George, 2018; St. Louis et al., Chapter 16). As noted earlier, several studies of speech-language pathology students have been carried out to document the extent to which the knowledge and experiences they receive affect their beliefs about, reactions to, and knowledge of stuttering (Reichel & St. Louis, 2004, 2007; Węsierska et al., Chapter 13).

In a recent study of college students in the United States and Poland, St. Louis et al. (2014) found that a "halo effect" influenced attitudes of SLP students versus non-SLP students in both countries. In other words, majoring in speech-language pathology versus other fields was associated with better stuttering attitudes in both countries. Training added to this effect such that American SLP graduate students had better attitudes than SLP undergraduates, more so than being a graduate versus undergraduate student in another major. Further, stuttering attitudes of Native American undergraduate students, who were older than the other American non-SLP undergraduate students, were similar to those of non-SLP graduate students. Finally, stuttering attitudes of the American students in general were more positive than attitudes of the Polish students. Similar to results shown earlier from database profiles, this study adds evidence that public attitudes in general are not as positive as SLP students' attitudes, but other cultural factors play important roles as well.

Several studies have demonstrated that coursework in fluency disorders has a positive effect on stuttering attitudes of SLP students (e.g., Junuzović-Žunić, Weidner, Reichel, Cook, St. Louis, & Ware, Chapter 14; St. Louis, Reichel et al., 2009; St. Louis, Williams et al., 2014). Other, unpublished works have been included in the *POSHA–S* database. Gottwald, Warner, Hartley, Fraas, Hawver, and St. Louis (2011) reported similar improvement in attitudes of SLPs and SLP students after watching a video about stuttering.

Information about Fluency Disorders

If public attitudes are to be changed by accurate information about stuttering, it must be shown that the information affects the attitudes of those whose professions or personal lives are ordinarily little affected by stuttering (Abdalla, Chapter 5; see also Boyle & Blood, Chapter 2; Gabel, Chapter 4; Langevin, Chapter 3). As noted earlier, Flynn and St. Louis (2011) demonstrated that a talk by a person who stutters or a video about the experience of stuttering can have a strong positive effect on *POSHA–S*-measured attitudes in high school students. Using the same video they used for SLPs and SLP students, Gottwald et al. (2011) reported no change in clinical SLPs' attitudes, presumably because their attitudes were extremely positive before watching the video (OSSs pre- and post- were 55 versus 56). With the same video treatment, however, Gottwald, Kent, St. Louis, and Hartley (2014) demonstrated that university professors did improve (OSSs 36 versus 47). Abdalla and St. Louis (2014) carried out a comparable study in Kuwait and found that education students improved their measured attitudes after viewing a video, but experienced teachers did not. Similarly, but using a semantic differential scale, McGee, Kalinowski, and Stuart (1996) found more negative attitudes in high school students after watching excerpts from a professionally prepared video on stuttering. For an unpublished student project in the *POSHA-S* database, Kestenbaum and Khnonov (2011) administered the *POSHA–S* to 51 students before and after watching the award-winning movie about the British King George VI who stuttered, *The King's Speech*, shortly after it had been released. Their OSSs increased from 21 to 32.

In another unpublished student project, Holcombe and Eisert (2012) carried out an experiment wherein two groups of participants (1) filled out the *POSHA–S* and another implicit attitude measure; (2) read either a one-page paper with information about stuttering or about stress and bullying; (3) watched a person stuttering while talking about a struggle with the problem or a person not stuttering but talking about a struggle with stress and bullying; (4) filled out the attitude measures immediately; and (5) filled them out again a week later. They found that the stuttering information and speaker occasioned a positive effect on their *POSHA–S* ratings that persisted one week, whereas the stress/bullying condition had little effect on their *POSHA–S* scores. Finally, Węsierska and St. Louis (2014) reported that a short information sheet debunking myths about stuttering resulted in improved ratings of students in both the UK and Poland on various *POSHA–S* items more than a similar information sheet about attention-deficit/hyperactivity disorder given to other groups of students. In contrast to these studies that produced improvements in attitudes, Puglik (2010) asked 15 students to read a brochure about stuttering and another group of 15 to read a brochure about dysarthria. There was little difference in their subsequent *POSHA–S* OSSs, 27 versus 25, respectively.

Systematic studies designed to change public attitudes are appearing. Most have showed that attitudes can be changed with increased information. Still, there are numerous variables as carefully outlined by Abdalla (Chapter 5) requiring further study.

Familiarity or Experience with Stuttering and Other Negative Attributes

It appears that experience with stuttering, even if one does not stutter, has the potential to be identified as a predictor of better than average attitudes. Klassen (2002) demonstrated that attitudes of the non-stuttering public who knew a specifically identified friend or family member who stuttered were more positive than those without such person identification. Langevin and Prasad (2012) reported that children who had previous associations with someone who stuttered manifested better peer attitudes than those without such associations. As reviewed by St. Louis et al. (Chapter 16), Daniels and Hughes (2011) demonstrated that parents of children who stutter have among the most positive attitudes sampled to date on the *POSHA–S*, with an OSS of 58. St. Louis et al. showed that family members or close friends of adults who stutter have more positive attitudes than adults who have no such known associations.

St. Louis and Rogers (2011a) confirmed this finding by sorting all the 3,751 respondents in the *POSHA–S* database in February 2011 on the "personal experience [with stuttering]" item. It is calculated according to a formula applied to the general section item containing an "all that apply" checklist of "persons known" who stutter. The six choices are weighted by the formula as follows: "me" = 60, "close friend" = 20, "relative" = 10, "acquaintance" = 5, "other" = 5, and "nobody" or nothing checked = 0. Any respondent's rating will therefore range from 0 to 100 (later converted to -100 to +100). After all *POSHA–S* ratings were rank-ordered according to "personal experience," the respondents were divided into four quartile groups: 0–25th percentile 25–50th percentile, 50–75th percentile, and 75–100th percentile. In addition, the authors performed the same procedures for "personal experience" with obesity and "personal experience" with mental illness. Figure 1.10 shows the OSS values for the four quartiles for each of the three sorts, i.e., familiarity with stuttering, obesity, and mental illness. It can be seen that the *least familiar with stuttering quartile* had a mean OSS of 2 while the *most familiar quartile* had a mean OSS of 26. The two middle quartiles were equal at 17 or very near the median for the database. The uneven improvements followed by declines in attitudes toward stuttering as a function of familiarity with obesity and mental illness indicate that such familiarity has less direct influence on attitudes toward a different attribute, i.e., stuttering, in this study. A mean of 15% of the 60 pair-wise *t*-tests typically carried out for *POSHA–S* comparisons for stuttering were significant, with a range of 5-47% and a mean Cohen's $d = 2.57$ or "very large." Thirty percent (range 7–73%) were different for obesity, with the mean d = .43 or "small" to "moderate." For mental illness, 15% were significant (range = 0–58%), and mean $d = 0.66$ or "moderate." Given the lack of consistent improvements in attitudes by quartile, especially for obesity and mental illness, the percentages are not particularly meaningful. However, the dramatically large effect sizes for stuttering familiarity provide support that such familiarity had a positive effect on stuttering attitudes (but see Boyle & Blood [Chapter 2] for a different perspective).

It is likely that carryover from stuttering experience to other negative attributes do not occur as well. Inspection of the subscores for obesity/mental illness in dozens of studies using the *POSHA–S* suggests that relatively little variability has been observed and that the ratings have been quite uniformly negative. It is interesting that Beste-Guldborg, St. Louis, and Campanale (Chapter 11) found that mean ratings for mental illness items among mental health professionals

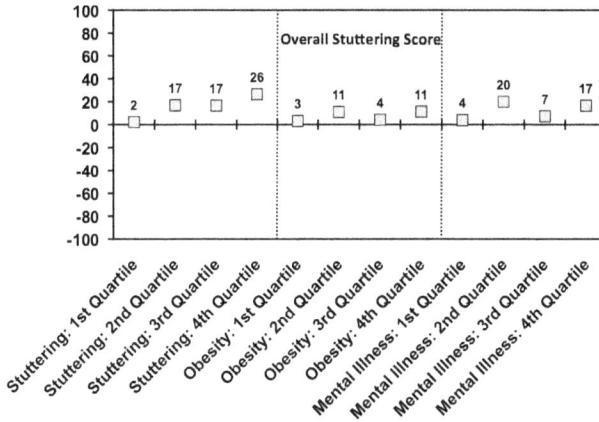

Figure 1.10: Changes in *POSHA–S* measured attitudes toward stuttering as a function of familiarity with stuttering, obesity, and mental illness.

were better than average but not the most positive (least negative) compared to other database samples analyzed to date.

Characteristics of the Stuttering

SEVERITY. St. Louis, Abdalla, Burgess, and Kuhn (Chapter 8) modified the *POSHA–S* such that "stuttering" was changed to either "severe stuttering" or "mild stuttering." In both the United States and Kuwait, hypothetically severe stuttering was rated more negatively than hypothetically mild stuttering. Nevertheless, the differences were not large. OSSs on the modified *POSHA–S*s favored mild stuttering by three points in the United States, 24 versus 21. In Kuwait, mild stuttering was rated 10 points more positively, i.e., 19 versus 9. Only 7% of the American *POSHA–S* ratings were significantly different, and 15% of the Kuwaiti ratings were significant. Most, but not all, of these favored mild over severe stuttering. This study suggests that greater stuttering severity is associated with more negative attitudes, but at least without visible or auditory exemplars of mild versus severe stuttering (e.g., Collins & Blood, 1990), its predictive potential is not large.

SEX OF THE PERSON WHO STUTTERS. St. Louis, LeMasters, and Poormohammad (Chapter 9) carried out a similar study in the United States and Iran, but modified the *POSHA–S* to read "male who stutters" or "female who stutters" rather than "person who stutters." They found no differences in attitudes toward males versus females who stutter in either country in English or Farsi.

29

Demographic Variables of Respondents

SEX. St. Louis (2012a) carried out a study designed to determine whether or not the sex of respondents made a difference in attitudes toward stuttering (the first study featured in Table 1.2 in the discussion of *t*-tests and Cohen's *d* analyses). Results of previous research were conflicting with some studies showing females had better attitudes (e.g., Burley & Rinaldi, 1986; Langevin, Kleitman, Packman, & Onslow, 2009) and others showing no sex differences (e.g., Patterson & Pring, 1991; Langevin, 2009). From one adult male and one adult female selected at random from 50 different samples in the *POSHA–S* database, St. Louis (2012a) found no significant differences for any of the 60 comparisons. As noted in the previous section, the study by St. Louis et al. (Chapter 9) found no *POSHA–S* differences as a function of the sex of the hypothetical stutterer. The authors also did not find differences in attitudes toward male or female stutterers when they subdivided their American and Iranian *respondents* according to male versus female. Based on these studies, it can be concluded with some confidence that neither the sex of the respondent nor the sex of the hypothetical stutterer makes a difference in measured attitudes on the *POSHA–S*. By inference, therefore, since most samples contain more females than males, the evidence suggests that this makes no difference in attitudes compared to equal sex representation.

AGE. Özdemir et al. (2011b) discovered that the attitudes of 11- to 12-year-old students were no different than those of their parents, grandparents or adult relatives, and neighbors. (See the next section on socioeconomic status for a full description.) Flynn and St. Louis (2011) found that high school students' attitudes were less positive than most studies of college students, and St. Louis, Przepiórka et al. (2014) reported that attitudes of graduate students were better than those of undergraduate students. No systematic studies have been carried out with *POSHA–S* ratings that systematically varied the age of respondents, but the database could be sorted to determine if age of adults makes a difference in attitudes.

SOCIOECONOMIC STATUS (EDUCATION, INCOME, AND OCCUPATION). The predictive potential of socioeconomic status (SES) in stuttering attitudes has been explored in a few studies. St. Louis and Rogers (2011b) carried out a study that was analyzed by quartile comparisons like the familiarity study, described above. The SES study investigated three derived measures of socioeconomic status: (1) years of education reported by the respondents; (2) the composite score for relative income (i.e., one's income compared to family and friends as well as to all

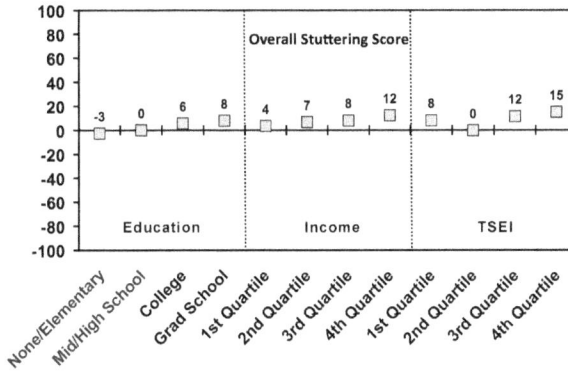

Figure 1.11: Changes in *POSHA–S* measured attitudes toward stuttering as a function of socioeconomic variables of education, relative income, and occupational status (TSEI).

the people in one's country); and (3) the Hauser and Warren (1997) Total Socioeconomic Index (TSEI). The TSEI is one of several measures used by Hauser and Warren to compare various American occupations taken from the U.S. Census in terms of their status in American society. All the database respondents who could be so classified by their occupations were assigned the TSEI number for their occupational status, with higher numbers representing higher socioeconomic status. Figure 1.11 shows the results of the quartile comparisons. Small but relative uniform improvements in attitudes occasioned higher quartiles for education and relative income. There was a greater overall difference among quartiles for occupational status (TSEI), but not in a uniform pattern. Mean percentages of statistically significant differences (and mean Cohen's d values) associated with the sorts for education, relative income, and occupational status were, respectively, 65% ($d = 0.36$), 21% ($d = 0.29$), and 33% ($d = .32$).

This study is hard to interpret and, like the companion study for familiarity, should await confirmation with the larger database using a statistical procedure such as regression analysis. It does suggest, however, that education and relative income might provide better predictive potential for better stuttering attitudes than occupational status.

Unpublished studies in India (Treasa & Kanaka, 2013; Usmani, Kanaka, & Rajashekhar, 2012) investigated public attitudes toward stuttering in the Hindi and Kannada languages, respectively, of either mid-SES or high-SES people. SES was not defined for individual respondents; instead, respondents in each of the two groups were recruited from regions known for moderate versus high SES. Usmani et al.'s study of 60 male and female adults in Hindi, 30 in each SES group, lived in the city of Allahabad in the Uttar Pradesh state in northern India. Treasa and Kanaka surveyed mothers living mostly in the seaside city of Mangalore in the Karnataka state in southwestern India. The OSSs for the mid-SES and high-SES groups in the Uttar Pradesh study were, respectively -10 (the lowest sample mean observed to date) and 0. Nevertheless, none of the *t*-test comparisons were significant between the two groups, quite likely influenced partly by modest sample sizes. In the Karnataka study, the 60 mid-SES mothers' OSS was -6 compared to the 60 high-SES mothers' OSS of -2. In this case, 8% (5/60) of the *t*-test comparisons were significant, with a mean $d = 0.77$ or "large."

Özdemir et al.'s (2011b) probability study of sixth-graders, parents, grandparents or adult relatives, and neighbors based on random selection of a representative region and schools within that region was not designed as an SES study, but clearly the individuals sampled in that study were of lower SES, according to education and relative income metrics, than the convenience sample to which the neighbors were compared in the Özdemir et al. (2011a) study as well as two previous convenience samples of Turkish adults (St. Louis, Andrade, Georgieva, & Troudt, 2005; St. Louis et al., 2011). The *POSHA–S* data of the second probability sample from the Özdemir et al. (2011b) study are shown in Table 1.3 and juxtaposed against the three earlier probability samples. The adults in the probability sample had only 4.8 to 8.2 years of education compared to 12.4 to 14.0 years for the three convenience samples. Relative incomes were very different as well, i.e., -15 to -7 for the probability samples versus 9 to 10 for the convenience samples. (The income items were not yet included in the *POSHA–S* for the first Turkey sample [St. Louis et al., 2005].) Surprisingly, attitudes of the children, parents, grandparents/adult relatives, and neighbors in the probability sample were very similar. Only 1% of the total pair-wise *t*-tests were significant between all the items, components, subscores, and OSS. The similarities in these values are apparent in Table 1.3. In the previous discussion of probability versus convenience sampling featuring these same studies, it was shown that, whereas OSSs did not differ, the various items, components, and subscores did. From the perspective of SES, therefore, it is reasonable to conclude that SES differences between the convenience and probability samples were substantial. They very likely made a difference in the results, but in ways that are not yet well understood.

Taken together, these studies of effects of SES on stuttering attitudes are

Table 1.3: Mean *POSHA–S* Ratings of Components, Subscores, and OSS for Seven Turkish Samples and the Median Values from the *POSHA–S* Database

	Adults[b]	Adults[c]	Adults[d]	Sixth-Grade Children[e]	Parents[e]	Grandparents / Adult Relatives[e]	Neighbors[e]	Database Median
Number	25	90	50	50	50	50	50	57
Mean Age (year)	29.3	31.2	27.5	11.8	37.6	62.8	34.5	36.1
Mean Education (year)	12.5	12.4	14.0	5.0	7.1	4.8	8.2	14.6
Mean Relative Income (-100 to +100)	—	10	9	-10	-13	-15	-7	1
OVERALL STUTTERING SCORE	*-1*	*-2*	*2*	*5*	*1*	*-2*	*-2*	*16*
Beliefs About People Who Stutter	*17*	*17*	*16*	*16*	*12*	*7*	*3*	*33*
Traits/Personality	6	-2	9	-13	-28	-26	-39	18
Help Source	-6	6	3	10	6	-4	0	19
Cause	20	7	11	-1	4	-2	4	34
Potential	48	57	43	67	67	60	45	62
Self Reactions to People Who Stutter	*-18*	*-21*	*-12*	*-6*	*-10*	*-12*	*-7*	*-1*
Accommodating/ Helping	14	26	47	23	27	18	31	47
Social Distance/ Sympathy	-7	-18	-3	-16	-18	-17	-15	4
Knowledge/Experience	-58	-64	-72	-41	-53	-42	-46	-36
Knowledge Source	-22	-28	-20	9	3	-6	1	-18
Obesity/Mental Illness	*-28*	*-38*	*-32*	*-53*	*-46*	*-53*	*-48*	*-34*
Impression	-7	-28	-10	-33	-28	-45	-34	-15
Want to Have	-85	-74	-85	-80	-71	-68	-68	-84
Amount Known	8	-12	-2	-45	-40	-46	-41	1

[a] Circa July, 2013, the *POSHA–S* database contained 8,144 respondents from 29 countries and in 20 languages. The median reflects the middle value of 188 sample means.
[b] St. Louis et al. (2005).
[c] St. Louis et al. (2011) (Contained a written definition of stuttering).
[d] Özdemir et al. (2011a).
[e] Özdemir et al. (2011b).

equivocal. It is likely that other uncontrolled factors may have affected the results, and future research will be required to elucidate the effects of SES more clearly.

Written Definition of Stuttering

The Turkish convenience samples shown in Table 1.3 provide further evidence regarding the effects of providing a written definition of stuttering as a correlate of measured attitudes on the *POSHA–S*. Coşkun carried out the Turkish component of a four-country study of cluttering and stuttering attitudes (St. Louis et al., 2011). The *POSHA–S* was modified in terms of order of items for that study, but importantly, it included written definitions of cluttering and stuttering. The stuttering definition was:

> Stuttering is a speech problem in which a speaker typically repeats or prolongs (draws out) parts of words, or gets stuck or blocked on words. Sometimes stuttering consists of strategies that try to reduce or avoid repeating, prolonging, or blocking. Stuttering is often associated with psychological stress or unpleasant feelings. Finally, the person who stutters often experiences a loss of voluntary control in saying certain words.

As seen in Table 1.3, the stuttering attitudes appeared to be generally unchanged, whether preceded by this definition in the second convenience sample or by the standard undefined presentation of the "disorder of stuttering" in the first and third convenience samples. Similar results have been found comparing the U.S. cluttering/stuttering study using written definitions with American studies of stuttering employing the *POSHA–S* without a definition.

Geographic Region and Language

Figure 1.12 divides the diverse samples in the *POSHA–S* database into geographic regions arranged from lowest to highest OSS. The mean of samples from Asia obtained as of July 2013 (India, Sri Lanka, and China) resulted in the lowest *POSHA–S* OSSs, followed by Africa (Cameroon and South Africa), the Middle East (Turkey, Lebanon, Syria, Jordan, Kuwait, and Iran), Central America/Caribbean/South America (Nicaragua, Puerto Rico, and Brazil), Eastern Europe (Bulgaria, Bosnia-Herzegovina, Croatia, Russia, and Poland), Western Europe (Norway, Denmark, Sweden, Germany, the United Kingdom, Ireland, and Italy), and North America (United States and Canada).

Figure 1.13 categorizes the samples in the database according to language of the questionnaire, similarly arranged from least positive to most positive. The

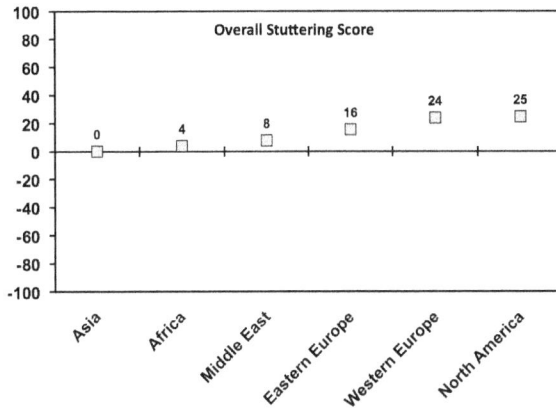

Figure 1.12: Mean Overall Stuttering Scores of samples from different geographic regions in the *POSHA–S* database.

languages of the *POSHA–S*s mostly parallel the countries and regions sampled. The differences are likely due primarily to geography rather than linguistic factors or differences in translations. Scandinavian languages, German, Bosnian/Serbian/Croatian, and English represented the highest language-associated attitudes, while Hindi, Italian, Kannada, Bulgarian, and Russian represented the lowest. Importantly, languages did not always parallel the regions shown in Figure 1.12. Samples in English have been used in non-native English-speaking areas, such as Denmark, the KwaZulu-Natal region of South Africa, Sri Lanka, and India. French has been used in both Canada and Cameroon. Interestingly, relatively large samples in Italian from three regions of Italy had some of the least positive OSSs, ranging from -6 to 0 (Tomaiuloi, Del Gado, Capparelli, & St. Louis, 2013).

A study carried out by St. Louis and Roberts (2010) explored the interaction of language and geography. Adults were recruited to fill out the *POSHA–S* in either French or English, whichever was their stronger language, in two countries where both languages were used officially, Canada and Cameroon. The authors found that attitudes were more positive in Canada (and similar to those in the United States) than in Cameroon, regardless of whether the respondents rated their attitudes in French or English.

Demographic Variables Not Yet Studied or Well Understood

Other demographic items appear in the *POSHA–S* that might be correlated with stuttering attitudes. These include completion time, parental and marital

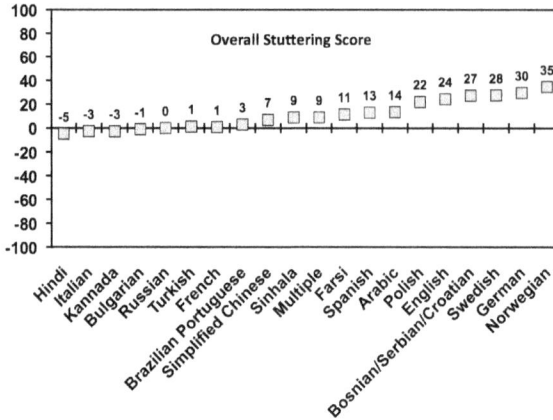

Figure 1.13: Mean Overall Stuttering Scores of samples from different language translations used in the *POSHA–S* database.

status, number of languages known, occupations (other than speech-language pathology and teaching), race, religion, health/ability items (i.e., physical health, mental health, ability to speak, and ability to learn), and life priority items. The life priority items were the last additions to the *POSHA–S* and, until recently, have not been completed by enough respondents to determine the extent of their potential association with *POSHA–S* ratings. They comprise 12 items, i.e., "being safe and secure, being free to do what I want, spending quiet time alone, attending parties or social events, imagining new things, helping the less fortunate, having exciting but potentially 'dangerous' experiences, practicing my religion, earning money, doing my jobs or my duty, getting things finished, and figuring out how to solve important problems."

Of course, virtually any ratings on various items, or combinations of items, could be evaluated as potential correlates of better attitudes between or among groups. To suggest an outlandish example, it would be easily possible to sort the *POSHA–S* database and compare stuttering attitudes of mothers versus fathers who all rate themselves as left-handed, intelligent individuals with good health. So far, however, none of these demographic variables have been noticed in the nearly 200 samples analyzed to be consistently associated with more or less positive *POSHA–S* ratings. For example, as noted, completion time of the final *POSHA–S* averages about 10 minutes, but considerable variability has occurred. For samples, the median completion time is 10.8 minutes, with a range of 4.8

minutes to 4.7 hours, and for individual respondents, 12.0 minutes with a range of 1.0 minute to 72.0 hours (c.f., St. Louis & Roberts, 2010). Neither race nor religion have appeared to be related to *POSHA–S* ratings as well. Descriptors of race are often reported as one's nationality or some other designation of political heritage. Additionally, both race and religion can be politically controversial in some countries and thus have been omitted entirely by a number of investigators.

In two studies, a number of these variables were inspected at the request of journal editors, but with little elucidation of their predictive potential. First, in an attempt to assure that demographic differences did not affect overall results between large samples from Hong Kong and China, Ip et al. (2012) compared the following demographic pairs for both samples since respondents differed in percentages represented by each pair: married versus unmarried; parents versus non-parents; students versus non-students; and respondents with higher versus lower than average relative income; higher versus lower than average physical health; and higher versus lower than average mental health. No more than 1% of any of the 60 t-test comparisons for any of these demographic variables was significant for either the Hong Kong or mainland China samples. Second, in a study of public attitudes in Poland, Przepiorka et al. (2013) sorted the respondents into halves according to the highest (best) OSSs versus the lowest (worst) OSSs. Then pair-wise t-tests were run between the high versus low halves for all the rated variables in the *POSHA–S*, including a number of demographic items. As expected, all stuttering attitude items were more positive for the best half, but so too for all obesity or mental illness items, with 68% of the total of 60 ratings being statistically significant. Age, education, relative income, sex ratio, health rating, ability ratings, and 11 life priority items were not significantly different. Of particular interest were demographic variables that were different as a function of the OSSs. Surprisingly, only the following three variables significantly favored the best OSS values, i.e., life priority of "getting things done," knowledge of intelligence, and knowledge of left-handedness. How to interpret this puzzling finding is not apparent and illustrates the difficulty in identifying potentially effective, logical predictors.

What Have We Learned?

Since the inception of IPATHA in 1999, a great deal about the epidemiology of public attitudes toward stuttering has been learned. Obviously, solid science must take account of all the evidence available. In this chapter, I have attempted to provide a state of the science that has evolved in this area by focusing almost exclusively on the *POSHA–S*, leaving the other chapters to focus more broadly on the diverse literature in the areas of stigma, teasing and bullying, discrimination, and changing attitudes.

At the risk of oversimplification, the following are concluding statements about public attitudes that can be drawn from the *POSHA–S* epidemiological findings:

1. "The public" encompasses a very broad array of populations, yet similarities in public attitudes outweigh differences in samples around the world. The current, but limited, data available suggest that there are probably geographic differences. Attitudes that are more accurate, sensitive, and in accord with current research appear to be more prevalent in North America and Northern Europe than in Eastern and Southern Europe, the Middle East, Central and South America, South or East Asia, and Africa, yet exceptions have been documented (e.g., Valente et al., 2014). Language differences are probably slight since sample differences appear to be better explained by geography.

2. Personal experience with, exposure to, and focused information on stuttering and/or speech-language pathology are associated with better than average stuttering attitudes. People who stutter—even those who have never had speech therapy—also have better than average attitudes. Leaders in the stuttering self-help movement, most of whom also stutter, have the most positive attitudes observed so far, but fluency specialists' attitudes are also very positive. Together, these two groups probably set the "gold standard" beyond which it may not be reasonable to try to change public attitudes. Also, limited evidence suggests that parents, family members, and close friends of people who stutter have more positive attitudes than those without such associations. Weak evidence exists suggesting that even experience or familiarity with other stigmatizing conditions such as obesity and mental illness can have a slight positive effect on stuttering attitudes.

3. Characteristics of stuttering, or the way "stuttering" is presented to respondents, no doubt have important influences on measured stuttering attitudes. Even a careful definition, written for laypeople, appears not to make a difference in public attitudes of a hypothetical stutterer on the *POSHA–S*. Consistent with the equivocal evidence in the literature regarding the effect of stuttering severity on public attitudes (e.g., Collins & Blood, 1990; Gabel, Hughes, & Daniels, 2008; Logan & O'Connor, 2012; Turnbaugh, Guitar, & Hoffman, 1979), stated severity of a hypothetical stutterer had only a limited effect on public attitudes in one study.

4. Sampling characteristics affect the attitudes results that are obtained. Clearly, past research has shown that different measures beget different results (see Hughes, Chapter 21). Yet, even with a standard measure such as the *POSHA–S*, probability sampling that assures more representative sampling of an entire population generated different results than the convenience sampling that has characterized virtually all of the past research on public attitudes.

5. Treatments aimed at improving attitudes generally, but not always, have at least some of their desired effects. Such treatments have included personal presentations by—or interactions with—people who stutter, specially constructed videos, films, information sheets, and coursework in fluency disorders (see Abdalla, Chapter 5). Limited evidence suggests that interaction with a live person who stutters might have more dramatic influence on attitude change than a video or film, even though the challenges of replicating such an effect are daunting.

6. Among the public, males and females rate stuttering virtually the same. Moreover, it does not appear to matter if the person they are rating is male or female.

7. It is not clear when attitudes are established, although limited evidence suggests they are present in childhood. In at least one study, 11- to 12-year-old children's attitudes toward stuttering are virtually the same as those of their parents, grandparents and adult relatives, and neighbors.

Required Epidemiological Research

Many more comparable broad-based samples across different populations locally, regionally, nationally, and internationally are needed. For future studies, I suggest that some kind of representative sampling of targeted populations should be used if possible. Further, I suggest that investigators should consider using the *POSHA–S* along with other desired measures because, with its growing database, the instrument has been documented as a solid measure that can provide meaningful sample comparisons across wide-ranging populations. If possible, as well, there should be collaborations with and participation by stuttering self-help organizations in future research. The primary value of carrying out multiple research studies in this way is that, when combined across studies, the research has the potential to identify the complex range of variables that influence any given population's attitudes toward stuttering. Obstacles do exist, of course. Getting the research results out quickly is an important challenge to overcome. Editors or reviewers of respected, peer-reviewed journals may become increasingly reluctant to publish many more studies of public attitudes around the world because (1) they may believe that the current number of such published studies is already sufficient or excessive and/or, more serious; (2) they believe that this line of research is irrelevant. It might be possible that Web site publishing by a reputable group, perhaps an arm of a working group to grow out of the effort initiated at the Stuttering Attitudes Research Symposium (St. Louis, Weidner, Gabel, Hughes, & Coleman, 2014), could launch such a Web site that would peer-review and publish good studies in this area. Another future obstacle to be overcome is the maintenance of the *POSHA–S* database. For more than a dozen years, I have continually worked on developing, updating, reorganizing, and maintaining the database. For that effort to continue into the next generation, when the value of the database will be much greater than its current value, someone or some group will need to take over the effort.

Another epidemiological research need is to identify predictors of positive and stigmatizing attitudes. Appropriate but user-friendly strategies must be developed to analyze database variables. Obviously, sophisticated statistical procedures will be necessary, but researchers must be cognizant that beginning researchers, such as master's students, will not be comfortable with many of those procedures. We need to pilot and develop new demographic variables that might be associated with better or worse public attitudes in order to identify populations that can be studied further with in-depth quantitative and qualitative methods. Evidence of potential predictors of stuttering attitudes would also foster the identification of isolated groups, e.g., those who hold especially negative attitudes toward stuttering, that could be targeted in efforts to change attitudes. Perhaps the most daunting obstacle to these efforts, one that may never be completely overcome, is that "attitudes" (i.e., beliefs, reactions, thoughts, and knowledge) about anything will not easily be—and probably never completely—captured by any algorithm. Another obstacle is that this kind of research is time-consuming, difficult, and complex.

New and better ways of measuring attitudes need to be developed. For reasons hopefully made clear in this chapter, it makes sense to utilize the *POSHA–S* as part of this effort. It should be compared to implicit attitude measures, such as the *Implicit Association Test* (Greenwald, McGhee, & Schwartz, 1998), physiological measures (e.g., Guntupalli et al., 2007), or qualitative analyses (e.g., Schlagheck, Gabel, and Hughes (2009). Also, and ultimately central to the societal impact of this research, we need to develop ways to validate self-reported attitudes with actual behavior. Developing new and better ways to measure attitudes will permit a fuller understanding of how attitudes are acquired, maintained, and changed. Practical obstacles exist in designing studies that will motivate careful and high levels of subject participation while protecting human participants and maintaining informed consent.

There is an omnipresent need for systematic studies designed to change and improve public attitudes toward stuttering. I suggest that future investigations employ both new and documented strategies, as well as control groups. When multiple strategies are employed, ideally, they should be used in non-overlapping regions. One critical need is for studies that document the permanence of change, or lack thereof, induced by the treatments. The value of such research is obvious: changing public attitudes over the long term could be expected to result in more stutterers seeking treatment, less stigma experienced by them, and overall enhanced quality of life. The obstacles, of course, are large. This kind of long-term research is expensive, time-consuming, and difficult.

Finally, there is a need to develop clinical tools and strategies that are informed by epidemiological studies. One suggestion is to measure the attitude environment in which individual stuttering children and adults live (c.f., St. Louis et al., Chapter 16). If such clinical measures could be developed, then individual attitudes could meaningfully be compared to sample-measured attitudes. Additionally, a logical next step would be to develop strategies to alter individual attitude environments, such as attitudes of stuttering clients' families and friends. Another would be to measure the effects of individual attitude environments on clinical outcomes, or vice versa. Obstacles include getting the families and friends of people who stutter to agree that their own attitudes may be a part of the problem and the required paradigm shifts from stuttering treatment involving change on the part of the client to involving change on the part of everyone in the client's environment.

A Concluding Challenge

As a final challenge to researchers, clinicians, teachers, and "the public," I offer the following model for an "ideal" social environment for people who stutter. The six dimensions are goals that might be achieved. If achieved, the social environment would be:

1. *enlightened:* having current and accurate knowledge about stuttering;
2. *understanding:* able to understand and appreciate what the person who stutters experiences;
3. *accommodating:* willing and able to make allowances—when necessary—for people who stutter;

4. *assisting:* willing and able to help, offer sensitive advice, or needed support a person who stutters;
5. *sympathetic:* feeling genuine concern for people who stutter; and
6. *accepting:* not being bothered by stuttering even when confronting it personally.

Chapter 2

Stigma and Stuttering: Conceptualizations, Applications, and Coping

Michael P. Boyle, Gordon W. Blood

ABSTRACT

Stuttering is a disorder of communication that for many people extends far beyond overt instances of disfluent speech. The multidimensional nature of the disorder includes cognitive, affective, and social components. Because stuttering manifests mostly in social situations, there are bound to be social consequences, many of which are negative and may impact the individual who stutters. The public's negative reactions toward stuttering and people who stutter are relevant to the concept of stuttering being classified as a stigmatized disorder. This chapter will focus on the stigma of being a person who stutters. We will first review various conceptualizations and models of stigma, and how these notions of stigma are relevant for people who stutter. Then we will detail various coping mechanisms that people who stutter employ to deal with a stigmatized condition, and conclude with ideas for reducing the stigma experienced by people who stutter.

Conceptualizations of Stigma

Perhaps the most general and simple definition of stigma is that it is a "mark of shame" or "disgrace" (Link & Phelan, 2006). Goffman's (1963) book, *Stigma: Notes on the Management of Spoiled Identity*, was a seminal work in the area of stigma and provided a more concrete definition. Many authors continue to use his definition, which describes stigma as an "attribute that is deeply discrediting" and that reduces the individual with the stigmatized condition "from a whole and usual person to a tainted, discounted one" (Goffman, 1963, p. 3). Goffman wrote about the link between attributes and stereotypes and about the distinction between stigmas that are "discredited" (when one's differentness is known about and visible) and "discreditable" (when one's stigmas are not immediately noticeable). Since the time of Goffman's publication, the topic of stigma has become a popular research topic that has been applied to many different groups of individuals, including people of color, women, lesbian-gay-transgender individuals, obese or overweight individuals, people with HIV-positive status, people with intellectual disabilities, and people with mental illness, among others (Corrigan, Larson, & Kuwabara, 2010). Stigmatizing conditions can manifest in the form of physical appearance, behaviors, or group memberships (Crocker, Major, & Steele, 1998).

Other authors have added to the concept of stigma with modified definitions over the years. Jones and colleagues emphasized the notion of stigma being a "mark" or attribute that links an individual to undesirable characteristics (Jones, Farina, Hastorf, Markus, Miller, & Scott, 1984). The presence of the undesirable characteristic then discredits the individual in the eyes of others. Their model follows from the work of Goffman (1963), and highlights the idea that stigma is both a trait and the outcome of being known to possess the trait. They described how stigmatized traits vary on different dimensions, including concealability (the extent to which the stigma can remain hidden from other people), course (whether the stigma is reversible or irreversible), disruptiveness (the extent to which the stigma interferes with social interactions), aesthetics (whether the stigma triggers a reaction of disgust), origin (how the stigma came into being), and peril (the extent to which the stigma represents a danger or threat to other people).

Link and Phelan (2006) added to the conceptualization of stigma offered by Jones et al. (1984) by describing in detail the process by which a "mark" or stigmatized attribute leads to negative consequences for the individual with the trait. Link and Phelan described how labeling a trait or difference leads to stereotypes and separation from the non-stigmatized group. Stigmatized conditions engender negative emotional responses from the public, and then the stigmatized individual experiences a loss of status in society and subsequent discrimination. Link and Phelan's model also states that this process happens in the context of a power imbalance, wherein stigmatized groups have reduced social, economic, and political power.

Corrigan and colleagues conceptualize stigma as having both public stigma and self-stigma elements (Corrigan, Rafacz, & Rüsch, 2011; Corrigan & Watson, 2002). Public stigma refers to what society believes about and how they act toward a stigmatized group; these include stereotypes, prejudice, and discrimination. Stereotypes are knowledge structures learned by a group that provide shortcuts for classifying individuals and making sense of the world. Not all stereotypes necessarily refer to negative/undesirable characteristics, and not all members of a societal group will agree with stereotypes they hear about other groups of people. Prejudice, however, represents agreeing with a stereotype and concurrently experiencing a negative emotional response (e.g., a feeling of discomfort around someone else). Stereotypes and prejudiced reactions can lead to discrimination, which is the behavioral outcome (e.g., not hiring someone for a job).

Corrigan and colleagues (2011) go on to describe how such public stigma can be internalized in the process of self-stigma. In this model, perceived stigma (awareness of negative stereotypes) leads to self-stigma in which the individual applies the stigma to others with the condition in general (stereotype agreement) and to himself or herself personally (self-concurrence). This process includes negative beliefs about the self, negative emotional reactions to the self, and self-discrimination in which the individual fails to participate in desired activities. The process leads to what Corrigan and colleagues call the "why try" effect (e.g., "Why should I try to get a job that requires lots of talking? I am not worthy of that.") (Corrigan, Larson, & Rüsch, 2009), and finally to detriments in psychological well-being, including reduced self-esteem and self-efficacy. Critically, this model of stigma separates *perceived stigma* (awareness of being stigmatized) and *self-stigma* (internalization and application of stigma to others or to the self personally).

Stigma has also been conceptualized in terms of a distinction between "felt" stigma and "enacted" stigma (Jacoby, 1994). In this dichotomy, enacted stigma refers to actual episodes of negative reactions and discrimination from the public toward individuals with stigmatized traits; felt stigma refers to shame associated with the stigmatized trait and the fear of being evaluated negatively by other people. Although this conceptualization may seem similar to that of Corrigan and colleagues, it allows for the possibility of felt stigma to occur independently of—or even precede—any enacted stigma. In fact, some individuals with a high amount of felt stigma may experience very low levels of enacted stigma due to concealment of the stigmatized trait in order to protect themselves. In addition, felt stigma relates more to feelings of fear and dread about others' perceptions and reactions and anticipation of social rejection due to the stigmatized condition, whereas self-stigma refers more to accepting negative societal reactions and incorporating them into one's own values and beliefs about the self (Livingston & Boyd, 2010).

Another aspect of stigma, known as "structural" stigma (or "institutionalized" stigma) deals with the rules, policies, and procedures of entities of public or private power that can restrict rights and opportunities of individuals with stigmatized conditions (Herek, 2007). Although similar to public stigma previously described, it is considered to exist primarily at the macro level of cultural ideology. Therefore, stigma can be thought of as existing at the systems or macro level (structural or institutional stigma), the group or meso level (social, public, or enacted stigma), and the individual or micro level (felt or self-stigma) (Livingston & Boyd, 2010).

Although there are many variations in the conceptualization of stigma summarized above, it is important to note that current models of stigma acknowledge the critical role of social and cultural processes in stigmas (Herek, 2007; Weiss, Ramakrishna, & Somma, 2006). This contemporary conceptualization emphasizes that a stigma is not an inherent or intrinsic quality of an individual, but rather it is identified in particular social contexts and relationships (Barreto & Ellemers, 2010; Shelton, Alegre, & Son, 2010). It has been stated that "stigmatized individuals possess (or are believed to possess) some attribute, or characteristic, that conveys a social identity that is devalued in a particular social context" (Crocker et al., 1998, p. 505), which emphasizes the critical role of sociocultural processes. For example, if an individual with a trait typically considered stigmatized were to be found in an environment where everyone else exhibited the same trait, it would no longer be viewed as stigmatizing in that context.

Synthesizing all of these different components of stigma leads to a general working definition. Livingston and Boyd (2010) defined internalized stigma as it relates to mental illness as "a subjective process, embedded within a socio-cultural context, which may be characterized by negative feelings (about the self), maladaptive behavior, identity transformation, or stereotype endorsement resulting from an individual's experiences, perceptions, or anticipation of negative social reactions on the basis of their mental illness" (p. 2151). This definition captures the interaction between societal and individual levels of stigma and emphasizes the notion of internalized stigma as a subjective or individual process.

Research has shown that living with a stigmatized condition may result in negative consequences. Public stigma may lead to fewer opportunities in vocational, educational, and social dimensions of life, leading to reduced quality of life and psychological well-being (Corrigan et al., 2010; Major & O'Brien, 2005;

Steele, 1997). Hiding a concealable stigma may lead to reduced overall mental and physical health, including hypertension (Link & Phelan, 2006) and negative affect (Frable, Hoey, & Platt, 1998). Self-stigma, or internalization of stigma, is related to increased anxiety and depression (Mak, Poon, Pun, & Cheung, 2007; Yen, Chen, Lee, Tang, Yen, & Ko, 2005), lower self-esteem, hope, empowerment, and self-efficacy (Corrigan, Watson, & Barr, 2006; Livingston & Boyd, 2010), lower quality of life and well-being (Kellison, Bussing, Bell, & Garvan, 2010), and difficulties in social functioning (Berger, Ferrans, & Lashley, 2001). Self-stigma is also related to decreased use of clinical services and decreased adherence to treatment (Corrigan, 2004; Sirey, Bruce, Alexopoulos, Perlick, Friedman, & Meyers, 2001). It is critical to note that many individuals with a condition that is stigmatized in society do not experience detriments to certain aspects of well-being such as self-esteem (Crocker & Major, 1989), and there seem to be many variables affecting why certain individuals display lower well-being in response to stigma and certain individuals do not (Mak et al., 2007).

Public Stigma and Stuttering

In light of the definitions and conceptualizations of stigma above, it is not difficult to see how stuttering can be classified as a stigmatized disorder. The "mark" or trait that signals the stigma is the actual stuttering, i.e., the overt behaviors (both primary symptoms and secondary manifestations that call attention to it). The signal of overt stuttering leads to the perception that people who stutter possess negative or undesirable personality characteristics. Extensive research collected over decades indicates that people who stutter are perceived as having undesirable personality attributes such as being introverted, shy, anxious, nervous, quiet, tense, guarded, fearful, embarrassed, and frustrated (Kalinowski, Stuart, & Armson, 1996). Similar findings have been observed regarding perceptions of children who stutter. Betz, Blood, and Blood (2008) reported that university students perceive preschool and kindergarten children who stutter as more guarded, nervous, shy, self-conscious, tense, withdrawn, avoiding, afraid, insecure, self-derogatory, and quiet compared to controls who do not stutter. In many different societies across the world, these beliefs about the undesirable characteristics of people who stutter have been recorded among the general public (Craig, Tran, & Craig, 2003; de Britto Pereira, Rossi, & Van Borsel, 2008; Ip, St. Louis, Myers, & An Xue, 2012), college students (Boyle, Blood, & Blood, 2009; Hughes, Gabel, Irani, & Schlagheck, 2010a), teachers (Abdalla & St. Louis, 2012; Dorsey & Guenther, 2000), special educators (Ruscello, Lass, Schmitt, & Pannbacker, 1994), health care professionals (Beste-Guldborg, St. Louis, &

Campanale, Chapter 11; Silverman & Bongey, 1997), employers (Hurst & Cooper, 1983a), vocational rehabilitation counselors (Hurst & Cooper, 1983b), and speech-language pathologists (Cooper & Cooper, 1996; Maviş, St. Louis, Özdemir, & Toğram, 2013; Węsierska,Węsierska, St. Louis, & Beste-Guldborg, Chapter 13).

Some caveats should be mentioned. Recent findings that teachers' and speech-language pathologists' stereotypical views of stuttering people may not be as strong as in the past (Cooper & Cooper, 1996; Irani & Gabel, 2008; Swartz, Gabel, & Irani, 2009), potentially representing a positive shift in attitudes about stuttering; however, evidence of teachers' stereotypes being no better than those of the general public does exist (e.g., Arnold & Goltl, 2013). In addition, mixed methods research examining why laypeople provide certain descriptions of people who stutter may indicate that listeners may use terms like "shy," "anxious," or "frustrated" to describe reactions to living with stuttering and negative societal responses, rather than being perceptions of inherent personality characteristics of people who stutter (Hughes et al., 2010a).

Previous research theorized that negative personality characteristics in people who stutter were inferred from the observation of a seemingly anxious and tense state during speaking. In other words, members of the public look at stuttering individuals struggling with excessive tension during speech, and they infer that these must be character traits of the individual rather than simply symptoms of a disorder (Doody, Kalinowski, Armson, & Stuart, 1993; Kalinowski, Lerman, & Watt, 1987; Kalinowski et al., 1996; Woods & Williams, 1976). In addition, most people who do not stutter have experienced moments where their fluency breaks down and usually this happened during situations in which they were anxious, tense, or nervous. From their own experiences with momentary disfluency resulting from nervousness, it has been shown that these speakers conclude that nervousness is a constant personality characteristic of people who stutter (i.e., "I stutter when I am nervous, and that person stutters all of the time; therefore, that person must be nervous all the time") (White & Collins, 1984; MacKinnon, Hall, & MacIntyre, 2007). It is also possible that portrayal of stuttering people with negative characteristics in the print media (Johnson, 2008), children's television (Johnson, 1987), and literature (Logan, Mullins, & Jones, 2008) provides some basis for negative opinions on the personality characteristics of people who stutter.

Another negative perception of people who stutter that has been identified is that they are somehow less capable or competent than their fluently speaking peers. Physicians who stutter are viewed as less intelligent, educated, and competent than those who do not stutter (Silverman & Bongey, 1997). University students perceive both lawyers and factory workers who stutter to be less competent than their fluent counterparts (Silverman & Paynter, 1990). Despite the public's many negative perceptions of people who stutter, there are also some positive attributes as well. People who stutter can be reported as nice, patient, friendly, cooperative, pleasant, and trustworthy while at the same time being considered nervous, tense, shy, incompetent, and unemployable (Boyle et al., 2009; Hughes et al., 2010a). This profile of characteristics is what Cuddy, Fiske, and Glicke (2008) would label "high warmth" and "low competence." Such a profile may elicit pity and avoidance from the general public.

In addition to negative beliefs about people who stutter, there is also evidence of physiological reactions (skin conductance and heart rate changes) that signify discomfort in hearing a person stutter (Guntupalli, Kalinowski, Nanjudeswaran, Saltuklaroglu, & Everhart, 2006). Also, the seeds of discrimination can be inferred from findings that employers, vocational rehabilitation counselors, and highly educated university students (who will likely be in positions of power after graduation) believe that stuttering is an obstacle for attaining employment, particularly for those positions that require a great deal of speaking (Hurst & Cooper, 1983a, 1983b; Schlagheck, Gabel, & Hughes, 2009). University students, teachers, and speech-language pathologists have reported that certain jobs requiring frequent oral communication are less appropriate for people who stutter as viable career options (Gabel, Blood, Tellis, & Althouse, 2004; Irani, Gabel, Hughes, Swartz, & Palasik, 2009; Logan & O'Connor, 2012; Swartz, Gabel, Hughes, & Irani, 2009). Finally, stuttering can lead to an increase in victimization and being bullied (Blood & Blood, 2004, 2007; Blood, Blood, Tramontana, Sylvia, Boyle, & Motzko, 2011) as well as leaving individuals vulnerable to rejection academically (Davis, Howell, & Cook, 2002), socially, and romantically (Van Borsel, Brepoels, & De Coene, 2011). Clearly, this accumulation of evidence regarding public perceptions supports the notion of stuttering being classified as a publicly stigmatized disorder.

Other variables supporting this finding include factors largely out of control of the person who stutters such as stuttering severity. More severe stuttering, in terms of frequency of disfluent events, is often linked with more negative perceptions compared with milder stuttering (Gabel, 2006; Panico, Healey, Brouwer, & Susca, 2005; Susca & Healey, 2001, 2002; Turnbaugh, Guitar, & Hoffman, 1979), although this is not always the case (e.g., Gabel, Hughes, & Daniels, 2008). It is hypothesized that with increased speech disruptions and visibility of secondary characteristics, it is more difficult for the listener to follow what the speaker is saying, therefore making the listener's reaction more negative. It seems that negative reactions toward stuttering can begin at a young age, as it has been found that preschool-age children (Ezrati-Vinacour, Platzky, & Yairi, 2001) and school-age children (Evans, Healey, Kawai, & Rowland, 2008) have been observed to react negatively to stuttering. Langevin, Packman, and Onslow (2009) observed preschool children who stutter interacting with peers during play and found that in some cases they were interrupted, ignored, or mocked. Findings related to the effect of gender on people who stutter are equivocal with some research suggesting that males give more negative ratings of people who stutter than do females (Burley & Rinaldi, 1986), while other reports demonstrate no such effect (Patterson & Pring, 1991; St. Louis, 2012a). It does appear that there are no significant differences in perceptions of a person who stutters based on the gender (Burley & Rinaldi, 1986; Patterson & Pring, 1991; St. Louis, LeMasters, & Poormohammad, Chapter 9) or age of the stuttering individual (Lass, Ruscello, Pannbacker, Schmitt, & Everly-Myers, 1989; Woods & Williams, 1976). Finally, it appears that attributing stuttering to psychological causes leads to more negative perceptions and desired social distance from people who stutter compared with attributing stuttering to genetic or unexplained causes (Boyle et al., 2009).

Self-Stigma and Stuttering

Like public stigma, self-stigma is essential to consider. First, it is clear that many people who stutter are acutely aware of negative reactions they may receive from the public. Boyle (2012) interviewed 18 people who stutter to determine their perceptions of what other people think about their stuttering. A majority of the participants (61%) believed that the general public views stuttering individuals as less intelligent than others. Specific examples of words used were "less intelligent," "dumb," "stupid," "slow," "ignorant," "mental retardation," and "less capable." A majority of people who stutter interviewed (56%) also believed that the public views them as nervous. Specific terms used included "nervous," "anxious," and "uncomfortable." Fewer participants of those interviewed (28%) believed that the public views them as confused, with specific examples including "confused," indecisive," "don't know what they want to say," and "haphazard." A minority of participants (17%) believed that members of the general public view them as having a psychological disturbance, using words such as "psychological problem" and "unstable mentally."

Boyle (2012) also asked stuttering participants how they think most people in the general public feel when talking to people who stutter. A majority (61%) commented that people felt uncomfortable talking to individuals who stutter, using words like "uncomfortable," "anxious," "nervous," and "embarrassed." A minority of the participants (39%) believed that listeners were confused talking to people who stutter, using the words "confused," "don't know how to react," "uncertain," and "surprised." Finally, only about 33% of the participants believed that others were impatient when talking with people who stutter, using the words "impatient," "frustrated," and "annoyed." Overall, a majority of participants' answers to these open-ended questions regarding the public's perceptions and feelings toward people who stutter were judged to be negative and indicated awareness of stigmatizing attitudes and feelings from communication partners.

These findings support previous qualitative research that has reported people who stutter being afraid that communication partners will view them unfavorably because of their stuttering. Examples of words that have been reportedly used by people who stutter include being fearful that they will be seen as "mentally defective," "strange," "crazy," "incompetent," "inferior," and "stupid," among others (see Bricker-Katz, Lincoln, & McCabe, 2010; Corcoran & Stewart, 1998; Klompass & Ross, 2004; Plexico, Manning, & Levitt, 2009a; Whaley & Parker, 2000). Qualitative research has also illustrated that people who stutter internalize stigmatizing thoughts and apply them to themselves, rather than merely being afraid of what others think. Quotes from people who stutter illustrate that internalizing negative attitudes is related to poor self-perceptions and failure to participate in desired activities. Examples include "because I stutter, I don't deserve to say what I was going to say. I think it kind of brings down my self-worth at times. Like with looking for a job, that oh, I'm not worthy of that" (Plexico et al., 2009a, p. 98), and "If you thought about it, I'm sure you [could think of] a million things you could have done every day if you hadn't stuttered. The telephone calls you could have made. The times you could have gone out. You know, there's millions of them" (Corcoran & Stewart, 1998, p. 10).

In addition to qualitative evidence, quantitative data on a large group of adults who stutter have been recently obtained regarding the internalization of stigma related to stuttering. Boyle (2013a) reported on the development of the *Self-Stigma of Stuttering Scale* (4S), which measures multiple components of stigma (stigma awareness, stereotype agreement, and stigma self-concurrence). The scale has sound psychometric properties, including internal consistency, $\alpha = .87$, and temporal stability, $r = .80$. From a sample of 291 adults who stutter, 89% demonstrated high levels of awareness of public stigma related to stuttering (e.g., "Most people in the general public believe that people who stutter are insecure"). In addition, although only 18% agreed with negative stereotypes about other people who stutter (e.g., "I believe that people who stutter are nervous"), a substantial number (39%) of the sample exhibited high levels of stigma self-concurrence in which they applied negative stigmatizing thoughts to themselves personally. Examples of stigma self-concurrence include negative feelings about the self (e.g., "Because I stutter, I feel less capable than people who don't stutter") and self-discriminating thoughts (e.g., "Because I stutter, I stop myself from taking jobs that require lots of talking"). It is hypothesized that this internalized stigma is related to the many challenges experienced by people who stutter in many realms, including educational (Daniels, Gabel, & Hughes, 2012), vocational (Bricker-Katz, Lincoln, & Cumming, 2013; McAllister, Collier, & Shepstone, 2012), and social (Bricker-Katz et al., 2010; Lowe, Guastella, Chen, Menzies, Packman, O'Brian, & Onslow, 2012; Tudor, Davis, Brewin, & Howell, 2013).

In recent years there have been many findings reported in the literature related to negative psychological problems in people who stutter. Perhaps the two problems discussed most are anxiety disorders and compromised quality of life. As a population, people who stutter are reported to have higher levels of social and generalized anxiety disorders (Iverach, O'Brien, Jones, Block, Lincoln, Harrison, Hewat, Menzies, Packman, & Onslow, 2009; Iverach & Rapee, 2014), particularly in social evaluative domains (Bricker-Katz, Lincoln, & McCabe, 2009) and lower quality of life than people who do not stutter (Craig, Blumgart, & Tran, 2009). In addition, people who stutter have demonstrated more negative affect (Iverach, O'Brian, Jones, Block, Lincoln, Harrison, Hewat, Menzies, Packman, & Onslow, 2010) and higher levels of psychological distress (McAllister, Collier, & Shepstone, 2013) than control groups of individuals who do not stutter. These negative reactions are linked to reduced communication attempts in daily situations and restriction in participation in life activities (Bricker-Katz et al., 2009; Plexico et al., 2009a). Manning and Beck (2013) suggested that the anxiety and quality of life deficits reported and/or experienced by people who stutter are entirely natural reactions that develop as a consequence of stuttering. Although there is debate about the prevalence of personality disorders in people who stutter, it has been proposed that their presence in some individuals is likely due to negative feedback they received as children regarding their speech disfluencies (Iverach et al., 2009).

When increased anxiety and personality disorders do occur in people who stutter, we postulate that negative social evaluation (i.e., stereotyping, prejudice, and discrimination) is instrumental in the development of increased anxiety and personality disorders when they do occur in people who stutter. The concept of being evaluated negatively due to a certain characteristic or trait is clearly relevant to the development of self-stigma. If so, it would then be anticipated that internalizing stigmatizing attitudes is related to lower psychological well-being in people who stutter. In fact, Boyle (2013a) reported data from a large group of adults who stutter demonstrating a strong negative correlation between stigma self-concurrence (i.e., internalized stigma) and self-esteem, and medium negative correlations between stigma self-concurrence and both self-efficacy and life satisfaction. These data show a link between internalized stigma and important aspects of well-being. Stigma self-concurrence was also negatively related to perceived stuttering severity using a 9-point self-rating scale (Boyle, 2012).

In recent years, it has become clear that addressing quality of life and well-being in clients who stutter should be considered an integral part of assessment and treatment (Craig et al., 2009; Cummins, 2010; Yaruss, 2010). The American Speech-Language-Hearing Association (ASHA) (2014b) has adopted the terminology of the International Classification of Functioning, Disability, and Health (ICF) for disability and health-related domains described by the World Health Organization (WHO). This model emphasizes personal and environmental factors in addition to structural or biological deficits. Although some authors have consistently focused on reductions in the structural impairment (i.e., stuttered speech) and question the relevance of social, emotional, or cognitive components in improving treatment outcomes (e.g., Ulliana & Ingham, 1984; Ingham, 2012), it is clear, using the framework of the WHO and ICF adopted by ASHA, that a variety of outcomes are important and worth measuring as outcome variables. It has been argued previously that the only relevance of cognitive and social variables to treatment outcomes is that they represent speech behavior of people who stutter in specific situations and therefore if speech is modified, then so too will attitudes and emotions (Ingham, 1979; Ryan, 2001; Webster, 1977). However, the findings that stereotype agreement (a measure of attitudes toward other people who stutter) was a predictor of self-esteem, self-efficacy, and life satisfaction (Boyle, 2013a) challenges that notion because agreeing with stereotypes for other people who stutter is independent of one's perceived stuttering severity (Boyle, 2012). These findings support the idea that negative beliefs about stuttering, apart from one's perceptions and feelings about one's own stuttering, can predict well-being.

Another finding of note from the Boyle (2013a) study is that merely being aware of societal stigmatization against people who stutter is only weakly related to well-being. This finding appears to reduce support for the "looking glass–self hypothesis" that many researchers proposed long ago—namely, that if people who stutter are aware of negative perceptions about them, they will internalize this to the detriment of their self-concept (Turnbaugh et al., 1979). This means that assessment of awareness of stigma only will not provide an adequate picture of the effect of stigma on an individual who stutters. Just because a person is aware of stigma does not mean that he or she will automatically internalize those attitudes. This is an encouraging finding because it implies that even if total eradication of negative public attitudes about people who stutter is not possible, stuttering people can work on other coping strategies to buffer themselves from these negative perceptions. It appears that many people who stutter are resilient and have developed many adaptive ways of coping with stuttering (Craig, Blumgart, & Tran, 2011).

Coping with Stigma

Stuttering is a disorder particularly prone to stigma because of the great variability from fluent moment to disfluent moment, the uncertainty of the cause of the condition, and the randomness of stuttering episodes, all of which can make communication partners and bystanders feel uneasy, apprehensive, concerned, or helpless. The feeling of being stigmatized, discredited, disliked, dissimilar, and part of an ostracized and devalued group can be a daily occurrence for people who stutter every time they speak. As explained earlier, this may result in reported psychological distress and lower quality of life in some people who stutter (Iverach, Jones, O'Brian, Block, Lincoln, Harrison, Hewat, Menzies, Packman, & Onslow, 2009; Iverach, O'Brien et al., 2009; Plexcio et al., 2009a; Tran, Blumgart, & Craig, 2011). Also, as discussed earlier, stigma in stuttering has been clearly established in a wide variety of populations (Boyle et al., 2009).

The pervasive nature of stuttering and resulting stigma can contribute to feelings of devaluation, alienation, sadness, and unworthiness in people who stutter. It may also lead to avoidance, social withdrawal behaviors, and lower self-esteem (Blood, Blood, Dorward, Boyle, & Tramontana, 2011; Blood, Blood, Tellis, & Gabel, 2003; Blood, Blood, Wertz, Wade, & Mapp, 1997; Blood & Conture, 1998; Boyle, 2013a; Bricker-Katz et al., 2013; Craig et al., 2009; Cummins, 2010; Daniels & Gabel, 2004; Koedoot, Bouwmans, Franken, & Stolk, 2011; Klompas & Ross, 2004; Plexico, Manning, & DiLollo, 2005; Plexico et al., 2009a; Plexico, Manning, & DiLollo, 2009b). A former client of one of the authors very eloquently described the stigma of stuttering over 15 years ago when he stated simply, "It's all about just trying to live with this stuttering." That statement sums up the stigma—the devaluation, the discrediting, the feelings, and the attitudes. The stuttering speech behaviors are only part of the condition and often desired speech changes can and do occur. However, it is the living with the "mark" of stuttering that needs to be addressed and dealt with so people who stutter can successfully adapt, maintain positive self-esteem, develop a helpful life outlook, and build or expand functional social connections, all while bearing the "mark."

It is important to understand that like other groups who are stigmatized, people who stutter respond and react to stigma in a variety of ways depending on their core values, adaptive and learned resources, and situational context. A range of coping and managing strategies can be used for dealing with stigma. This section reviews methods for dealing with both public stigma and self-stigma. Strategies for dealing with both types of stigma include: problem-focused and emotion-focused strategies, engagement and disengagement strategies, and proactive and reactive strategies. As mentioned earlier, Goffman (1963) described two types of individuals who were stigmatized: the "discredited" (when one's differentness is publicly recognized and visible), such as an individual who is blind, a person who has lost a limb, or a person who stutters severely, and the "discreditable" (when one's stigmas are not necessarily noticeable), such as a survivor of cancer, an individual with a mild form of epilepsy, or the person who stutters very mildly. Those with discredited stigma must learn ways to deal with the reactions of others and themselves (including tactics of disclosure, protest, education, and contact), while those with discreditable stigma need to make decisions about concealment, selective disclosure, education, and selective contact (Chaudoir, Earnshaw, & Andel, 2013).

In stuttering, not only does the type, visibility, and severity of stuttering impact ways of dealing with stigma, but so do specific social contexts, previous interactions, and the speaker's desire for secrecy or privacy. Individuals coping with the negative effects of chronic illness or disability need to make decisions regarding the best strategic options for behavior across various contexts (Earnshaw & Quinn, 2012). Often people with concealable stigma adopt the coping tactics of selective disclosure or concealment. Ragins (2008) has developed a model for those with concealable stigmas to disclose their condition in a systematic manner. There are many documented strategies for coping with public stigma. These strategies will be reviewed in the following sections.

Coping with Public Stigma

St. Louis (2010, Chapter 1) and others have stated the time has come to develop a science of public attitude change regarding stuttering, negative attitudes, stereotypes, and stigma. Similarly in the mental health field, Corrigan and Kosyluk (2013) echoed this call in an article about the processes for erasing public stigma. From different disciplines, they both espouse a common idea that science must meet advocacy efforts if stigma reduction and erasure are to be successful. This section of the chapter presents several tactics and strategies that people who are stigmatized publicly have used successfully in specific situations and contexts where they feel threatened. The reader will recall that public, enacted, or interpersonal stigma refers to the experiences of individuals who are stigmatized regarding their interactions with members of the stigmatizing group. Strategies for managing and coping with public stigma have been derived from Corrigan and O'Shaughnessy (2007), Schmader, Croft, Whitehead, and Stone (2013), and LeBel (2008) and include concealment, protest, education, and contact.

1. CONCEALMENT. Often the decision is made to conceal an invisible stigmatizing condition (Goffman, 1963; Corrigan & Lundin, 2001; Jones, Farina, Hastorf, Markus, Miller, & Scott, 1984; LeBel, 2008). Some people who stutter are able to hide their stuttering or cover stuttering by using multiple averting or distraction tactics. These may include avoiding specific words, sounds, or syllables; substituting words; using analogies to explain topics; pretending to be lost in thought; feigning the search for a word; deliberately providing false information; using diversion; agreeing or disagreeing nonverbally; circumlocuting; or electing silence (Clair, Beatty, & MacLean, 2005; Sheehan, 1970, 1975). Some individuals may consciously decide to avoid the social identity of a person who stutters and reject the identity in all interactions by acting as if they were a fluent speaker. In this case, concealing may not simply be a technique to avoid stuttering but rather a strategic choice to benefit these stigmatized individuals by eliminating perceived stigma and/or anticipated stigma as well as any degrading, limiting, and unfair negative stereotypes.

Based on these choices, Douglass and Quarrington (1952) classified stuttering people as exteriorized (overt) and interiorized (covert). They defined the covert person who stutters as someone intentionally trying to conceal his or her stuttering at all costs to avoid any negative reactions from conversational partners and the general public. These individuals never admit publicly to having a stuttering condition. Covert stuttering was also reviewed by Murphy, Quesal, and Gulker (2007), who shared their own personal clinical views about the behavior and the current lack of research on this topic. People who stutter may choose this concealing strategy to manage their stigma and potential social threats, maintain their self-esteem, and avoid unwanted negative interpersonal conflicts. However, many researchers have suggested that living a life of avoidance may be harmful to long-term psychological adjustment and well-being (Barreto & Ellemers, 2010; Brekhus, 2003; Eribon, 2004; Kelly, 2010; Shelton et al., 2010).

Butler (2013) conducted focus groups and semi-structured interviews to examine how 38 people who stutter coped with the intermittent and variable public stigma of stuttering. She reported that stuttering people "grudgingly report their management approaches include concealing, drafting in unwitting others, role-playing and segregating self from their stammer" (p. 1113). She referred to this concealment as "identity cloaking," which is similar to "passing" (i.e., portraying oneself as a "normal" fluent speaker). "Identify cloaking" also describes a range of other approaches. She described six emergent themes from the data. The first theme was concealing as a "hiding space" due to experienced and anticipated social stigma and exclusion. Participants also expressed an "understanding" of why people found it difficult to converse with them as a person who stutters and expressed a need to avoid contact. Butler suggested this showed loss of individuality, acceptance of blame, and a resulting lack of social inclusion. The second theme was labeled "mental space to exchange words" to describe those who found switching words and sentences as a form of social control while concealing stuttering to reduce possible offenses and disappointment. Just over 15% of the sample labeled themselves as covert.

The third theme was labeled "social space as a prop cupboard," which included 20% of Butler's sample who defined themselves as "persons who sometimes stammer showcasing the contextual and variable nature of stuttering where they appeared to accept the identity conflict and were proud of their ability to heed and to be reactive to societal cues" (p. 1119). The fourth theme, labeled "bodily space," described the experiences of low status and accompanying embarrassment, shame, guilt, and anger. This was precipitated by their perceptions of fluent speakers' perceptions of people who stutter and that they "hated," "despised," or "couldn't stand" their own stuttering and would "try anything that's out there," usually including physical and bodily changes to increase fluency (p. 1120). The fifth theme was categorized as a "space for 'it,'" which highlighted the ability in some people who stutter to separate their stuttering from their self-identity and the tendency to view the recurrence of their stuttering as the arrival of "it." About 20% of the sample described stuttering as "it" in an attempt to gain separation from stuttering. Butler referred to this as a form of dis-identification as people who stutter attempt to distance themselves from any perceived or anticipated stigma, stereotypes, prejudice, and discrimination. The last theme that surfaced from her study was identified as "space as place to perform," which dealt with "the influence of role and the narration involved in the playing of a part," "putting on another hat," or performing for others to avoid a destructive identity (p. 1121). Butler's discussion of stigma in people who stutter focused on identity cloaking, identity conflict, the context of concealing, the need for normalizing, covering, and accentuating other attributes or deflecting.

From the above review, it is clear that for those who can conceal their stuttering, one of the first decisions in managing a discredited social identity and resulting stigma may be the use of concealing stuttering to protect self-esteem and general well-being. The situation may also exist where a person who stutters discloses his or her stuttering in some situations, but not in other situations based on the context and anticipated stigma. This has been referred to as *negotiated concealment* in stigmas associated with health-related issues (e.g., epilepsy, asthma, and multiple sclerosis) (Green, 2009; Grytten & Måseide, 2005). Hiding stuttering or passing as a fluent speaker to avoid negative social penalties, disadvantages, and listener reactions has been reported in the literature (Corcoran & Stewart, 1998; Crichton-Smith, 2002; Klompas & Ross, 2004; Plexico et al., 2005; Plexico, Manning, & Levitt, 2009a, 2009b).

In one of the first studies examining perceived stigma, disclosure practices, and self-esteem of adolescents who stutter, Blood, Blood, Tellis, and Gabel (2003) found that stuttering did not present a stigmatizing condition for the majority (65%) of adolescents who stutter. The authors of the study developed the *Stigmatization and Disclosure in Adolescents Who Stutter Scale*, a seven-item scale using a 4-point Likert scale format, confirmed the structure and validity of the scale and asserted that 60% of adolescents who stutter rarely or never discussed or disclosed their stuttering, a clear form of concealment. This suggested that hiding or selective concealment of stuttering was used as a coping strategy for these adolescents. The results regarding disclosure and concealment of stuttering in this age group were confirmed by Hearne, Packman, Onslow, and Quine (2008) using qualitative methods and most recently by Erickson and Block (2013), who replicated the Blood et al. (2003) study. Erickson and Block (2013) reported that 62% of their adolescents also responded to keeping their stuttering "a secret often and/or sometimes," while only 28% claimed to "never keep it a secret." Less than half of the adolescents claimed that all of their friends knew they stuttered, and 73% "rarely or never" talked about their stuttering. These are examples of deflecting, concealing, and discrediting the stigma of stuttering.

Disclosure of stuttering in adults who stutter was traditionally perceived as having a positive impact on reducing perceived stress in conversational partners (Collins & Blood, 1990), but now only appears to have a positive impact on perceptions when the listener has the opportunity to compare conditions of disclosure and non-disclosure, which is not applicable to everyday situations (Healey, Gabel, Daniels, & Kawai, 2007; Lee & Manning, 2010). It may be possible, however, that the type of disclosure (i.e., positive and affirmative versus apologetic) could explain differences in listener responses across studies.

Concealment is not always seen as a negative avoidance technique but may be a way that individuals who are unjustly refused their rights and privileges because of stigma attempt to "level the playing field" (Kroeger, 2003). Individuals who elect to conceal their condition often strategically plan to conceal their condition to maintain their privacy, self-esteem, and well-being. These individuals regard the concealing, not as a passive act, but a deliberate action and a precaution to protect privileges and rights they believe have been unjustly deprived (Beals, Peplau, & Gable, 2009; Clair et al., 2005; Goffman, 1959, 1963; Jones et al., 1984; London, Downey, Romero-Canyas, Rattan, & Tyson, 2012; Phillips, Rothbard, & Dumas, 2009; Quinn & Chaudoir, 2009; Vescio, Gervais, Heiphetz, & Bloodhart, 2009).

The context and the intention to conceal are also important in coping when dealing with stigma. There is an important differentiation between "secrecy" and "privacy" with respect to concealing a stigmatized identity. The former suggests shame and embarrassment about the condition (e.g., internalizing negative stereotypes of others, afraid to lose current acquaintances/coworkers, embarrassment about living with the condition, or humiliation about being discovered). Shame and embarrassment have been reported in people who stutter (Ginsberg, 2000; Plexico et al., 2009a). The latter suggests the people have a self-identity that they do not wish to share for their own personal reasons (e.g., their right to share information about themselves, current understanding of negative stereotypes of their condition, perceived changes in comfort level with friends/coworkers, or concerns about others' ignorance about their condition). This suggests that even though they may be covert in their stuttering, they have maintained their positive self-esteem and general well-being.

2. EDUCATION. Education as a strategy refers to approaches to dealing with public stigma by replacing false information with factual data. Stigma and negative attitudes are very resistant to change, although educational and information management programs have shown positive outcomes for stigma associated with HIV/AIDS (Greene & Banerjee, 2006; Sengupta, Banks, Jonas, Miles, & Smith, 2011), racism (Dovidio, Gluszek, John, Ditlmann, & Lagunes, 2010; Sanchez & Garcia, 2009), religious differences (Herzig, Roysircar, Kosyluk, & Corrigan, 2013), sexism (Swim, Hyers, Cohen, & Ferguson, 2001; Swim, Mallett, & Stangor, 2004), homosexuality and other gender differences (Bockting, Miner, Swinburne, Hamilton, & Coleman, 2013; Goldberg, Kinkler, & Hines, 2011; Preston, D'augelli, Kassab, & Starks, 2007), substance abuse (Livingston, Milne, Fang, & Amari, 2012; Livingston, Tugwell, Korf-Uzan, Cianfrone, & Coniglio, 2012), and mental illness (Corrigan & Shapiro, 2010; Corrigan, Morris, Michaels, Rafacz, & Rüsch, 2012).

In a recent systematic review of 72 articles representing 38,364 research participants from 14 countries, Corrigan et al. (2012) provided evidence of stigma reduction in adults and adolescents regarding mental illness through educational programs. The authors also indicated that another strategy, "interpersonal contact," was even more effective than educational programs at reducing stigma for adults. However, for adolescents, educational campaigns and programs were more effective than interpersonal contact. Parallel research could be conducted examining the comparisons of educational campaigns and personal contact campaigns for adolescents and adults who stutter.

Regarding attitudes toward stuttering, The Stuttering Foundation, National Stuttering Association, Friends: The National Association of Young People Who Stutter, and similar groups have used educational approaches to address their goals of stigma erasure and attitude change of the public. Members of these organizations and others have employed education approaches to changing attitudes and stigma with informational books, pamphlets, DVDs, and posters aimed at specific audiences (e.g., classroom teachers, pediatricians, or parents). The rationale is that accurate and factual information about stuttering and people who stutter will counter current negative stereotypes and promote understanding of stuttering. Although subjective and personal stories about the success of these educational strategies are common in stuttering, few empirical studies or reviews in the area of stuttering research have tested/demonstrated how education and information management reduce stigma. This situation is improving however, as planned and documented improvements in attitudes or lessened stigma have been documented at least temporarily (e.g., Abdalla, Chapter 5; Abdalla & St. Louis, 2014; Flynn & St. Louis, 2011).

3. CONTACT. Contact involves members of the public spending time with people with targeted stigmatized conditions and interacting with them. Optimally, this method involves people with the stigmatized condition who are leading successful lives. This may reduce the perceived differences of the individual with the stigmatized condition. As mentioned previously, contact appears to be the strongest and most effective means of reducing public stigma toward individuals with mental illness (Corrigan et al., 2012). The results of studies on the effect of familiarity with stuttering individuals (not personal contact per se, but reported associations) are equivocal with some studies showing that familiarity and social closeness may be related to more positive perceptions about people who stutter (Klassen, 2001, 2002; Langevin, 2009; Langevin, Kleitman, Packman, & Onslow, 2009), and others showing no such effect (Boyle et al., 2009; Doody et al., 1993; Fowlie & Cooper, 1978; Gabel et al., 2004).

Recently, Flynn and St. Louis (2011) reported on a study presenting live oral or recorded video presentations on stuttering to 83 high school students to determine the extent to which their attitudes toward stuttering could be changed. Using the *Public Opinion Survey of Human Attributes-Stuttering* (*POSHA–S*) as a pre-test and post-test measure, they examined two educational conditions: (1) a 45-minute oral live presentation by a person who stutters during health classes; (2) an MTV (Music TV) *True Life®: I Stutter* 45-minute video (Schneider, 2007) presentation with the person who stutters in the oral condition as one of three people featured in the video. Using an adapted version of the *POSHA–S* (St. Louis, 2011a, 2011b, 2012b, 2012c), the authors reported that attitudes improved overall on the *POSHA–S*. They concluded that high school students' attitudes toward stuttering and people who stutter can be improved, at least temporarily, by a professionally prepared video on stuttering and even more so through a live presentation by a person who stutters. This type of research could pave the way for continued studies examining stigma reduction and attitude change through educational campaigns presented by people who stutter. Anti-stigma campaigns and research must address what maintains the stigma against stuttering and what may reduce it.

Importantly, the Flynn and St. Louis (2011) study contrasts with previous studies designed to lower negative public attitudes toward stuttering because it involved a speaker who stuttered, who was relatively close in age to the intended audience, and who also spoke about stuttering in a lighthearted and sometimes humorous manner. These components may have been critical in improving attitudes toward people who stutter. It is puzzling to note, however, that two-thirds of the high school students wrote in a follow-up procedure that they believed the stuttering speaker was "faking" his stuttering. Previous studies that have used education but no contact with stuttering people (e.g., McGee, Kalinowksi, & Stuart, 1996; Snyder, 2001) produced far less favorable results with little notable attitude changes. Obviously, determining what the optimal strategies are for reducing public stigma toward stuttering is an important area of future research.

4. PROTEST. One common management strategy for public stigma is protest (Corrigan & Kosyluk, 2013). Where education is considered a proactive tactic only, protest efforts are considered to be both a proactive and reactive tactic. Protest may include: public expressions of unfairness and injustice; calling out the non-stigmatized person for his or her behavior, attitudes, and feelings; and social activism activities. For example, a campaign aimed at Warner Brothers a number of years ago to stop having actors play nervous, bumbling, incompetent stereotypes of stuttering people, as well as cartoon characters laughing and mocking people who stutter (e.g., "Porky Pig") fall under this strategy. Milder forms of protest for stigma reduction can also occur. Gently confronting and correcting a member of the non-stigmatized group about false statements during a private conversation or even in public forums (e.g., classroom, civic debate) are subtle forms of protest and education.

Protest activities are usually the response to an obvious public victimization or stigmatization of a condition. The use of protest provides opportunities for teachable moments for members of the stigmatizing group and also empowers the members of the stigmatized group. For example, a young stuttering female in speech therapy was conducting stuttering attitude surveys on a university campus. The first few exercises went well until she approached two female students, who asked numerous questions like "Is this really happening to me?" or "Are you for real?" The stuttering speaker took a moment, composed herself, disclosed that she stuttered, and then asked them what they found amusing. They continued to smirk until she stated, "Does it really make you feel better to put me down?" As she walked away with her clinician, she explained that she felt sorry for them because they were so ignorant and uninformed. Significantly, at this point, she said, "Let's do some more of these surveys; I've got a lot of work to do for myself and for them." Her disclosure, followed up with protest, had a favorable impact on her self-esteem and acceptance of her identity as a person who stutters.

Although such clinical anecdotes are common, little empirical evidence has been provided in the area of stuttering that systematically demonstrates the use and/or benefit of these strategies. Craig et al. (2011) highlighted the importance of empowerment and resilience in people who stutter, and this may be a fine example of client resilience, a "fighting spirit," and hardiness. If these types of skills can be taught or encouraged in treatment protocols, research studies could determine if such skill sets could act as a defense and safeguard against stigma for people who stutter.

Coping with Self-Stigma

Stigmatizing views toward individuals with disabilities are a reality of society. Accordingly, since it is society that generates stigma, it is important to remember that individuals should not be made to feel guilty about having stigmatizing thoughts about themselves. Although a primary aim of the aforementioned strategies is to change the public stigma associated with stuttering, it is perhaps not realistic to expect that all or even most of the public's responses to stuttering will be positive in the immediate future, especially if people who stutter manifest self-stigma. Therefore, based on recent research, it will be potentially beneficial to provide people who stutter with strategies and resources to minimize or reduce self-stigmatizing thoughts, feelings, and behaviors as well. Whereas public stigma deals more with interpersonal relations, self-stigma deals more with intrapersonal issues. The following section discusses some potential strategies and tactics for coping with self, internalized, or intrapersonal stigma. These strategies are similar to those reported with other self-stigmatized disorders such as mental illness (Corrigan et al., 2010) and chronic illnesses (Earnshaw & Quinn, 2012), which include disclosure and acknowledgment, peer support, and cognitive restructuring.

1. DISCLOSURE AND ACKNOWLEDGMENT. The decision about disclosing a stigmatized condition is also a decision about authenticity, an analysis of the cost and benefits, and the critical context of disclosure (Corrigan & Matthews, 2003). In many ways, the choice is a two-edged sword. Disclosing eliminates one's constant fear of exposure, need for secrecy, and double-identity dilemma, as well as increases one's access to new levels of personal and organizational social support. Simultaneously, however, it also may expose the individual to increased rejection, isolation, negative bias, and inaccurate generalizations about capabilities, skills, and potential (Clair et al., 2005).

There can be many potential degrees of disclosure, and disclosure of a stigmatizing condition can be considered on both a micro and macro level. On the micro level, people who stutter may have specific contexts or situations (e.g., work, school, or social) where they may choose to disclose their identity as people who stutter (i.e., selective disclosure). They may adopt the persona of a fluent speaker in certain social contexts but not others (e.g., with friends versus employers). Other individuals who stutter may choose to disclose stuttering indiscriminately to anyone in any situation. Still others may "broadcast" their stuttering to others using advertising and pseudo-stuttering. Disclosure and acknowledgment are not simple decisions. Discussing the false-role conflict of a person who stutters, Sheehan (1970, 1975) suggested that stuttering individuals should accept their role as a person who stutters and not try to "fake" or "pass" as a fluent speaker. He believed that the optimal way to address the stuttering problem (behaviors and potential stigma) was to acknowledge to oneself and others a true identity as a person who stutters. Anti-avoidance therapies have been developed on the acceptance of the role and social identity of being a person who stutters (Sheehan, 1970; 1975; Van Riper, 1971). The acceptance of the identity of a stuttering person can be acknowledged in public situations and interactions (Van Riper, 1971).

In the stuttering literature, an excellent example of this strategy is provided by Sugarman (1980), who discusses "coming out" as a two-stage process. This includes "acknowledgment," which is the beginning of self-discovery and learning about the problem, and then "admission" and "owning the problem" of "I am a stutterer" (p. 155). Owning the problem means taking responsibility and admitting to oneself and others that one stutters. Murphy, Yaruss, and Quesal (2007b) highlight the benefits of role-playing and self-disclosure via education of classmates with a nine-year-old child who stutters. Trichon and Tetnowski (2011), reporting on the benefits of participation in a self-help conference using a qualitative analysis approach, revealed several themes that minimized the negative impact of stuttering on the 12 stuttering participants. In addition to the positive benefits of experiencing a safer and "stutter-friendly" environment that supported friendship and community building, participants also reported increased social activity and "openness" about their stuttering (i.e., disclosure and acknowledgment) as positive outcomes of attending the conference.

Disclosure has the potential for increasing contact between people who stutter and members of the public, therefore reducing both public and self-stigma. Similarly, disclosure makes it possible for individuals with the same condition to meet and help one another (e.g., joining self-help groups, to be discussed later) and reap the benefits of social support and a sense of belonging to a larger group.

Strategies for facilitating disclosure have been documented in the stuttering literature. A major advantage of freely chosen disclosure is the potential for connection with an "authentic" self as well as access to treatment services, legal mandates or protections (e.g., Americans with Disabilities Act) (Mackelprang & Salsgiver, 1999), and social support from other stigmatized members. The activation of social and political assistance and social support networks can be used to address academic and occupational discrimination for acknowledged and disclosed disabilities. Anti-avoidance therapies have been developed to counter the desire or need to conceal stuttering and are outlined and discussed in detail by numerous authors (Guitar, 2013; Manning, 2010; Van Riper, 1973; Sheehan, 1970, 1975; Shapiro, 2011; Yairi & Seery, 2011).

Cautions must be considered as well. Disclosure may not always be the best choice for people who stutter, depending on their perceived, enacted, or anticipated stigma. If the clear benefits of this approach are not recognized, appreciated, and endorsed by the stutterer, the tactic may not be successful or may backfire. Even though "approach-oriented"—as opposed to "avoidance-oriented"—coping seems to be important for some people who stutter in improving quality of life and overall well-being (Plexico et al., 2009b), a developmental process appears to guide these decisions. Additionally, caution should be considered in accepting one's condition and acknowledging it as it relates to self-stigma. It is possible that while in the process of accepting the stuttering or the stigmatizing condition, the individual may begin to "use" the condition to attribute educational, social, and vocational failures to the stigma (Major & O'Brien, 2005). This kind of self-handicapping self-stigma can have another set of harmful negative consequences for the individual who is stigmatized.

2. PEER SUPPORT. The next stigma-management strategy discussed here is the participation in—and use of—support, self-help, or mutual-aid groups and self-help advocacy efforts. Elafros, Mulenga, Mbewe, Haworth, Chomba, Ata-dzhanov, and Birbeck, (2013) suggested that peer-support groups are an effective way to decrease epilepsy-associated stigma while Chou, Robb, Clay, and Chronister (2013) reported on the beneficial and positive effects of social support to buffer individuals with substance-abuse problems from self-stigma. Demissie, Getahun, and Lindtjørn (2003) reported on the positive benefits of support groups for individuals with tuberculosis as a means of increasing group members' knowledge and reducing their personal negative feelings and beliefs. The self-help meetings provided assistance in addressing common problems, shared concerns, and enhancing individual social support. The authors found that the mutual support component improved the attitudes of the majority of participants.

Typical support group models incorporate both information and support services, are led by a member of stigmatized group, and are often open to members of both stigmatized and non-stigmatized groups. These models have reported success not only in increasing knowledge and services for individuals with specific conditions (e.g. diabetes, cancer, or asthma), but also in providing ways to reduce stigma through peer bonding and new partnerships in advocacy efforts. Some (Corrigan & Kosyluk, 2013; Corrigan & Lundin, 2001) refer to the value of support groups for managing stigma as a by-product of bonding with other individuals who are stigmatized and the attendant social support. Public endorsement of a stigma in a group offers a community for fellowship and acceptance. Studies have shown that individuals who are members of stigmatized groups (e.g., serious mental illness) and who participate and identify with mutual self-help groups report less social stigma than those who do not identify with these groups. It has also been suggested that the social support from these self-help groups actually buffers participants from public and self-stigma and contributes to better overall adjustment, well-being, and self-esteem.

Corrigan, Sokol, and Rüsch (2013) recruited 85 people with schizophrenia or other psychiatric disorders who completed psychological self-report measures, including a measure of self-stigma, during face-to-face interviews. Participants also completed self-report of mutual-help activities (e.g. membership in a group for people with mental illness that is run by people with mental illness), the satisfaction rating of the experiences, a group identification rating, and a social support rating. Results suggested involvement in mutual-help programs decreased participants' perceptions of self-stigma. Although preliminary in nature, the authors suggest that high group identification and perceived positive social support (components of mutual-help programs) positively influence the overall quality of life for individuals who are stigmatized.

Support groups also offer another possible advantage to assist stigma reduction. They provide individuals with the opportunity to "re-define" themselves and their identity. Nario-Redmond, Noel, and Fern (2012) suggest that "re-defining" disability and "re-imaging" the self not only protect—but actually enhance—self-esteem while managing stigma. They reported on two surveys with 93 and 268 adults with disabilities, respectively, about the impact of group identification. The results suggested that identification with a group in a formalized manner (e.g., a self-help group) was self-protective both in terms of dealing with stigma and maintaining general well-being. They speculated that belonging to advocacy or social activism groups empowered the members of the group. This type of management actually negates the stigma by replacing it with positive attributes, that is, attributes that redefine the stigmatizing condition. Additionally, Baretto and Ellemers (2010) suggest that group identification with a stigmatizing condition can be a source of resilience to combat public stigma.

Support groups, self-help groups, mutual-aid groups, and self-help advocacy efforts are not new in the area of stuttering as a way to manage negative attitudes and stigma (Ramig, 1993; Reeves, 2006, 2007; Trichon, 2007; Trichon & Tetnowski, 2011). Reporting on the experiences of 71 people who stutter who completed detailed questionnaires, Yaruss, Quesal, Reeves, Molt, Kluetz, Caruso, and Lewis, (2002) found that the 57.1% of people who stutter described the support group experience as having a "very positive impact" on their self-image and acceptance of their stuttering. An additional 36.7% of the people who stutter reported support group participation had a "somewhat positive impact."

Boyle (2013b) published a study reporting on the relationship between support group membership for stuttering and internalized stigma in 279 adults who stutter. One-hundred seventy-five of the participants (63%) had current or prior support group experience and 105 (37%) had no such experience. Participants completed a series scales measuring self-esteem, self-efficacy, life satisfaction, self-stigma, perceived stuttering severity, and other stuttering-related perceptions. Boyle found that people who stutter who had experience participating in support groups for stuttering reported lower self-stigma scores, were more likely to believe that they would stutter for the rest of their lives, and placed less importance on fluent speech than functional communication when talking to other people. Individuals who joined support groups to help other people feel better about themselves (81 participants, 46% of the sample) reported significantly higher self-esteem, self-efficacy, and life satisfaction compared to people who stutter with no support group experience. These findings showcase the positive benefits of support groups with people who stutter in terms of stigma management and support those of Yaruss et al. (2002) in that the majority of participants perceived support groups for stuttering to be extremely helpful (45%) or moderately helpful (29%).

3. COGNITIVE RESTRUCTURING. A person who stutters who demonstrates negative thoughts and beliefs about himself or herself (e.g., "No one will like me if they know that I stutter") has a major challenge and barrier to participation in desired activities and achievement of life goals. Qualitative research has demonstrated that people who stutter can indeed demonstrate negative attitudes toward themselves to the detriment of their psychological well-being and quality of life (Crichton-Smith, 2002; Plexico et al., 2009a). Over the past several years, increasing interest has been given to therapies that target negative thoughts of people who stutter.

Cognitive behavioral therapy (CBT) is a treatment that identifies unhelpful negative thoughts in clients and then tests these negative assumptions and potentially challenges their accuracy. The goal is for the client to modify or replace negative thoughts or negative "self-talk" with positive self-talk. For example, if a client thinks "I will never be successful and people do not like me," the thought can be identified and modified to something like "I can and will be successful and many people do like me." Blood (1995a, 1995b) developed the *POWER2* program, a CBT-based treatment for adolescents and adults who stutter that focuses on how people who stutter speak, think, and feel while decreasing their stuttering severity. The *POWER2* (Permission, Ownership, Well-being, Esteem of One's Self, Resilience, and Responsibility) program was based on Bandura's (1994) classic self-efficacy model. Blood reported positive changes in self-attitudes of stuttering participants through the use of counseling and psychotherapy techniques drawn from CBT. Blood (2003) later published a communication and social skills workbook for adolescents and adults who stutter dealing with attitudes and feelings about stuttering based on CBT. Other authors (e.g., Botterill, 2011; Menzies, Onslow, Packman, & O'Brian, 2009) have also embraced similar methods to assist clients who stutter. Constantino, Eger, and Matthies (2013) reported on a pilot study using self-reports to measure the effectiveness of a CBT treatment program with 11 stuttering participants. At the conclusion of the CBT program, seven participants reported more positive speaker experiences with various audiences, particularly with strangers and authority. In addition to facilitating cognitive restructuring, CBT can also help with exposure and desensitization to perceived or anticipated negative situations (see Menzies et al., 2009, for a review). This type of therapy has been tested with people who stutter, and data show that participation in CBT improves global life functioning and entry into fear situations, even more so than therapy focused on speech change only (Menzies, O'Brian, Onslow, Packman, St. Clare, & Block, 2008).

In addition, the use of "mindfulness" practice is relevant to the management of negative thoughts and feelings that can be associated with stuttering (Boyle, 2011; Silverman, 2012). Unlike CBT, mindfulness does not aim to change or replace negative thoughts with positive thoughts. Instead, the intent is to develop a broader understanding of the thought process itself, resulting in a person feeling less trapped and controlled by his or her thoughts. The person can cultivate mindfulness through activities and practices designed to enhance awareness and attention, emotional regulation, and acceptance (see Boyle, 2011, for a detailed review). Mindfulness practice has been applied to stuttering treatment with programs such as *Mindfulness Based Stress Reduction* (de Veer, Brouwers, Evers, & Tomic, 2009) and *Acceptance and Commitment Therapy* (Beilby, Byrnes, & Yaruss, 2012), results of which demonstrate that mindfulness therapy can be helpful in improving psychological well-being and quality of life in people who stutter.

Finally, assertiveness-based treatment programs can be helpful in modifying self-stigma in people who stutter. Many stutterers do not speak up for themselves when someone violates their expectations for how they would like to be treated. Of course, many people in the general public have difficulty being assertive (e.g., returning food at a restaurant or telling audience members in a movie theater to be quiet); however, this reticence in stuttering people is often compounded because of the anticipated difficulty of physically producing the speech necessary to communicate the message (Yairi & Seery, 2011). Clinicians find that some clients who stutter complain that others respond negatively to their speech difficulties, e.g., interrupting them, completing thoughts for them, or even mocking them, but they did nothing in response. More subtle examples of a lack of assertiveness include clients saying things like "I would like to participate in class, but I don't want to take up the valuable class time" or "I don't feel comfortable using my speech techniques with other people because I don't want to bother them with how I am talking." These examples illustrate that people who stutter can sometimes fail to assert their own rights and preferences in deference to their listeners, and relinquish their power to speak.

Strategies in therapy can be used to increase a client's sense of power and assertiveness. Role-playing situations in which clients reported they have deferred to someone else or been made to feel negatively about themselves can be practiced in therapy. Blood's (2003) therapy program includes this critical component of helping the client to differentiate between responding in a "powerful" versus a "powerless" manner to hypothetical challenging situations, all within the context of a game. Such activities can be very helpful in providing the stutterer with multiple options for responding to challenging circumstances and initiating a cognitive change that promotes a sense of confidence and control in all aspects of life.

Conclusion: Understanding Stigma Will Bring About Change

This chapter examined conceptualizations of stigma, reviewed applications of public and self-stigma to people who stutter, and discussed several potential strategies for stigma reduction. It also highlighted the need to conduct well-designed, methodologically sound studies to determine the benefits and advantages of using specific strategies aimed at stigma management. Important issues that clinicians and researchers addressing stuttering stigma face include:

1. assessing short-term and long-term stigma-reduction programs using specific strategies;
2. differentiating between subjective self-stigma and societal public stigma;
3. understanding the roles of professional organizations, the health care industry, academic, business, and government institutions in reducing stigma against stuttering and people who stutter;
4. measuring the effects of anti-stigma interventions that decrease perceived public or social stigma with standardized reliable instruments for post-program outcomes;
5. assessing the effects of public awareness campaigns on stigma reduction;
6. isolating the roles of culture, age, and gender in specific stigma-reduction strategies;
7. exploring the role of contact with other people who stutter sharing and telling their stories about living and managing stigma on stigma reduction;
8. determining the roles of job, school, or social life contexts in disclosing or concealing stuttering;
9. assessing the effects of educational programs and differences between educational information and direct contact that have been observed in other health-related disabilities;
10. exploring the effects on family and friends living with people who stutter who feel stigmatized;
11. comparing the integration of systematically designed anti-stigma programs with more behaviorally based fluency-shaping methods; and

12. comparing advantages of changing public attitudes toward stuttering versus changing individual attitudes of people who stutter.

The battle against stigma in stuttering has been raging for centuries (Blood, 1999). With renewed focus and increased research and clinical attention, the power and "mark" associated with the stigma of stuttering may begin to be reduced. In the meantime, while society offers no cure for stuttering stigma, as researchers and clinicians, we can continue to support, lead, and design scientific initiatives aimed at interpersonal, intrapersonal, community, and government levels to mitigate the stigma associated with stuttering.

_____

Chapter 3

Bullying Experienced by Youth Who Stutter: The Problem and Potential Intervention Strategies

Marilyn Langevin

ABSTRACT

Personal characteristics, social factors such as peer rejection, coping styles, and exceptionalities such as stuttering place children at risk for bullying. This review brings together the literature on bullying in youth in the general population and those who stutter. It also discusses potential coping strategies and their evidence base, which can be considered when helping children with and without exceptionalities who are victims of bullying.

Bullying is a ubiquitous problem that affects a minority of typically fluent children but a majority of children who stutter who present for therapy. As background to discussing teasing and bullying experienced by children and adolescents who stutter, I will first present what is known about bullying in general. Thereafter, I will discuss potential interventions with victimized children at the client-centered (e.g., individual) and universal (e.g., classroom or school-wide) level. Although preschool children are also teased because of their stuttering (Langevin, Packman, & Onslow, 2009, 2010), this chapter focuses on school-age children.

Bullying in Youth

Definition

Bullying is conventionally defined as a subtype of aggression that has three key elements: an intent to harm, repetition over time, and a power differential in which children who are bullied have difficulty defending themselves against a more powerful individual or group (Salmivalli & Peets, 2009). The requirements of a power differential and repetition over time distinguish bullying from other forms of peer aggression such as physical and verbal fights between children of equal power in terms of size, psychological prowess, or social status (Baly & Cornell, 2011; Dooley, Pyzalski, & Cross, 2009; Olweus, 1993). However, recent research suggests that students may apply the term "bullying" more broadly to include social conflicts that do not include a power differential (Baly & Cornell, 2011). A concept of social bullying that includes conflicts in which there is no power differential likely results in somewhat inflated self-reports of being bullied and calls for education about what bullying is and is not (Baly & Cornell, 2011). Despite the need for such distinction and education, particularly in research, it remains that a student who experiences social conflict that causes social or psychological harm, whether or not there is a real or perceived power imbalance, may still need help from adults. The same also applies to some students who experience one-time or limited-time aggression who may consider the event to be bullying (Guerin & Hennessy, 2002). Although such experiences of aggression do not meet the repetition criterion, it is recognized from a life events model that children who suffer peer aggression for a limited time can endure long-term negative consequences (Kochenderfer-Ladd & Wardrop, 2001). It can also be argued that repeated reliving of the one-time event and associated feelings of stress can be considered repetition of the event. Cyberbullying (discussed below) is another form of a one-time event that can have devastating effects for which the requirements of repetition by the perpetrator and a power differential do not strictly apply.

Conceptualizations—and Cognitive, Emotional, and Behavioral Sequelae—of Bullying

The conceptualization of bullying and understanding of its consequences have undergone a paradigm change over the years. From the seminal work of Olweus (1993) in which the core features of bullying were defined, the conceptualization of bullying progressed to understanding it as a relationship problem in which children who bully use power and aggression to control others, from which escape for the victimized child is difficult (Craig & Pepler, 2008). More recently, bullying is being viewed as a significant social, mental, and physical health problem (Lester, Cross, Dooley, & Shaw, 2013; Vaillancourt, Duku, Becker, Schmidt, Nicol, Muir, & MacMillan, 2011) with neurobiologic effects and genetic influences (Vaillancourt, Clinton, McDougall, Schmidt, & Hymel, 2010). Bullying is also being viewed from a socio-ecological perspective as it affects the school climate, which in turn influences victims and bystanders (see Cornell, Gregory, Huang, & Fan, 2013).

SOCIAL, MENTAL, AND PHYSICAL HEALTH. Historically, being victimized by bullying (hereinafter referred to interchangeably as "victimization," "being bullied," the "child who is bullied," and "children who are bullied") has been linked to diminished psychological well-being, including low self-esteem, negative emotional stress, poor social adjustment, including school avoidance and rejection by peers, and psychological distress. Psychological distress can include high degrees of anxiety, depression, and suicidal thoughts. Children who are bullied can also experience physical ill-health symptoms such as medically diagnosed illnesses and psychosomatic symptoms, and poor academic performance (Rigby, 2003; Schwartz, Gorman, Nakamoto, & Toblin, 2005). (See Boyle and Blood, Chapter 2, for a detailed discussion of issues related to stigma.)

More recent research into the effects of bullying on social and mental health, including depression, hopelessness, and physical ill health, provides further evidence of the negative consequences for victims. For example, Lester et al. (2013) compared mental and social health outcomes of adolescents transitioning from primary to secondary school. They defined social health as the "ability to get along with others, dealing with social institutes and societal mores" (p. 109). Indicators of social health were measures of loneliness at school, peer support at school, connectedness to school, and safety at school. Mental health indicators were measures of depression and anxiety. Regarding social health, Lester et al. (2013) found that feeling lonely at school or being less connected to school was associated with being in the group of children who experienced stable or increasing levels of bullying over the period from the end of Grade 7 to the end of Grade 9. They also found that feeling safe at school was protective for males but not females, and having high peer support was protective for females but not males. Regarding mental health, Lester et al. found that bullied children reported higher levels of depression and anxiety at the end of Grade 9 than the non-bullied group.

Hopelessness is regarded as a predictor of depression (Siyahhan, Aricak, & Cayirdag-Acar, 2012). It was defined by Siyahhan et al. (2012) as the "cognitive dimension of depression . . . associated with individuals' perceptions of lacking control over future event outcomes" (p. 1053). These authors found hopelessness to be higher in victimized children than non-victimized children. Additionally, boys reported higher levels of hopelessness than girls.

Recent research into the physical effects of bullying has viewed bullying as a chronic stressor that may affect brain function, notably, cognition, the sympathetic nervous system, and the immune system, including cortisol production

(Rex-Lear, Knack, & Jensen-Campbell, 2012). In an investigation of effects of bullying on health and cortisol levels in adolescents, Knack, Jensen-Campbell, and Baum (2011) found that more frequent peer victimization predicted more frequent and more severe health problems, more visits to the school doctor or nurse, and more abdominal pain. They also found that victimization was associated with decreased cortisol levels and a flattened cortisol-awakening response in victimized as compared to non-victimized children. The cortisol-awakening response is believed to mobilize the body's resources for the day (e.g., Tops, Riese, Oldehinkel, Rijsdijke, & Ormel, 2008). In a two-year longitudinal study of children who were 12 years of age at the start of the study, Vaillancourt et al. (2011) also found associations between peer victimization, symptoms of depression, and cortisol production that in turn had deleterious effects on memory functioning. Peer victimization predicted poorer visual pattern recognition; however, it also predicted better spatial recognition memory. Based on similar findings in research into social stress experienced by adults, Vaillancourt and associates speculated that bullying-related stress could lead to increased vigilance resulting in enhanced spatial attention. Although a review of the neurobiological effects of chronic stress is beyond the scope of this chapter (e.g., research that documents changes in gray matter volume, hippocampal size, loss of neurons in the hippocampus, and impairments in memory and learning [Rex-Lear et al., 2012]), research into bullying as a chronic stressor is vitally important to our understanding of the neurobiological effects of bullying and their link to poor academic performance and mental, social, and physical health (Vaillancourt et al., 2010).

GENETIC AND ENVIRONMENTAL INFLUENCES ON PEER VICTIMIZATION. Related to the need to understand bullying as a chronic stressor is the need to understand genetic and environmental factors that influence risk for victimization and differential responses to victimization. Two studies provide conflicting evidence of genetic and environmental influences on peer victimization; however, the difference in findings may relate primarily to differing age characteristics of the samples. In a study of victimization of 9- and 10-year-old children in just over 1,000 twin pairs, 73% of the variance in being a victim of bullying was due to genetic influences with the remainder due to non-shared environmental factors (Ball, Arseneault, Taylor, Maughan, Caspi, & Moffitt, 2008). In discussing the nature of genetic influences on victimization found in their study, Ball et al. make the distinction that victimization is an exposure rather than a direct behavior. Accordingly, they posited that genetic influences found in their study could reflect heritable traits that "influence children's vulnerability" (p. 108), such as personality traits, social cognitive deficits, and difficulties with emotional regulation that have been shown to mediate genetic influences on victimization. With regard to environmental influences, Ball et al. describe non-shared environmental factors as those that are unique to each twin, for example, different groups of friends, random experiences that impact each twin differently, including bad luck, and different maternal treatment. Shared environmental factors are those that are common to the twin set that impact each twin equally, for example, family income.

In contrast to the findings for predominantly genetic influences on victimization in older school-age children, a study of victimization in kindergarten children with 253 twin pairs revealed the opposite. Rather than being due to genetic factors, variance in victimization was almost completely due to shared (29%) and non-shared (71%) environmental factors (Brendgen, Boivin, Vitaro, Girard, Dionne, & Pérusse, 2008). Thus, as Brendgen et al. state, these findings suggest that victimization in kindergarten is primarily "driven" by environmental variables.

Implications of large genetic influences such as those reported by Ball et al. (2008) suggest that heritable traits that mediate victimization (e.g., emotional dysregulation) may need to be targeted in client-centered interventions with victimized children. On the other hand, large environmental influences suggest that broad school-based (i.e., universal) interventions that address the school's climate need to be targeted. A further contribution of gene-environment research to our understanding of bullying elucidates why some bullied children may develop mental health problems while others will not. In an investigation of the same population of children reported on in Ball et al. (2008) referred to above, but with additional measures of victimization and emotional problems obtained at 12 years, a serotonin transporter gene was found to moderate the development of emotional problems for frequently victimized children who were short-allele carriers as compared to children who were long-allele carriers (Sugden, Arseneault, Harrington, Moffitt, Williams, & Caspi, 2010). A short allele has been associated with dysregulation of serotonergic neurotransmission. See Sugden et al. (2010) for a detailed description.

IMPACT ON SCHOOL CLIMATE. Bullying affects all children whether they are directly or indirectly involved in bullying. In a recent study of the impact of teasing and bullying in predicting high school dropouts, Cornell, Gregory, Huang, & Fan (2013) found that higher rates of reported teasing and bullying in school were associated with increased dropout rates. Interestingly, reports of personal victimization were not correlated with dropout rates. These findings lead the authors to suggest that school climate measures rather than personal reports of victimization may be a better gauge of the seriousness of the bullying problem in schools. They speculated that pervasive teasing and bullying may lead to disengagement, avoidance, distraction, inattentiveness, and ultimately poor academic performance. Indeed, evidence of the effects of bullying on cortisol production and the influence of environmental factors (i.e., non-shared environment) provide empirical support for these speculations.

Types of Bullying

Bullying is typically described as verbal, social or relational, physical, and cyberbullying. Verbal bullying includes name-calling, ridicule, insults, and hurtful teasing. Social or relational bullying is intended to harm a child's self-esteem, social status, or peer relationships by, for example, spreading nasty rumors or lies, ignoring or purposefully leaving a peer out, preventing peers from joining, and attempting to make other students dislike the target child. Physical bullying involves hitting, kicking, taking money or possessions or breaking possessions, and threatening to hurt. Cyberbullying, defined below, involves the use of electronic media to bully. The most frequently experienced bullying behavior appears to be verbal bullying, followed in order by social or relational bullying, physical bullying, and cyberbullying (Siyahhan et al., 2012; Wang, Iannotti, & Nansel, 2009). In general, boys tend to be more involved in physical or verbal bullying, and girls tend to be more involved in social and relational bullying. The terms "direct bullying" and "indirect bullying" are also used. Direct bullying generally refers to bullying that is directly enacted on the victim by the perpetrator. Indirect bullying refers to bullying that is carried out by a perpetrator through a third party (e.g., spreading lies and rumors through peers) in which it may be difficult or impossible for the perpetrator to be identified.

Although it is clear that electronic media (e.g., text messaging, fake Internet sites, and chat rooms) can be used to carry out traditional forms of verbal and relational bullying and can include threats to physically harm a target, there is debate about how to define cyberbullying. Wingate, Minney, and Guadagno (2013) defined cyberbullying as the "intentional and habitual use of fear or humiliation to intimidate a victim and demonstrate superiority over electronic mediums" (p. 89). Embedded within this definition are the three key features of bullying: intent to harm, repetition or chronicity, and a power differential (Wingate et al., 2013). However, it can be argued that repetition is not relevant because the technology allows multiple victimizations through forwarding and through the permanence of the aggressive postings (e.g., Internet sites on which it is impossible to delete postings) (Wingate et al., 2013). It can also be argued that the imbalance in power may be the most relevant feature of cyber-bullying due to the victim's loss of power and inability to respond immediately and effectively as is possible in bullying delivered in traditional (e.g., face-to-face) ways (Dooley et al., 2009; Wingate et al., 2013). Research has also shown that the anonymity of the Internet makes it possible for students of high power to be targeted (Vandenbosch & van Cleemput, 2008); such students are generally insulated from being victims of traditional forms of bullying. Regardless of whether there is a real or perceived power imbalance, cyberbullying has the potential to be more damaging than face-to-face bullying (Wingate, Minney, & Guadagno, 2013) given the victim's loss of control and permanence of Internet-based aggressive acts (e.g., pictures and videos). Of great concern is that 38% of adolescents who self-identified as perpetrators of cyberbullying thought that those who commit cyberbullying do it "for fun" (Raskauskas & Stoltz, 2007).

Bullying Participant Roles

Participant roles include those who bully, are victimized, are dually involved, and those who are bystanders (sometimes described as those who are not involved). Each role is described below.

- VICTIMS OF BULLYING. According to an ecosystem model, a dynamic relationship exists between a child's personal characteristics and the characteristics of his or her social environment (Andreou, Didaskalou, & Vlachou, 2008; Bronfenbrenner & Ceci, 1994). Well-known predictors of bullying include social anxiety, peer rejection, and social withdrawal (Cook, Williams, Guerra, Kim, & Sadek, 2010; Salmivalli, 2010); however, victimization is less likely to occur in classrooms that have peers who defend victims or challenge bullying (Salmivalli, 2010). According to typical youth, being different or standing out in some way also invites victimization (Guerra, Williams, & Sadek, 2011). Sadly, victims are often blamed for their victimization, particularly when they are the only victim in the class and when victimization continues over a prolonged period (Guerra et al., 2011; Salmivalli, 2010). Victims tend to have fewer friends and be less accepted than non-victims (Card & Hodges, 2008). With prolonged bullying, victims of bullying can seemingly fulfil a "social role" in the classroom or social environment (Salmivalli, 2010).

- CHILDREN WHO BULLY. Perpetrators of bullying have been described as those who bully proactively or reactively; however, some children engage in both proactive and reactive aggression (Marini & Dane, 2008). Children who proactively bully do so in a planned way to gain and maintain social status within their peer groups (Craig & Pepler, 2007; Salmivalli, 2010; Salmivalli & Peets, 2009). They are often highly socially skilled individuals who have power as a result of age, size, and psychological or social status. They may have heightened abilities to read peers' intentions and emotions. Children who engage in proactive bullying are often perceived by the peer group to have high self-esteem, to be popular and "cool" (even though they may be disliked by peers), and to be perceived as leaders in school (Craig & Pepler, 2007; Guerra et al., 2011; Marini & Dane, 2008; Salmivalli, 2010). Children who bully reactively do so in response to real or perceived provocation and may do so as a result of having difficulty with emotional regulation (Card & Hodges, 2008; Marini & Dane, 2008). Finally, some perpetrators are described by peers as "wannabes," who bully to try to gain popularity and power, but are relatively unsuccessful in doing so (Guerra et al., 2011).

- CHILDREN WHO ARE DUALLY INVOLVED. Children who are dually involved bully in some situations and are victims in other situations. In addition to having difficulties with emotional regulation, these children may have more internalizing problems than children who bully only; they may be more anxious, more submissive, and, as a result, are easy targets (Marini & Dane, 2008). In comparison to children who bully only, dually involved children may be at greater risk for emotional maladjustment and may have more trouble fitting in at school (Nansel, Overpeck, Pilla, Ruan, Simons-Morton, & Scheidt, 2001; Juvoven, Graham, & Schuster, 2003; Perren & Alsaker, 2006).

- BYSTANDERS. Bullying is also traumatic for peers who witness bullying. Bystanders participate in bullying in different ways. They can assist or reinforce bullying, even through subtle behaviors such as smiling (Salmivalli, Lagerspetz, Björkqvist, Österman, & Kaukiainen, 1996; Salmivalli, 2010). Observational research revealed that peers reinforced the behavior of bullies 85% of the time by assisting or watching (Craig & Pepler, 1998). Other peer-participant roles include defenders, who try to stop the bullying and/ or support the victim, and outsiders (also called bystanders or uninvolved children), who passively allow bullying to continue (Salmivalli, Lagerspetz et al., 1996; Salmivalli, 2010); approximately one-third of the peer group may be outsiders and up to 20% could be defenders (Salmivalli, 2010). Intervening is a challenge for bystanders. They may be caught in the dilemma of knowing that bullying is wrong (Salmivalli, 2010), but are hesitant to intervene because they are uncertain about what to do, afraid that intervening will cause more problems, or are afraid that intervening will cause them to lose social status or be bullied themselves (Andreou et al., 2008; Salmivalli, 2010). Other factors that reduce children's willingness to defend a victim or intervene are diffusion of responsibility and pluralistic ignorance. Diffusion of responsibility occurs when children do not take responsibility for their part in the action (Salmivalli, 2010) or believe that other witnesses will intervene. Pluralistic ignorance occurs when group members maintain silence because they believe that intervening would not be in keeping with the group norm (Wingate et al., 2013). Defending in the case of cyberbullying is particularly problematic given that the bystander group size often increases exponentially and contributes to the diffusion of responsibility.

Frequency of Bullying Involvement among Youth

Estimates of bullying involvement among youth in general vary across studies, due in part to differing definitions of bullying and differing methods of data collection (e.g., self-report as compared to peer and teacher nomination). The most often used method is self-report of victimization and perpetration of bullying, which may result in overestimates as discussed above.

Between 30% and 60% of typically fluent children are bullied at some time during a school semester or year, with between 6% and 15% of children being bullied chronically (i.e., once a week or more often) (Card & Hodges, 2008). More recently, Vaillancourt et al. (2011) found that 35.4% of their sample reported having been bullied in the two months prior to the first data collection point. With regard to frequency subgroups, in their study of the trajectories of bullying over transition from primary to secondary school, Lester et al. (2013), found that only 40% of their sample of 3462 children were *not* involved in bullying. Of the 60% who were involved, 52% were in the low stable victimization group (i.e., students who consistently reported low victimization across primary and secondary school), 4% were in the low increasing victimization group (i.e., students whose victimization increased from low levels at the end of primary school and the beginning of secondary school to high levels of victimization by the end of the second year of secondary school), and 4% were in the medium stable victimization group (i.e., students whose levels of bullying were medium at the end of primary school and during the first two years of secondary school).

Estimates of children who bully range from 5% (Craig, 1998) to13% (Nansel et al., 2001), with a recent study (Langevin & Prasad, 2012) indicating that 12.1%

of students admitted to perpetrating bullying once a week or more often. Estimates of children who are dually involved range from 6.3% (Nansel et al., 2001) to 19% (Craig, 1998; Schwartz, Proctor, & Chien, 2001).

Bullying Involvement of Youth Who Stutter

Frequency of Bullying Experienced by Children Who Stutter

In what appears to be the first investigation of bullying involvement of children who stutter, Langevin, Bortnick, Hammer, and Wiebe (1998) investigated the frequency and nature of bullying in a convenience sample of 28 children (24 males and four females; seven to 15 years of age). Using the *Teasing and Bullying Questionnaire (TBQ)* that was developed for the study, Langevin and colleagues asked children if they were teased or bullied about their stuttering, how frequently it occurred, where it occurred, and the degree to which children were upset by it. In addition to teasing and bullying related to stuttering, children completing the *TBQ* were also asked if they were teased and bullied about things other than their stuttering. Langevin et al. (1998) found that 59% of participants were bullied about their stuttering, with 56% reportedly being bullied once a week or more often. Sixty-nine percent of children were bullied about other things, for example their name, hair, weight, clothes worn, or things liked, with 55% being bullied once a week or more often. Children appeared to be more upset with the bullying that related to their stuttering (81%) than other things (67%). Children reported that peers most frequently imitated or made fun of their stuttering and called them names. They also reported that bullying most frequently occurred on the playground followed by the classroom.

The definition of bullying used in the *TBQ* incorporated the key features of bullying, i.e., intent to harm, repetition over time, and a power imbalance. However, the definition used in the *TBQ* also included "hurtful teasing" as a bullying behavior. This was because children who stutter who participated in focus groups with the author did not categorize teasing about their stuttering as bullying. Thus, the definition of bullying used in the *TBQ* referred to teasing as a bullying behavior in a more salient way than the definition of bullying that was generally being used by researchers at the time. This raised concern that children may have been overreporting bullying.

The salience of teasing as a distinct form of bullying, however, is reflected in the more recently developed *Perceived Prevalence of Teasing and Bullying* scale, which is being used in investigations of school climate (Bandyopadhyay, Cornell, & Konold, 2009; Cornell et al., 2013), and in other measures used in research into genetic and environmental influences on bullying (e.g., Ball et al., 2008). Although Langevin et al.'s 1998 findings yielded frequency data that were higher than the range reported in the bullying literature for samples of children without specified exceptionalities at that time (9% to 35%), they are closer to the high end of the range (60%) more recently reported by Card and Hodges (2008) for bullying in general and Wang et al. (2009) for verbal bullying (53.6%). Further, the finding that 81% of children reported being bullied (either about stuttering only, other attributes only, or both stuttering and other attributes) is consistent with the retrospective study of Hugh-Jones and Smith (1999) in which 83% of adults reported that they were bullied in childhood. At present, an investigation is underway to update data from children who have received therapy at the Institute for Stuttering Treatment and Research (Langevin & Gervais, 2013). Preliminary analysis of frequency data in a subsample of 31 of the children suggests that findings are similar to those reported in Langevin et al. (1998).

In a series of three comparative group studies, using two different measures of bullying, Blood and colleagues consistently found that children and adolescents who stutter were at higher risk for being bullied than their matched controls. In two studies, Blood and Blood (2004, 2007) used the *Life in School* checklist (Arora, 1994). Six of its 39 statements measure direct and physical bullying that occurred during the week in which the questionnaire was completed. As Blood and Blood (2004) noted, forms of bullying that include name-calling and laughing at someone were not included in the index of bullying because developers found that fewer than 30 % of children in their sample categorized these behaviors as bullying. In their 2004 sample of 53 adolescents who stutter and 53 matched adolescents who do not stutter (age 13 to 18 years), Blood and Blood found that 43% of the adolescents who stutter compared to 11% of the matched fluent peers were at significantly greater risk for being bullied. In their 2007 study with 18 boys who stutter aged 11 to 12 years and 18 matched fluent peers, Blood and Blood found that 61% of the boys who stutter compared to 22% of the boys who did not stutter were at significantly greater risk for being bullied.

In a more recent study with adolescents aged 13 to 18 years who do and do not stutter, Blood, Blood, Tramontana, Sylvia, Boyle, and Motzko (2011) used the *Bully-Victimization* scale (Reynolds, 2003), which has separate *Bully* and *Victimization* scales. The *Bully* scale measures perpetration of overt aggression physical (e.g., hitting or fighting) and relational aggression and harassment (e.g., verbal threats, name-calling, or teasing). The *Victimization* scale measures being the recipient of peer aggression and relational aggression. Compared to 27% of the non-stuttering participants, 44% of the adolescents who stutter were in the clinically significant range for victimization. The difference in mean scores between the groups was statistically significant with children who stutter being at greater risk than fluent peers. In addition, Blood, Blood, Tramontana, et al., (2011) found that two students who stuttered compared to eight students who did not, representing 3.7% and 7.4% of the sample, respectively, were classified as bullies.

The self-report findings of Langevin et al. (1998) and Blood and colleagues (Blood & Blood, 2004, 2007; Blood, Blood, Tramontana, et al., 2011) are supported by peer-nomination findings reported by Davis, Howell, and Cook (2002). In their sample of 403 children (aged eight to 14 years) in which 16 children stuttered (i.e., one in each of 16 classes), children were asked to nominate peers who fit eight behavioral descriptions, two of which related to being a perpetrator or a recipient of bullying. Compared to 11% of the fluent children, 38% of children who stutter were nominated as victims. As well, 13% of children who stutter were nominated as perpetrators of bullying compared to 13% of fluent children.

In summary, evidence from studies using self-report and peer-nomination methodologies indicate that children who stutter who are in or are seeking therapy appear to be at higher risk for victimization than their fluent peers. The findings of Blood, Blood, Tramontana, et al. (2011) and Davis et al. (2002) indicate that children who stutter are also sometimes perpetrators of bullying. Future research is needed to determine the extent to which children who stutter perpetrate bullying and are dually involved.

Social and Mental Health Consequences of Bullying for Children Who Stutter

Like their fluent counterparts, children who stutter experience short- and long-term social and mental health consequences of bullying. In their retrospective study, Hugh-Jones and Smith (1999) reported on the short- and long-term effects of bullying. Short-term consequences included loss of self-confidence, low self-esteem, withdrawal, feelings of guilt, shame, embarrassment, frustration, depression, difficulty in making friends, negative effects on schoolwork, and increased stuttering. Many of the short-term consequences (e.g., low self-confidence or low self-esteem) persisted into adulthood. Other long-term effects included continued difficulty in recovering from childhood experiences and negative effects on vocational choices and achievement of potential (Hugh-Jones & Smith, 1999). These findings are supported in the more recent investigations of Blood and Blood (2004, 2007) and Blood, Blood, Tramontana, et al. (2011) into the links between bullying in children who stutter and anxiety, self-esteem, optimism, and life satisfaction. Blood and Blood (2007) found significant correlations between the risk of bullying and anxiety measures for children who do and do not stutter; children who were at greater risk for bullying were more likely to have higher anxiety scores. These data are consistent with research that shows that anxiety is associated with bullying in typically fluent children and suggests that elevated levels of anxiety experienced by adults who stutter may begin in childhood. As Blood and Blood (2007) noted, there is likely a bidirectional relationship between high anxiety and bullying in children who stutter.

With regard to self-esteem, Blood and Blood (2004) found that adolescents who were at risk for bullying (whether or not they stuttered) had poorer self-esteem scores than adolescents who were not at risk for bullying. Similarly, Blood, Blood, Tramontana, et al. (2011) found that children who stutter and who were bullied had poorer levels of self-esteem than children who stutter and who were not bullied. They also found the same results for measures of optimism and life satisfaction.

Individual and Environmental Factors That May Contribute to Bullying of Children Who Stutter

There is little doubt that stuttering is a noticeable difference that invites bullying and places children at risk for having difficulty "fitting in" at school (Evans, Healey, Kawai, & Rowland, 2008). As well, there is little doubt that the environment plays a role in the exacerbation or mitigation of bullying. Given that negative attitudes toward an individual or group of individuals is a predictor of bullying (Cook, Williams, Guerra, Kim, & Sadek, 2010), the literature evidencing negative peer attitudes toward children who stutter (Langevin, 2009; Langevin & Hagler, 2004; Langevin, Kleitman, Packman, & Onslow, 2009) and peer rejection (Davis et al., 2002; Hartford & Leahy, 2007) suggests that intervention at a universal level is required. Universal interventions, the major foci of anti-bullying work in the schools, target the student population at the classroom, school-wide, or district-wide level. Indeed, within the field of stuttering there have been persistent calls over many years for universal-level education about stuttering in schools (see Langevin, Chapter 20; Langevin & Prasad, 2012) and in other sectors of the population.

A Universal Intervention to Improve the Classroom and School Environment for Children Who Stutter

Langevin and Prasad (2012) reported on a universal intervention that used *Teasing and Bullying: Unacceptable Behaviour* (*TAB*) (Langevin, 2000), a bullying-prevention program that also aimed to improve attitudes toward children who stutter. *TAB* is comprised of six teaching units, one of which is devoted to educating students about stuttering. It also includes a video that depicts a girl who stutters who co-narrates the video and a boy who stutters who is teased in classroom scenes. *TAB* was intended to be used by speech-language pathologists, educators, and allied professionals who work with children and was intended to be used as a classroom-level resource for children in grades 3 to 6 in school-wide bullying intervention programs. Although *TAB* can and has also been used in client-centered interventions (i.e., with individual children and in small group treatment programs for children) as described in Langevin, Kully, and Ross-Harold (2007), its effectiveness in reducing bullying in client-centered interventions with children who stutter has not been empirically investigated.

As a by-product of using *TAB*, it was anticipated that speech-language pathologists, teachers, and other adults who work with children also would acquire a better understanding of stuttering and teasing and bullying in general. Indeed, Blood, Boyle, Blood, and Nalesnik (2010) and Blood, Robins, Blood, Boyle, and Finke (2011) documented a need for speech-language pathologists to learn more about bullying, in particular relational and verbal bullying. Further, Ostrov and Godleski (2007) suggest that speech-language pathologists have an important role to play in bullying prevention, in particular with children who have language disorders who are involved in being victims and perpetrators of relational aggression.

In their feasibility study with 608 children in grades 3 to 6, Langevin and Prasad (2012) used the *Peer Attitudes Toward Children who Stutter Scale* (*PATCS*) (Langevin, 2009; Langevin & Hagler, 2004; Langevin et al., 2009) to measure change in peer attitudes and the *Pro-Victim Scale* (Rigby & Slee, 1991, 1993) to measure changes in attitudes toward bullying. The *PATCS* has three subscales that measure positive social distance, social pressure, and verbal interaction. The *Pro-Victim Scale* also has three subscales that measure approval of bullying, rejection of weak kids, and support for victims. Findings suggest that *TAB* has the potential to be effective in improving attitudes toward children who stutter for students in general, and in particular in children who do not know someone who stutters. More specifically, results suggest that after being involved in the *TAB* intervention, based on their self-reports, children who do not know someone who stutters may be more inclined to associate with children who stutter, resist social pressure that intends to limit social interactions with or ostracize children who stutter, and experience less frustration due to interruptions in communication caused by stuttering. As the authors noted, these findings are encouraging because it is the children who do not know someone who stutters who typically have the least positive attitudes toward peers who stutter. In addition, items that had the highest change scores included "Kids who stutter are like normal kids," "I would like a kid who stutters to talk for our group in class," and "I would walk in the hall with a kid who stutters." The improvement in mean scores of these items suggested that children who stutter are more likely to be accepted among a peer group who has experienced education about stuttering due to a fundamental change in understanding commonalities among children who do and do not stutter. These results are encouraging given that they suggest higher levels of peer support for children who stutter. As a result, children who stutter may feel safer and more connected at school. Importantly, Lester et al. (2013) reported that peer support was a protective factor for girls who were bullied and feeling safe at school was a protective factor for boys, while feeling lonely at school and less connected at school was associated with being subjected to stable or increasing levels of bullying. The findings of Langevin and associates also suggest that children who are not involved in bullying (i.e., bystanders) may be more inclined to affiliate with children who stutter after participating in *TAB*. Again, this is a positive finding given that children who are not involved in bullying, who comprise the largest proportion of the student body, have the potential to have substantial influence in creating a more supportive environment for children who stutter and have the potential to become defenders. Future research is needed to investigate the degree to which participation in *TAB* has the potential to influence uninvolved children to become defenders.

Research into Client-Centered Interventions with Children Who Stutter

Reports of client-centered interventions with children who stutter are few in number. Typically such interventions aim to improve problem-solving strategies through discussion and role plays that help the child develop and choose appropriate responses to bullying. Classroom presentations about stuttering are also typically carried out by the child with or without the support of the speech-language pathologist (e.g., Langevin et al., 2007; Murphy, Yaruss, & Quesal, 2007b) or made solely by the child's speech-language pathologist (Turnbull, 2006). These reports have documented positive outcomes. Langevin et al. (2007) reported on two children who had been teased and who had participated in teasing and bullying discussions during their intensive treatment program. In follow-up, one child's teasing ended when his friend defended him. The second child's teasing stopped when he sought help from the teacher, who then intervened. Murphy et al. (2007b) and Turnbull (2006) reported on the use of classroom presentations in their case studies: the child who stutters in Murphy et al. (2007b) made a classroom presentation about stuttering, whereas in Turnbull's (2006) study, two speech-language pathologists made the presentation. In both studies the authors reported that the children who stutter were pleased with the presentations and classmates responded positively. At follow-up, the child in Murphy et al. (2007b) was no longer concerned about bullying. More recently Langevin (Chapter 20) reported on comments made by children involved in a stuttering education and bullying-prevention program (reported on in Langevin & Prasad, 2012). Results indicated that peers of school-age children who stutter were interested in learning about stuttering. These results provide further support for the long-held calls for education about stuttering in the schools.

Options and Considerations for Responding to Bullying

Research is beginning to accumulate on coping strategies that children used in response to bullying. Based on a national online survey with 1,852 youth who ranged in age from four to 19 years (mean 12.6) Craig, Pepler, and Blais (2007) provide a thorough overview of the response strategies used by youth. The authors asked participants what type of bullying they experienced, what they did to stop the bullying, how effective their strategies were in stopping the bullying, and what motivated them to do something about the problem. Participants were given the following list of strategies from which they could select: telling someone (parent, sibling, school staff, or student), verbal counter-aggression, physical counter-aggression, standing up for self, joking, using revenge, using distraction, doing nothing, ignoring, getting help, and an "other" category. Effectiveness ratings ranged from 1 (the strategy did not work) to 3 (the strategy worked really well).

Findings revealed that all strategies received effectiveness ratings greater than 1.5, indicating that they worked to some extent at least some of the time. The strategy that received the second-highest effectiveness rating in Craig et al. (2007) was standing up for oneself, followed by getting help and talking to parents. Although not the most effective, ignoring was the most frequently endorsed strategy. The "other" category received the highest effectiveness ratings even though it was the least used strategy. These findings suggest that youth can be very resourceful in determining a strategy that might work best for them in a particular situation. The following is a discussion of the evidence base for each of these strategies and additional considerations that warrant attention when preparing to intervene in bullying and help all children develop response strategies that are appropriate.

Standing Up for Oneself

It is important to help all children develop assertive behavior because it develops their sense of social mastery and facilitates peer acceptance (Mahady Wilton,

Craig, & Pepler, 2000). Camodeca and Goossens (2005) also found that assertiveness was perceived by all children in their study (whether victim, bully, defender, follower, outsider, or not involved) to be the most effective strategy for stopping bullying; however, children who bullied thought that retaliation was the best way to stop bullying. The authors surmised that this may be because retaliation works for children who bully and, consequently, do not believe that assertiveness would stop them from engaging in bullying. As well, it is very possible that they do not want their victims to become more assertive and thereby cause them to lose their power.

The importance of being able to stand up for oneself must be viewed within the context of children's motivation for doing so. Craig et al. (2007) found that factors that spurred respondents to do something were *not* concern for their academic, psychological, or emotional health (which adults believe to be important) and *not* education or information campaigns about bullying. Rather, participants were motivated by their need to "exert control and be assertive." They were also motivated by their emotional reactions to the bullying (e.g., anger) and the escalation or persistence of bullying. Because children who are victimized tend to have internalizing problems that make them appear anxious, depressed, or withdrawn, they become easy targets. Thus, it is vitally important that children be helped to identify and practice assertive behaviors so that they can be successful in being assertive in peer interactions. It is also important to help children remember that standing up for oneself does not imply that confrontation is the only way to do so. Brainstorming different ways of being assertive and choosing options that suit the child is critically important, particularly in view of findings of Smith, Talalmelli, Cowie, Naylor, and Chauhan (2004), who used logistic regression to study strategies for escape from victimization (as well as continuing victimization and new victimization). They showed that "sticking up for self" was not associated with escape from victimization.

Getting Help/Telling Someone

In contrast to standing up for oneself, Smith et al. (2004) found that "talking to someone" and "getting more/different friends" were associated with escape from victimization. Although respondents in the Craig et al. (2007) investigation rated telling parents as being slightly more effective than talking with school staff or other students, it was clear that talking with someone was helpful some of the time.

Research indicates that having friends, making new friends, having quality friendships, and being accepted by one's peer group protect against victimization (Bollmer, Milich, Harris, Maras, 2005; Boulton, Trueman, Chau, Whitehand, & Amatya, 1999; Hodges, Boivin, Vitaro, & Bukowski, 1999). However, in order for friendship to be a protective factor, friends must have the capacity to be able and willing to stand up for the victimized child (Hodges et al., 1999; Smith, Shu, & Madsen, 2001). Unfortunately, some victimized children tend to affiliate with children who also tend to be victimized or have internalizing problems (Hodges et al., 1999). Craig et al. (2007) emphasized the importance of helping children to recognize healthy relationships and develop skills to enable them to be appropriately assertive in their relationships.

Ignoring the Bullying, Walking Away, and Avoiding the Child Who Bullies

Passive coping strategies that include ignoring, walking away, and avoidance have also been associated with the de-escalation or resolution of bullying (Mahady Wilton et al., 2000). However, it is possible that these strategies may also perpetuate the problem if they reinforce the bully's behavior (e.g., the bully achieves social gain) or if the victim avoids only to feel temporary relief. Ignoring, walking away, or avoiding is even more complex when environmental supports and the age of the bullied child are considered. For example, Smith et al. (2001) caution that ignoring bullying in an unsupportive environment may be relatively successful; however, in supportive environments, ignoring the bullying can serve to conceal the child's distress when in fact supports are available to help the child. On the other hand, Smith et al. (2001) also argue that because the use of ignoring as a coping strategy increases with age, ignoring is a socially skilled coping strategy that older children develop.

Nonchalance

Acting nonchalant is another strategy that could be categorized as a form of ignoring. Salmivalli, Karhunen, and Lagerspetz (1996) reported preliminary evidence that nonchalance was the most constructive response to aggression for 12- to 13-year-old boys and girls. They describe nonchalance as staying calm, acting as if the bullying is not being taken seriously, and acting as if one does not care. In so doing, the victim does not give the bully the desired emotional response and is actively engaging in a behavior to protect himself or herself; this could be interpreted as a form of self-reliance (next section).

Self-Reliance and Problem-Solving

Baldry and Farrington (2005) discussed a variety of coping strategies that included problem-focused coping and emotional-focused coping. In problem-focused coping, people actively try to face the problem, solve it, and ask for help if they need it. In contrast, in emotion-focused coping, people concentrate more on themselves than the problem and they react emotionally, for example, by crying or venting. Using a modified version of Causey and Dubow's (1992) *Self-Report Coping Measure*, Kristensen and Smith (2003) found that self-reliance/problem-solving was the most used coping strategy by their sample of 10- to 15-year-olds. Items included "Try to think of different ways to solve it," "Change something so things will work out," "Know there are things I can do to make it better," and "Try extra hard to keep this from happening again" (p. 481). Importantly, Baldry and Farrington (2005) found that problem-solving strategies buffered the negative impacts of emotion-focused coping styles and suggested that children who typically respond with emotional-focused coping can learn problem-focused coping skills.

Gender Differences

In terms of preferred responses to bullying, girls are more likely than boys to get help or tell someone (Craig et al., 2007) and to use assertiveness strategies that include pro-social and conflict-resolution strategies (Camodeca & Goossens, 2005). It is thought that girls prefer assertiveness strategies because they are not expected to fight back and because they are reared to be more empathetic and to reject violence. In contrast, boys are less likely than girls to use pro-social and conflict-resolution skills (Camodeca & Goossens, 2005), but tend to react with physical aggression, revenge, or humor (Craig et al., 2007). Craig et al. assert that boys' tendency to react with aggression has a negative effect. They point out that boys believe their "aggressive and confrontational strategies" are effective, yet research has shown that counter-aggression prolongs bullying and makes it more severe (Mahady Wilton et al., 2000). It appears that boys may need help in developing more adaptive pro-social responses to bullying that result in escape from bullying. Accordingly, it is encouraging that findings from Craig et al. (2007) suggest that boys are open to ignoring the bullying and to using humor and distraction strategies (Craig et al., 2007).

Age Differences

As a response to bullying, Camodeca and Goossens (2005) found that younger children preferred nonchalance; however, both these investigators and Craig et al. (2007) found that as children grew older, they tended to use counter-aggression more often. At the same time, Craig et al. (2007) found that older children were more likely to report ignoring and doing nothing.

Closeness of Peer Relationships

Craig et al. (2007) found that girls were more likely than boys to be bullied by a friend. However, as the degree of closeness in the relationship between the children who bullied and the children who were victimized increased, the victimized children were less likely to do something to stop the bullying. As the authors indicated, fear of losing the friendships likely accounts for this behavior.

Duration of Bullying

Children who are subjected to prolonged bullying are at risk for adopting the belief that they deserve the bullying and also are at risk for responding to bullying in habitually passive and accepting ways. Indeed, habitualized passive responding is a problem for both victims and bullies (Salmivalli & Peets, 2009) such that both groups of children may need the ongoing support of adults to help them replace habitualized maladaptive responses with more socially, psychologically, and emotionally adaptive ones.

Conclusion

Many factors contribute to the cause of teasing and bullying. These include personal characteristics such as submissiveness and high levels of anxiety. They also include social factors such as having few friends or peer rejection, coping styles, and identifiable characteristics such as stuttering. We have at our disposal many options for client-centered and universal intervention. Ideally, client-centered interventions for bullied children will be undertaken within an environment in which universal interventions are concurrently in place. Different plans of action are needed that take into account the nature of the bullying, the personal characteristics of the bullied children, and the school or peer group climate. Research into the effectiveness of coping responses suggests that children who are bullied need to be able to effectively use a range of response options and need the support of adults.

Chapter 4

Job Discrimination Associated with Stuttering in Adults

Rodney Gabel

ABSTRACT

A significant body of research suggests that a pervasive negative stereotype of stuttering exists. Additionally, a growing body of research has found that stuttering may also lead an individual to face discrimination in occupational choices and experiences. The purpose of this chapter is to discuss research and connect it to theories describing the impact of stuttering on employment issues. Among these are role entrapment, marginalization, paternalism, and stigma (both societal stigma and self-stigma). The chapter concludes with suggestions for future directions related to this research.

Introduction

Most definitions of stuttering outline the multifactorial nature of stuttering (Cooper, 1993; Yairi & Seery, 2011). Stuttering can have a profound impact on communication, thus affecting interpersonal relationships. Because stuttering affects an individual's ability to communicate with others, it is believed that the way a person copes with stuttering can be shaped somewhat by listeners' responses (Smart, 2001; Van Riper, 1982). In their discussion of the International Classification of Functioning, Disability, and Health (ICF), Yaruss and Quesal (2004a) discuss the impact of listeners' perceptions on the lives of people who stutter. The authors discuss the participation restrictions (also known as handicaps), which often lead to barriers to social, educational, and vocational endeavors. In many ways, these societal barriers have the potential to impact the person more profoundly than the physiological symptoms of stuttering (Yaruss & Quesal, 2004a). They are often a result of how friends, family, employers, teachers, and others view or evaluate the individual who stutters. These evaluations often take the form of negative stereotypical attitudes toward stuttering and people who stutter.

Stereotypes and stereotypical attitudes may be positive, but are more often negative and detrimental to an individual because: (1) the individual is put into a category due to a singular characteristic; (2) the person is polarized by a clear demarcation between those who are in the category and those who are not; and (3) a stereotype of any kind leads to behaviors and actions that reduce options (Smart, 2001). A series of research studies have found that a variety of populations report negative stereotypes of people who stutter, including speech-language pathologists (SLPs) (Cooper & Cooper, 1985, 1996; Lass, Ruscello, Pannbacker, Schmitt, & Everly-Myers, 1989; Ragsdale & Ashby, 1982; Turnbaugh, Guitar, & Hoffman, 1979; Węsierska,Węsierska, St. Louis, & Beste-Guldborg, Chapter 13; Woods & Williams, 1971, 1976), educators (Crowe & Walton, 1981; Arnold & Goltl, 2013; Lass, Ruscello, Schmitt, Pannbacker, Orlando, Dean, Ruziska, & Bradshaw, 1992; Lass, Ruscello, Pannbacker, Schmitt, Kiser, Mussa, & Lockhart, 1994; Ruscello, Lass, Schmitt, Pannbacker, Hoffman, Miley, & Robison, 1990; Yeakle & Cooper, 1986), health care professionals (Beste-Guldborg, St. Louis, & Campanale, Chapter 11; Silverman & Bongey, 1997; Yairi & Carrico, 1992), college students (Ruscello, Lass, & Brown, 1988; Silverman & Paynter, 1990), laypeople (Crowe & Cooper, 1977; Ham, 1990), and college students (Ruscello et al., 1988, 1990; Silverman & Paynter, 1990). Additionally, negative stereotypes often lead to stigma. Goffman (1963), in his classic book, described stigma as the process by which a single attribute leads an individual to become discredited or seen as less of a person. Such an individual develops a negative social identity, and is less valued by society (Goffman, 1963). Wright (1983) discussed how this type of "spoiled identity" can damage the individual's self-esteem and self-concept and often limit the individual's access to many aspects of his or her life.

The purpose of this chapter is to discuss negative stereotyping and stigma related to stuttering and the impact that it might have on an individual's access to employment. First, the concept of stereotyping and the potential impact it might have on employment will be discussed. Basic research studies exploring the attitudes that the non-stuttering public has about stuttering people will be the focus. The important concepts of role entrapment and vocational stereotyping, and research bearing on these issues with people who stutter, will be examined, as will factors that might limit occupational stereotyping and role entrapment. Finally, ideas for future research directions will be explored.

The Impact of Stereotyping

As discussed earlier, many potential issues relate to stereotyping. Attitudes and stereotypes are strong mediators for behavior and thus can lead to prejudice and discrimination (Allport, 1986). In this process, attitudes and stereotypes come to represent the beliefs about a group or person while prejudice reflects the feelings or affective response to the group or person, and these can lead to discrimination. Stated in another way, in this model, attitudes and stereotypes are the mediators for prejudice and discrimination (Allport, 1986; Smart, 2001).

The relationship between stereotypes and discrimination can lead to serious issues with employment opportunities for people who stutter. Smart (2001) described three concepts central to stereotyping and discrimination related to employment. The first is *marginalization*, which occurs when a person who stutters is not allowed to participate wholly in the community per his or her goals, abilities, or interests due to societal stereotypes toward stuttering. Marginality occurs because the dominant group holds a negative perception of stuttering and the person who is stuttering, even if this is counter to how the stuttering individual defines himself or herself. Thus, stuttering individuals, when entering an employment setting, might be defined as being unable to perform certain tasks or careers due simply to the presence of stuttering.

Stereotyping also can lead to Smart's (2001) second employment-related concept, *paternalism*. Paternalism is the process by which people without a disability will act upon their belief of what is best for disabled people without consulting them. Paternalism may be well intentioned or even helpful if the required work tasks are too difficult for the individual to achieve. In this scenario, people who do not stutter might suggest that certain careers or tasks are not appropriate for people who stutter. So, if in a position of power, people who do not stutter would then either not recommend or hire a person who stutters to work in certain careers or to assume specific responsibilities within a career. This behavior is both undesirable and unethical from the vantage point of individuals who are capable of making their own decisions (Smart, 2001; Wright, 1983).

Smart's (2001) third concept is role entrapment related to *disability*. As with marginalization and paternalism, role entrapment affects the social, academic, and employment experiences of stuttering people. Role entrapment occurs when a group in power defines the roles that a minority group or individual can or cannot assume. Role entrapment has been most often identified with occupational choices. For example, Hahn (1997) found that people with disabilities were often victims of role entrapment and restricted to lower-paying jobs. For people with disabilities (including people who stutter), role entrapment leads to being viewed with lowered expectations and an assumption that they may not be held to high standards. Consequently, role entrapment will keep individuals with a disability, including stuttering, in an inferior or undesirable position.

Studies Exploring the Impact of Stereotyping on Employment of People Who Stutter

As noted earlier, people who stutter are perceived negatively by society. As documented above, a variety of groups, including SLPs, educators, health care professionals, laypeople, and college students, have reported stereotypical personality characteristics of stuttering people. Among the characteristics often attributed to people who stutter are shyness, anxiousness, nervousness, self-consciousness, insecurity, and even lack of intelligence. As was discussed, these types of negative stereotypes related to stuttering can lead to discrimination in the form of paternalism, marginalization, and role entrapment. For the purpose of this chapter, discussion of the impact of stuttering attitudes and stereotyping will be limited to employment.

Hurst and Cooper (1983a) carried out the first study related to employment issues of attitudes of non-stuttering individuals toward people who stutter. Using an inventory developed to investigate the attitudes of employers toward stuttering, these researchers surveyed the attitudes of 644 personnel and industrial relations directors. Only 29% of the employers perceived that stuttering hindered job performance. Contrary to this finding, 50% of the employers reported that stuttering decreased employability. Of all the employers, 43% reported that people who stutter should seek employment that required little speaking, 40% agreed with the statement that stuttering would make it difficult for a person to gain a promotion, and 83% agreed with the statement that people who stutter made them feel uncomfortable.

In a related study, Hurst and Cooper (1983b) studied 152 vocational rehabilitation counselors' attitudes toward and knowledge of stuttering. Eighty-five percent of the rehabilitation counselors responded correctly to items related to knowledge of stuttering, such as the cause of stuttering, the need for therapy, and other factual questions. Nevertheless, 50% of the counselors believed that most stuttering individuals had a psychological problem. In addition, 78% of the counselors believed that stuttering was indeed vocationally handicapping. Finally, 88% of the counselors reported that they felt most individuals would be uncomfortable when speaking with an individual who stuttered. Together with the previous study, these findings suggest that vocational rehabilitation counselors and employers both had negative attitudes toward people who stutter.

Other research has explored how people who stutter are viewed while participating in certain careers. To study the influence of stereotypes of stuttering on employment, Silverman and Paynter (1990) studied the attitudes of 48 college students toward two careers for a non-stuttering and stuttering worker, i.e., a "factory worker," a "factory worker who stutters," a "lawyer," and a "lawyer who stutters." The participants were randomly assigned to each condition, with 12 participants responding to each scale. The participants rated an 81-item semantic differential scale to evaluate the four possibilities. The results of the study suggested that the factory worker who stuttered was rated significantly more negatively than his or her fluent counterpart on 16 of the 81 scales. The factory worker who stuttered was described as more afraid, insecure, tense, cowardly, and weak than the factory worker who did not stutter. This hypothetical worker was also judged to be less talkative, sociable, coordinated, dominant, affluent, aggressive, and confident than the factory worker who did not stutter. The construct of a lawyer who stuttered was viewed more negatively than was that of a factory worker who stuttered on 34 of the adjective scales. The lawyer who stuttered was evaluated as more afraid, confused, tense, discontented, frightened, lazy, dependent, uncomfortable, naive, and disorganized than was the lawyer who did not stutter. Additionally, the lawyer who stuttered was evaluated to be less intelligent, employable, competent, educated, confident, talkative, mature, secure, natural, witty, stable, dominant, rich, sane, alert, and aggressive than was the lawyer who did not stutter. These findings suggested that individuals who stuttered were evaluated less positively than individuals who did not when performing these two careers.

In a study designed to measure the influence that stuttering was likely to have on the perceptions nurses held toward a physician who stuttered, Silverman and Bongey (1997) surveyed the attitudes of 20 nurses toward a "doctor who stutters" and a "doctor who does not stutter." Ten nurses were randomly assigned to each condition. The respondents evaluated each scenario using a 20-item semantic differential scale, revealing significant differences for 12 of the 20 items. A "doctor who stutters" was evaluated more negatively than a "doctor who does not stutter," i.e., less competent, mature, intelligent, secure, competent, confident, educated, and reputable, as well as more afraid, tense, nervous, and aggravating. These findings suggest that nurses reported negative traits to describe both abilities and personality characteristics of doctors who stuttered.

Overall, these studies suggest that people who do not stutter reported negative attitudes toward people who stutter related to employment. Both employers and vocational counselors have reported that stuttering people are less employable and may have difficulties in different aspects of employment (Hurst &

Cooper, 1983a, 1983b). In other studies, people who stutter were viewed negatively when performing certain careers. The data also suggest that people who stutter are viewed as less capable of performing certain tasks related to work (Hurst & Cooper, 1983a), less employable (Hurst & Cooper, 1983b), and are viewed less positively than people who do not stutter working in the same careers (Silverman & Paynter, 1990; Silverman & Bongey, 1997). Across all of these studies, there appears to be some evidence that societal attitudes will lead people who stutter to become marginalized in the work arena and experience difficulties in employment.

Studies Exploring Role Entrapment

Several research studies have explored whether stuttering individuals experience role entrapment in the form of occupational stereotyping. Most of these studies utilized the *Vocational Advice Scale (VAS)* (Gabel, Blood, Tellis, & Althouse, 2004). The *VAS* is a scale developed to measure the attitudes that non-stuttering people have toward appropriate career choices for people who stutter and people who do not stutter. Measuring differences in advice provided to individuals who speak fluently and individuals who stutter provides an indication of role entrapment and vocational stereotyping. The *VAS* was informed by a previous measure, the *Decaro Attitude Scale (DAS)* (Decaro, Evans, & Dowaliby, 1982), which has been utilized to explore role entrapment and stereotyping of individuals with severe hearing impairments. (The *DAS* was found to have satisfactory validity and reliability.) Results from the 43-item *VAS* can be interpreted to represent the advice one might give to an individual, with the proper training, to pursue one of the most desirable careers projected for the twenty-first century (Krannich & Krannich, 1993). These careers represented a variety of different fields, including health care, technology, science, engineering, and service professions. Obviously, the careers were also expected to vary in the amount of communication skill necessary to be successful. Respondents are requested to rate their advice to people who either do or do not stutter with regard to pursuing each of 43 careers by indicating their agreement with each item using a 5-point Likert-type scale from 5 ("strongly agree") to 1 ("strongly disagree").

In Gabel et al's (2004) initial field study of the *VAS*, its psychometric properties of content validity, internal consistency, and test-retest reliability were reported to be satisfactory. In the study, 385 university students completed the *VAS*, with 197 students completing the questionnaire for a person who stutters and 188 responding to the questionnaire for a person who does not stutter. A one-way analysis of variance (ANOVA) was utilized to identify differences between responses for the two groups. There was no significant difference found for 23 careers, suggesting that these careers were no less appropriate choices for stuttering people. Twenty careers were identified to be less appropriate choices for people who stutter. In this study, it was suggested that these 20 careers required more communication ability compared to the 23 careers that were not found to be different for either type of speaker. Also, the five careers that were given the lowest mean for the person who stutters were attorney, judge, SLP, Protestant minister, and guidance/employment counselor.

Another study using the *VAS* by Irani, Gabel, Hughes, Swartz, and Palasik (2009) explored the presence of role entrapment and vocational stereotyping in 204 teachers. The respondents also completed an open-ended question asking them to report what had influenced their choices. Finally, the teachers completed a demographic questionnaire regarding their experiences in education and with stuttering. Eight careers were judged to be less advisable for people who stutter: judge, attorney, SLP, Protestant minister, guidance/employment counselor, psychologist, physician, and hospital administrator. Qualitative analysis of the open-ended question revealed three themes related to the teachers' ratings: (1) influence of the disorder (i.e., stuttering), (2) influence of the career, and (3) influence of the participants' personal views (e.g., being supportive). For the first theme, stuttering was the key factor in whether a career was advisable or not, such that people who stutter were viewed as unlikely to be able to carry out the career effectively. Interestingly, none of the demographic factors impacted the reports toward careers.

In a related study, Swartz, Gabel, Hughes, and Irani (2009) surveyed 158 SLPs regarding their attitudes toward career choices for people who stutter through completion of the *VAS*. The SLPs also completed demographic questions and an open-ended item to identify factors that influenced their ratings. The SLPs identified only two careers, SLP and attorney, to be less advisable for stuttering individuals than their reports for people with disabilities. Responses to the open-ended question suggested that many SLPs would advise people who stutter to pursue almost any career, while many reported that stuttering would impact career choices of people who stutter. Only the amount of professional reading had positive impact for the reports toward the career advice provided to items related to SLP and judge. The other demographic variables did not predict the SLPs' ratings of careers.

These three studies provide support that people who stutter do suffer from role entrapment in the form of vocational stereotyping. It varied across the three studies, with university students identifying 20 careers that were less advisable for people who stutter than people who do not stutter (Gabel et al., 2004), the teachers identifying the next highest number with 10 careers (Irani et al., 2009), and then SLPs the least with two careers (Swartz et al., 2009). Importantly, the same careers were identified as less advisable for stuttering individuals in all three studies. Specifically, it appeared that the greater the perceived need for communication in certain careers, the more likely participants were to regard that career as inadvisable for people who stutter. In the two studies that asked participants to provide reasons for their responses to the *VAS*, stuttering was stated as the major reason for why a career was less advisable for stuttering people than for those who do not stutter (Irani et al., 2009; Swartz et al., 2009).

Attempts to Change Role Entrapment and Occupational Stereotyping of People Who Stutter

The research reviewed above has consistently shown that the population who does not stutter report negative stereotyping related to employment and role entrapment related to occupational choices. These studies were motivated in part by research exploring factors that affect attitudes and stereotypes toward people who stutter. Historically, certain factors such as severity of stuttering (Gabel, 2006; Susca & Healey, 2002; Turnbaugh, Guitar, & Hoffman, 1979), therapy techniques or attending therapy (Gabel, 2006; Manning, Burlison, & Thaxton, 1999), gender (Burley & Rinaldi, 1986), disclosure or acknowledgment of stuttering (Collins & Blood, 1990; Healey, Gabel, Daniels, & Kawai, 2007; Silverman, 1988), and age of the participant (Patterson & Pring, 1991) have been explored to identify ways to positively impact attitudes toward people who stutter. Most of these variables, except for gender (e.g., St. Louis, 2012a; St. Louis, LeMasters, & Poormohammad, Chapter 9), appear to improve attitudes toward stuttering. Several research studies have explored whether these variables might impact attitudes and stereotyping related to employment and role entrapment.

Craig and Calver (1991) studied the effects of fluency-shaping therapy on the perceptions employers held of stuttering people. Thirty-four employers were surveyed regarding two groups of people who stutter who were employed at their companies. One group received therapy to speak more fluently, while the other group did not. The employers completed a 10-item Likert questionnaire assessing the communicative effectiveness of the employees who stuttered, both prior to and two months following treatment. The results suggested a significant difference between the perceptions of the treatment group prior to and following treatment. Employers perceived the speech of individuals who had completed treatment to be more acceptable because they believed the employees had improved their ability to communicate more effectively.

The perceptions toward the individuals who had not received therapy did not change over this time period. Results indicated that people who stutter were perceived more positively when they were able to improve their fluency. Aside from the documented reductions in stuttering, it may also be possible that the employers perceived these individuals more positively simply because they had attended therapy.

In the same study, Craig and Calver (1991) polled the 62 individuals who completed the same fluency-shaping therapy program. They were asked to complete a questionnaire regarding vocation and career change. The first question asked if they had been promoted since their completion of therapy. This question was not applicable for 19 of the subjects (i.e., job change or self-employed), but 19 of the 43 individuals who responded to this question reported a promotion following the completion of therapy. The second question asked if the participants had left their pre-treatment job and obtained another position. This item was not applicable for 12 of the participants (i.e., self-employed or promoted), yet 18 of the individuals responding to this item reported that a positive job change (i.e., an upgrade from their former position) followed treatment. Therefore, 60% of those individuals completing therapy reported a positive improvement in employment following treatment. Results of this study suggested that stuttering individuals were not only perceived in a more positive manner by employers following treatment to speak more fluently, but also experienced a positive change in career.

Gabel, Althouse, and Tellis (2002) completed a study exploring the potential impact of gender and familiarity with stuttering on role entrapment. To do this, 197 participants were surveyed regarding perceptions of employment options using the *VAS*. A 2X2 Multivariate Analysis of Variance (MANOVA) was completed to explore if gender and familiarity with stuttering people impacted participants' reports related to whether people who stutter should pursue any of the 43 items on the *VAS*. Neither variable was associated with improved attitudes toward any of the 43 careers indicating that these variables would not alter role entrapment. As with other studies utilizing the *VAS*, similar careers were rated as less advisable for people who stutter, especially those that required a higher degree of communication ability.

Gabel, Hughes, and Daniels (2008) administered the *VAS* to 260 university students to explore whether severity and involvement in speech therapy altered attitudes toward role entrapment related to employment. A 2X2 MANOVA was completed to identify whether these two variables impacted participants' ratings on the *VAS*. Neither factor improved attitudes, though certain careers were still seen as less advisable. These careers were the same set seen in past *VAS* studies, lending more support to the notion that certain careers appear less advisable for people who stutter, especially those that require a higher degree of speaking ability.

Schlagheck, Gabel, and Hughes (2009) conducted a mixed-method study of attitudes and role entrapment of stuttering people. The participants were 154 individuals from a community sample who completed a questionnaire with both forced choice and open-ended items exploring demographics, attitudes toward stuttering, and attitudes toward employment options for people who stutter. The open-ended items were analyzed qualitatively for emerging themes. The participants reported negative attitudes toward stuttering people. Interestingly, 82% of participants believed that stuttering would have a negative impact on employment. Themes for these reports included the communication disability, difficulty with certain tasks related to work, and a need to avoid certain careers. Careers that involved a significant amount of communication were reported to be less appropriate for people who stutter. Those participants who were familiar with males who stuttered were more likely to report that stuttering affected employment than participants who were not familiar. Thus, familiarity with a stuttering person and one's gender appeared to impact attitudes toward people who stutter as well as the attitudes toward employment of stuttering individuals.

Logan and O'Connor (2012) conducted two experiments using speech samples featuring levels of stuttering severity or pseudo-stuttering versus fluent speech and two questionnaires. One questionnaire was similar to the *VAS* and was designed to explore factors that affected perceptions of occupational advice. In the first experiment, 58 people who did not stutter listened to two audio samples, one sample with "more severe" stuttering and the other with acoustically modified "less severe" stuttering. The questionnaires determined if stuttering severity impacted reports of attitudes (measured on a personal attribute scale) and suitability of 32 careers for people who stutter. The study found that increased speaking demands of certain careers had a negative effect on attitudes toward stuttering people. The same variables negatively affected occupational suitability ratings for people who stutter. In the second experiment, 58 other individuals who did not stutter heard two audio samples, either an adult speaking fluently or an adult who was "stuttering" (i.e., a different sample of pseudo-stuttering similar to the "less severe" sample above) and then completed the same scales as in the first experiment. As with the first experiment, the authors found that decreased communicative functioning, in this case the presence of stuttering, decreased occupational suitability ratings and attitudes toward stuttering. In the first experiment, female participants' reports were more positive than reports made by males.

The studies reviewed (Craig & Calver, 1991; Logan & O'Connor, 2012; Schlagheck et al., 2009) did not find consistency as to the impact of severity on attitudes toward role entrapment of people who stutter. These findings differ from studies that have explored the impact of severity on general attitudes and stereotyping of people who stutter. The reason for such a discrepancy is unclear. The studies did find some support that female participants did report more positive reports than males related to role entrapment. Future research should explore whether severity of stuttering and other variables impact perceptions of occupational choices and role entrapment.

Studies Exploring Occupational Experiences of People Who Stutter

Compared to the extensive research exploring listener perceptions of people who stutter, fewer studies have focused on the work experiences of stuttering individuals. Rice and Kroll (1994) conducted one of the first studies to gather perceptions from people who stutter regarding their work experiences. The authors surveyed 282 stuttering people from Canada who responded to 10 5-point Likert scale questions that explored their experiences in the workplace. The study found that participants felt their performance reviews along with opportunities for advancement were negatively influenced due to their stuttering. Rice and Kroll also found just over 57% of participants agreed that (1) employers had misjudged their abilities because of their stuttering, and (2) they had not been asked to perform supervisory duties as a result of their stuttering. In a similar study, Rice and Kroll (1997) found that people who stutter face significant challenges and discrimination in the areas of job opportunities, evaluations of performance, promotion opportunities, social isolation, and limited occupational responsibilities due to their stuttering.

Klein and Hood (2004) explored the impact of stuttering on occupational choices and work performance of 232 stuttering individuals who completed a 17-item semantic differential scale. Over 70% of the participants believed that stuttering inhibited their opportunities to be hired or promoted, and 69% reported that stuttering had constituted a negative effect on their work performance in the past. Additionally, women perceived their stuttering to have less negative impacts than men. Those participants with more severe self-rated stuttering reported increased difficulties related to employment. Also, those participants with past therapy experiences reported that stuttering had less impact on employment than those reporting no previous therapy. Finally, non-Caucasians reported a greater impact of their stuttering on employment than Caucasians.

Palasik, Gabel, Hughes, and Rusnak (2012) explored the impact of stuttering on employment with instruments similar to those used by Klein and Hood (2004) and Rice and Kroll (1994, 1997). The participants were 184 people who stutter who completed a questionnaire that included 13 Likert-type items regarding employment experiences and demographic questions. Participants reported that stuttering affected some aspects of occupational experiences, and that their employers had both judged them negatively during interviews and limited promotional opportunities due to their stuttering. Participants reported that stuttering did not affect their choice of careers, that it did not inhibit whether they were asked to perform supervisory tasks, and that their coworkers appeared to accept their stuttering. Participants' reports were unaffected by stuttering severity, therapy experiences, type of employment, and income.

From a large general data set, McAllister, Collier, and Shepstone (2012) reported a cohort study that explored the occupational and educational impact of stuttering. Two hundred seventeen individuals who stutter were compared to a cohort of 15,694 individuals who do not stutter from survey and interview results. Respondents were asked to report on educational experiences and achievement, as well as the type of job they held and pay received at ages 23 and 50. Analysis suggested that the people who stutter were more likely to be bullied and score lower on cognitive tests than a matched control group. The authors did not find any significant effects of stuttering on educational achievement, which is contrary to findings of a study by O'Brian, Jones, Packman, Menzies, and Onslow (2011), who found that people who stutter did indeed score lower than people who do not stutter on tests of educational achievement. Finally, the study found that the only significant difference between the stuttering and non-stuttering groups occurred at age 50, whence the stuttering people had lower socioeconomic status and lower-status jobs. Though the authors interpreted these findings to support a lack of significant impact of stuttering on employment, it might also be argued that these findings do indeed support that people who stutter may experience issues with attaining equal pay and attractive job choices.

Bricker-Katz, Lincoln, and Cumming (2013) utilized a qualitative methodology to explore the work life experiences of people who stutter. Six male and three female adults who stuttered participated in an open-ended interview, and their narratives were analyzed phenomenologically. Four superordinate themes were identified by the authors: (1) stuttering is always there; (2) stuttering at work reveals a problem; (3) stuttering limits communication; and (4) stuttering limits occupational progression. Further, the authors identified self-stigma as central to how participants derived meaning from their experiences. Specifically, the participants reported fear of negative, stigmatizing public attitudes, and their internalization of such attitudes perpetuated their negative feelings about their abilities and self-esteem. Stuttering participants reported fear of negative evaluation, which appeared to be related to an increase in anxiety when approaching work. These findings identify the importance of self-stigma in understanding the work-life experiences of individuals who stutter.

A number of research studies reviewed in this section have found that adults who stutter report difficulties related to work experiences (Klein & Hood, 2004; Palasik et al., 2012; Rice & Kroll, 1994, 1997). Among the issues reported across these studies were difficulties in securing employment, in being promoted, and in performing communication tasks related to their jobs. The sole qualitative study that has been completed found that people who stutter attribute their difficulties with employment to their stuttering and speaking difficulties (Bricker-Katz et al., 2013). It is important to note that research suggests people who stutter may indeed experience these difficulties secondary to a process of self-stigma (Boyle & Blood, Chapter 2; Bricker-Katz et al., 2013; McAllister et al., 2012). The negative impact of stuttering on work experiences is most likely the result of a combination of negative societal attitudes (or public stigma) and self-stigma, since the two types are very closely related.

Summary

The purpose of this chapter was to discuss the potential impact that societal stereotyping of people who stutter has on employment opportunities and experiences. From the research reviewed, it is safe to assume there is ample evidence that stuttering people can very well encounter difficulties with employment as a result of their stuttering itself or their experiences as people who stutter. These difficulties are most likely related to negative stereotyping. When stereotyping leads to barriers to equal treatment and opportunities, it is suggestive of discrimination as a result of the stereotyping (Allport, 1986; Smart, 2001). The impact of discrimination can be quite broad-reaching and fits with recent research that has explored the global, negative impact of stuttering on quality of life (QOL) (Blumgart, Tran, & Craig, 2010; Craig, Blumgart, & Tran, 2009; Cummins, 2010; Yaruss, 2010).

As stated by the International Classification of Functioning, Disability, and Health (Yaruss & Quesal, 2004a), societal attitudes may very well have an impact on employment opportunities. Research suggests that employers (Hurst & Cooper, 1983a), vocational counselors (Hurst & Cooper, 1983b), university students (Silverman & Payner, 1990), and nurses (Silverman & Bongey, 1997) all viewed people who stutter negatively with respect to employability. This evokes what Smart (2001) referred to as marginalization, which occurs when the dominant group holds a negative definition of stuttering, even if this is counter to how the individual defines himself or herself. Thus, people who stutter may view themselves as capable of performing well in certain careers, but are seen as incompetent or unable to function in those careers due to the stereotype held by individuals who do not stutter. Additionally, these results can be explained by Smart's (2001) concept of paternalism, or the process by which a person without a disability will limit or protect a person who has a disability without consulting the individual about his or her goals.

The research discussed also suggests that role entrapment, in the form of occupational stereotyping, plays a key role in developing barriers for people who stutter in seeking employment. Every group surveyed so far has identified careers they would be less likely to advise stuttering individuals to pursue (Gabel et al., 2002; Gabel et al., 2004; Gabel et al., 2008; Irani et al., 2009; Schlagheck et al., 2009). These careers tend to be relatively prestigious careers (e.g., judge, lawyer, and SLP) and well paying. Additionally, the findings suggest that people who stutter are most likely going to interact with individuals who might view their prospects as limited because of their communication disorder and the amount of talking needed to perform well in certain careers (Irani et al., 2009; Schlagheck et al., 2009). To make the judgment that an individual is less able than normal to perform certain careers based solely on the presence of stuttering is not only role entrapment, but also a clear example of stigma (Goffman, 1963). The presence of stuttering appears to be guiding these decisions, despite the prospect that stuttering people may actually be fine communicators who just happen to stutter. More research is needed to study the presence of role entrapment in other populations such as employers or vocational counselors.

Discrimination, in the form of role entrapment, is not mitigated by factors that generally improve societal attitudes toward stuttering (Gabel et al., 2002; Gabel et al., 2008; Logan & O'Connor, 2012; Schlagheck et al., 2009). Only one study by Craig and Calver (1991) found that employer attitudes toward employees who stutter and job experiences (such as promotions and positive job changes) improved for people who stutter following successful treatment. Interestingly, studies have not explored the impact of disclosure or acknowledgment on the presence of role entrapment or occupational advice. Past research studies found that this technique or tactic positively impacted stereotyping of people who stutter (Collins & Blood, 1990; Healey et al., 2007; Silverman, 1988). Practically and clinically, this tactic would most likely be useful during a job interview or as a part of general communication with coworkers. Future studies should seek to explore the potential impact of disclosure on employment options and experiences for people who stutter.

Some research studies suggest that work-related difficulties experienced by stuttering individuals may be due self-stigma (Boyle & Blood, Chapter 2; Bricker-Katz, Lincoln, & Cumming, 2013; McAllister et al., 2012). Self-stigma occurs through a process by which societal attitudes are integrated into the personality of the individual. Thus, for people who stutter, negative societal attitudes and role entrapment might be internalized. In this way, individuals who stutter might begin to integrate barriers and discrimination into their belief systems about their own abilities and begin to hold back from pursuing certain types of careers. It is important to consider that the ICF model suggests the individual's beliefs about and reactions to stuttering can indeed form an activity limitation or handicap. More research should consider the impact on people who stutter that self-stigmatization can have on the opportunities related to employment.

In conclusion, the weight of the published evidence indicates that people who stutter will very likely experience discrimination related to employment. It is unclear how widespread this discrimination is in our society and the full extent of its impact on stuttering people. Large cohort studies, like the one completed by McAllister et al. (2012), would be helpful in further understanding these issues. Simultaneously, many issues that relate to role entrapment, the experience of discrimination, and strategies to change societal stereotypes should continue to be explored through a combination of quantitative survey designs and qualitative methods.

Chapter 5

Changing Attitudes Toward Stuttering

Fauzia Abdalla

ABSTRACT

This chapter critically reviews studies that have attempted to foster change in attitudes of fluent speakers toward stuttering. Although research on stuttering attitudes has been the subject of intense inquiry, only a handful of studies have documented ways to increase awareness and improve stuttering attitudes. Most of these investigations were based on samples gathered in Western nations. The studies varied in their target participants with a majority evaluating the attitudes of speech-language pathologists in training. Coursework and documentary videos were prevalent types of stimuli. Self-administered questionnaires were widely used to contrast pre- and post-intervention outcomes. Overall, the findings of the reviewed studies were inconclusive. Variables that may have contributed to this lack of consistency are explored. Areas for future research are noted, including the need for more rigorous methods of data collection, as well as exploring various types of interventions to effect lasting change in attitudes toward stuttering.

Introduction

Extant research has attested to the prevalence of unfavorable attitudes toward stuttering and people who stutter in populations from diverse geographic regions, cultures, ages, and professions (Abdalla & St. Louis, 2012; Betz, Blood, & Blood, 2008; Cooper & Cooper, 1996; Crichton-Smith, Wright, & Stackhouse, 2003; Crowe & Walton, 1981; Dorsey & Guenther, 2000; Ezrati-Vinacour, Platzky,

& Yairi, 2001; Hurst & Cooper, 1983b; Ip, St. Louis, Myers, & An Xue, 2012; Lass, Ruscello, Pannbacker, Schmitt, Kiser, Mussa, & Lockhart, 1994; Özdemir, St. Louis, & Topbaş, 2011a, 2011b; St. Louis, Andrade, Georgieva, & Troudt, 2005; St. Louis & Roberts, 2010; Van Borsel, Verniers, & Bouvry, 1999; Yeakle & Cooper, 1986). Lack of knowledge about stuttering may explain some of the misconceptions held by the general public, such as associating stuttering with emotional or psychological causes and ascribing stutterers with undesirable personality traits, such as being tense, reticent, embarrassed, anxious, nervous, shy, and fearful (e.g., Blood, Blood, Tellis, & Gabel, 2003; Craig, Tran, & Craig, 2003; Doody, Kalinowski, Armson, & Stuart, 1993; Klassen, 2001; Van Borsel et al., 1999; St. Louis, 2005). Moreover, the public may deem people who stutter as individuals "in need of help" (Mayo, Mayo, Gentry, & Hildebrandt, 2008) given that when interacting with people who stutter, fluent listeners often interrupt or complete the stutterer's utterance (Kamhi, 2003). Such negative misconceptions prevail despite the lack of empirical support for such contentions (Bloodstein & Bernstein Ratner, 2008) and regardless of exposure to or personal relationships with people who stutter (Doody et al., 1993; Leahy, 1994; McGee, Kalinowski, & Stuart, 1996). Conversely, Klassen (2001, 2002) found that some individuals' personal acquaintance with a person who stutters may have a favorable effect on their attitudes.

These negative stereotypes and their sequelae have detrimental consequences and can affect stutterers' quality of life and lead to social, academic, and vocational setbacks (Boyle, 2013a; Boyle & Blood, Chapter 2; Daniels, Gabel, & Hughes, 2012; Gabel, Blood, Tellis, & Althouse, 2004; Klompas & Ross, 2004; Yaruss, 2001). The following statement by a female teen who stutters clearly reveals the effect of such stigma on individuals who stutter. In recounting her classroom experience to Abdalla and Al-Saddah (2009), she recalled, "I raised my hand in class one time and the teacher interrupted me while I was speaking and told me I couldn't answer the question because I stutter. She embarrassed me further in front of the class by asking students to correct my speech. I wish my teacher would be patient and give me a chance to express my thoughts. I just want to be treated like other students in my class who do not stutter." Evidently, this youth's experience underscores the need for a greater understanding of her stuttering so she can receive equal opportunities to express herself as is the case for her fluent peers. Indeed over two decades ago, Crowe and Walton (1981) echoed a similar need when they recommended that "identification of undesirable teacher attitudes toward stuttering, coupled with a teacher education program, possibly could ensure that communicative interactions within the classroom complement the therapeutic process" (p. 167).

As a result of counterproductive experiences of many people who stutter, practitioners and researchers have continued to urge for campaigns to increase awareness and foster long-term change in attitudes toward stuttering. Organizations that advocate for people who stutter (e.g., Action for Stammering Children, 2014; International Project on Attitudes Toward Human Attributes, [St. Louis, 2014]; National Stuttering Association, 2014a; The Stuttering Foundation, 2014a) have contributed to this initiative by disseminating scientific information about stuttering to the public using varied resources like fact sheets, multimedia, conferences, and summaries of cross-cultural research. However, despite such efforts, recent research demonstrates the persistence of negative attitudes toward people who stutter (e.g., Van Borsel, Brepoels, & De Coene, 2011). Learning more about undesirable attitudes that stutterers confront would assist practitioners in dealing with their psychosocial difficulties, as well as determining effective methods for altering societal attitudes toward stuttering. Although research on stuttering attitudes has been the subject of intense inquiry, only a few studies have attempted to document and evaluate ways to reduce misconceptions about stuttering and tackle unfavorable attitudes toward people who stutter.

The purpose of this chapter is to: (1) review intervention studies aimed at improving fluent speakers' awareness and attitudes toward stuttering and people who stutter, and (2) examine factors that may have contributed to inconsistencies in their results. This review is general in the sense that it does not focus on the attitudes of a particular population since there are only a handful of studies on the topic. Studies on children, adolescents, and university students, as well as those of current and future service providers such as teachers and speech-language pathologists, have been included in the review. The intention is that this discussion will lead the reader to a better understanding of the complexities of changing attitudes, as well as to inform future endeavors aimed at improving public awareness and attitudes toward people who stutter. The chapter begins by providing a brief review of studies that have attempted to modify attitudes toward stuttering and people who stutter. It then examines possible factors that may have contributed to inconsistency in the findings. Future suggestions to make this line of research fruitful are discussed in the conclusion.

Attempts to Improve Awareness and Attitudes

Appendices A and B provide an overview of studies that have attempted to alter negative attitudes toward people who stutter. A search in several databases uncovered only 13 studies that have explored ways to improve awareness and change attitudes toward stuttering. Six of these studies have been published in peer-reviewed journals (Abdalla & St. Louis, 2014; Flynn & St. Louis, 2011; Langevin & Prasad, 2012; Leahy, 1994; McGee et al., 1996; Snyder, 2001) and eight are conference papers (Coleman, Weidner, Barney, Scott, Baker, Stephens, & Donsbach, 2013; Delaney, 2001; Gottwald, Warner, Hartley, Fraas, Hawver, & St. Louis, 2011; Gottwald, Kent, St. Louis, & Hartley, 2014; Hughes, Gabel, Roseman, & Daniels, Chapter 15; Junuzović-Žunić, Weidner, Reichel, Cook, St. Louis, & Ware, Chapter 14; Mayo, Mayo, Gentry, & Hildebrandt, 2008; Reichel & St. Louis, 2004, 2007). All the studies were based on samples gathered in Western countries (Ireland, the United Kingdom, and the United States) with the exception of Abdalla and St. Louis (2014) whose participants were from the Middle East (Kuwait). The studies vary in their target participants with a majority evaluating the attitude of student speech-language pathologists (SLPs), followed by adolescents, and recently teachers. Most of the studies have opted to use coursework to educate individuals, although documentary videos have also been used. Measurements to determine effectiveness of the intervention used mostly self-administered questionnaires such as a *Semantic Differential Scale* (Woods & Williams, 1976), the *Public Opinion Survey of Human Attributes–Stuttering* (*POSHA–S*) (St. Louis, 2005, 2011a) or *Clinician Attitudes Toward Stuttering* (*CATS*) inventory (Cooper, 1975), with a few incorporating qualitative analyses in the form of open-ended comments by the participants. The number of participants in the studies ranged from 10 to over 100.

Review of Research Studies

ALTERING ATTITUDES OF CHILDREN TOWARD STUTTERING. Measuring and attempting to alter fluent children's perceptions of stuttering is not as straightforward as those of older participants. Two studies have explored the possibility of using a special curriculum (Langevin & Prasad, 2012) or reading a story (Coleman et al., 2013) to modify school-age children's negative attitudes toward their peers who stutter. Langevin and Prasad (2012) used an educational program to stimulate changes in peer attitudes toward stuttering as part of a bullying awareness and prevention program in 608 young students toward school-age children who stutter in Canada. The program resulted in improvement in attitudes toward bullying and stuttering when children who watched the video (which was part of the curriculum) were compared with those who did not on the *Peer Attitudes Toward Children Who Stutter* (*PATCS*) (Langevin, 2009) scale and the *Provictim Scale* (Rigby & Slee, 1991). In particular, children with no previous involvement in bullying and those who did not know a person who stutters were found to display a greater improvement toward supportive attitudes following the training program than their counterparts who had previous experience with people who stutter or bullying.

Coleman and his colleagues presented four children aged four to six years with a video sample of a six-year-old child who stutters (Coleman et al., 2013). The children were asked nine questions to explore their perceptions of the child who stutters. A story about a character who stutters was then read to the four participants before asking them to review the video sample and answering the same series of questions again. A descriptive analysis of the children's responses to the questions demonstrated changes in their perceptions about stuttering following the story. In particular, they displayed improved attitudes, increased knowledge about stuttering, diminished listener avoidance, and a rise in objective responses.

ALTERING ATTITUDES OF ADOLESCENTS TOWARD STUTTERING. Two studies attempted to modify attitudes of fluent adolescents toward stuttering. In the first study, McGee et al. (1996) contrasted the perceptions of 36 fluent high school students (18 male, 18 female) aged 16 to 21 years toward two hypothetical male adolescents, one fluent and the other who stuttered. A 25-item semantic differential scale (Woods & Williams, 1976) was used to measure their perceptions prior to and after viewing a documentary videotape, *Voices to Remember* (Bondarenko, 1992b). The video features stories of a number of adults who stutter, most with positive outcomes. The post-viewing results showed no changes in the adolescents' negative stereotyping of stuttering. Prior to watching the video, the respondents rated the hypothetical adolescent who stutters as reflecting the "stuttering stereotype" on 44% of the items, e.g., being significantly more nervous, shy, guarded, and afraid than the hypothetical fluent counterpart. After the video, the students rated the male who stutters less favorably on three additional negative ratings, i.e., fearful, inflexible, and self-derogatory. About two-thirds (69%) of the students knew a person who stutters, and yet exposure did not seem to positively influence their perceptions of people who stutter. The authors noted that the videotape used in the study may have reinforced the respondents' preexisting negative stereotype rather than altering these attitudes. Consequently, the researchers concluded that viewing a videotape by itself may not be an effective method for sensitizing high school students toward people who stutter.

Flynn and St. Louis (2011) explored attitudes of 83 students (mean age 16.4 years) in a Mid-Atlantic high school in the United States to determine whether their perceptions could be positively influenced by using two types of presentations (live and video). The *POSHA–S*, supplemented with a few added items, was administered to the students before and after the presentations. One group of students (14 males, 26 females) listened to a 45-minute live oral presentation by a person who stutters and the other group (19 males, 24 females) viewed a 45-minute video, *True Life®: I Stutter* (Schneider, 2007). The content of the two conditions were slightly different, although both presented how people who stutter cope with day-to-day challenges they confront due to their stuttering. In the live oral presentation, Timothy Flynn (the author, a moderate-to-severe stutterer) provided facts and personal insights about stuttering, the impact of the disorder on his life, and how humor has been an effective coping mechanism. During the presentation, he recounted humorous stories about his stuttering from his childhood and school days. The professionally designed video separately featured three adults who stutter (Flynn and two females) dealing with their stuttering in varying situations: getting a job, competing for a pageant, and participating in speech therapy. A third condition involved a short 20-minute face-to-face presentation by Flynn after the second group of students viewed *True Life®: I Stutter*. The students in this condition completed a pre-*POSHA–S*, post-*POSHA–S* after the video, and a second post-*POSHA–S* after Flynn's 20-minute oral presentation. A comparison of the pre-test and post-test overall scores, as well as measures on selected items of *POSHA–S*, showed 32.8% (22 out of 67 comparisons) significant positive changes for the oral condition and 28.4% (19 out of 67 comparisons) changes for the video condition. Positive shifts in the combined video-oral condition were similar to the oral-only condition. These findings revealed that attitudes of adolescents can be improved, but more so through a live presentation by an individual who stutters than a professional video alone.

ALTERING ATTITUDES OF UNDERGRADUATE STUDENTS (NON-SLP MAJORS) TOWARD STUTTERING. Only one known study has focused on non-SLP university students. This particular study investigated the effect of watching a video on perceptions of undergraduate students who were not majoring in communication disorders. Mayo et al. (2008) used a 25-item semantic differential scale (Woods & Williams, 1976) in surveying 43 undergraduate students (15 males and 29 females) at an American university before and after watching a shortened version of the documentary video, *Speaking of Courage* (Bondarenko, 1992a), a companion video to the aforementioned *Voices to Remember* (Bondarenko, 1992b). This video, primarily featuring stuttering children, focused most dramatically on the struggles and triumphs of a middle-school-aged girl to overcome stuttering-related confusions and fears. The authors noted the overall tone of the edited version was positive. After viewing the video, the students exhibited significant positive shifts in attitudes on eight out of the 25 items. However, most of the shifts in the adjective pair ratings were not large. Four pairs related to cooperativeness, pleasantness, emotionality, and intelligence changed from "fairly" to "quite", flexibility remained within the "neutral" range, while openness, shyness, and daringness changed from "fairly" to "neutral," "quite" to "fairly," and "neutral" to "fairly," respectively.

ALTERING ATTITUDES OF PRE-SERVICE SLPS TOWARD STUTTERING. A majority of the literature on modifying attitudes has focused on speech-language pathology students not only because of easy availability for the instructor/ researchers but also because of the potential negative impact on future clients and the risk of the students developing and/or sustaining negative stereotypes toward people who stutter (Delaney, 2001). Leahy's (1994) study represents one of the earliest attempts to modify student SLPs' stereotypical attitudes toward people who stutter. She examined attitudes of third- and fourth-year under-graduate students in an SLP training program in Ireland toward a hypothetical male who stutters using a pre-/post-test design with an 11-item semantic differential scale adapted from Woods and Williams (1976). She provided the students with intensive coursework, simulated stuttering, and direct exposure to people who stutter in individual or group therapeutic interventions over the course of a year. The educational training included lectures on stereotype and exploring personal attitudes. In general, the training was found to have limited effectiveness in changing the attitudes of the pre-service clinicians. Although statistical analyses were not conducted to compare the pre- and post-test responses and only 13 of the 17 students completed the survey, these SLP trainees perceived people who stutter to be even more tense, reticent, and nervous than before the exposure. However, people who stutter were viewed in a positive light for three traits (pleasantness, quietness, and extroversion). Leahy hypothesized that the students' experience substantiated their previously established negative stereotype even after one year of coursework and clinical exposure designed deliberately to ameliorate their attitudes.

Seven years later, Delaney (2001) and Snyder (2001) explored attitude change in another group of SLPs in training. Delaney (2001) focused on involving the students in group therapy for adults who stutter, while Snyder (2001) relied on documentary videos. Participants in Delaney's study (2001) comprised 18 second-year undergraduate SLP students in a university in Wales, Great Britain. The students were divided into an experimental ($n = 8$) and a control group ($n = 10$). No details about their age, sex, and ethnicity were provided, yet none of the students received formal teaching on fluency disorders. The experimental group participated in the stuttering group sessions, while the controls did not receive exposure to people who stutter. The group sessions were 30 weeks in duration and aimed at decreasing fear and avoidance of stuttering and helping the clients appraise and develop a positive approach to stuttering and communication. Comparisons between the two groups in their ratings of three hypothetical stutterers (male child, male adult, and female adult) and two fluent speakers (child and adult males) were drawn using a 20-item semantic differential scale and a questionnaire the author adapted from several existing scales i.e., the *Attitudes Toward Stuttering* (*ATS*) scale. At the end of the year, no differences between the two groups emerged for most of the semantic differential scale comparisons. No statistically reliable differences were found for two subscales of the *ATS*: (1) generalizations and common perceptions of people who stutter and stuttering (24 items), and (2) attitudes related to listener responses to people who stutter (10 items). The pre- and post-treatment scores of the experimental participants were significantly better than those of the control group for the third *ATS* subscale, which pertained to responses of the person who stutters to his/her stutter. According to the author, the nature of the activities of the adult stuttering group sessions may have contributed to the significantly better attitudes for items concerning the stutterers' responses to his/her stutter in the experimental group than the control group. Also, overall, the experimental group was less likely to rate hypothetical people who stutter as being different than hypothetical fluent speakers.

Another study of university students was reported by Snyder (2001), who measured attitudinal change in two groups of graduate students enrolled in a fluency disorders class. One group watched a factual video, *Effects of Altered Auditory Feedback at Fast and Normal Speaking Rates* (Keith & Kuhn, 1996) while the other viewed *Speaking of Courage* (Bondarenko, 1992a; see above), an emotional video portraying some unfavorable social implications of stuttering. The former film was a clinical video showing severe stuttering that was greatly reduced by "singing" speech. The latter film chronicles the life of a young female who stutters and her experiences with the disorder. The students' pre- and post-test responses on the *Clinicians Attitudes Toward Stuttering* (*CATS*) inventory (Cooper, 1975) were contrasted. Post-test findings revealed that both types of documentaries were associated with subtle changes in perceptions of stuttering. A significant change was observed only in one item on the *CATS* for the emotional film. On the other hand, three items changed after the factual video. The changes were not necessarily in the desired direction, e.g., the statement "chances are that most stuttering is the result of multiple co-existing factors" changed from a median rating of "moderately agree" to "undecided." Snyder (2001) explained that the significant differences that emerged from the study were essentially artifacts of the *CATS*' lack of reliability and could not be viewed as authentic changes in perceptions. Nevertheless, the author interpreted these findings as confirming the fact that negative stereotypes toward people who stutter are resistant to change.

Reichel and St. Louis (2004, 2007) investigated the effects of a course in fluency disorders on attitudes of SLP graduate students toward stuttering. The 77 participants in the 2004 study were mostly female graduate SLP students approximately 28 years of age enrolled in two universities in New York. The experimental group ($n = 47$) received training in emotional intelligence and were exposed to about seven people who stutter who shared their emotional experiences. The control group ($n = 30$) did not receive such training. Four measures were used: (1) an experimental version of the *POSHA–S*; (2) the *Emotional Intelligence Scale* (*EIS*), a self-report tool that measures the ability to detect and express regular emotions in oneself and in others (Schutte & Malouff, 1999); (3) a 25-item bipolar adjective scale adapted with either/or choices from Woods and Williams (1976); and (4) qualitative responses.

There was a significant difference in the amount of knowledge about stuttering between the pre- and post-*POSHA–S* for both groups. No significant differences between the pre- and post-ratings for *EIS* were observed in either group of students. Interestingly, the bipolar adjective scale post-ratings were significantly more favorable for the experimental students (27% to 35% change) and the control group (27% to 33% positive shift). Only four paired adjectives changed positively in the experimental students while six shifted positively in the control group. It seems surprising to observe that the perceptions of the control group who did not receive training changed as a result of rating stutterers on the semantic differential scale before and after the semester.

In the 2007 study by Reichel and St. Louis, 20 graduate students from diverse cultures and ethnicity in a fluency disorders class participated in an intervention module that included short lectures, role-playing, student presentations, group discussions, and direct contact with five people who stutter. The same experimental version of the *POSHA–S*, administered at the beginning and end of the semester and responses to an open-ended questionnaire were analyzed descriptively. The results revealed that quantitative changes based on *POSHA–S* were more modest than the qualitative responses (i.e., comments of the students). Although 90% of the students reported improved attitudes and increased interest in treating people who stutter, 50% of the overall impression responses on *POSHA–S* remained unchanged, 40% showed a positive shift, and 10% were less favorable. Even though the *POSHA–S* results were mixed, the authors concluded that integrating a special training module on multicultural and multinational contexts into a graduate fluency disorders course can to an extent promote a better understanding of students' affective and cognitive bases of prejudice, as well as reduce stigma and negative stereotyping toward people who stutter.

Two other studies have reported favorable changes in attitudes of SLP students in the United States following fluency disorders coursework and practicum-related instruction. In one, Junuzović-Žunić, Weidner, Reichel, Cook, St. Louis, and Ware (Chapter 14) reported three coursework-related studies. The first found 13% positive shift in the pre- and post-comparisons of the *POSHA–S* in 86 graduate SLP students in New York City following a fluency disorders course (the aforementioned studies plus one more combined). The second from West Virginia University reported three sets of *POSHA–S* data (three months before the course, at the onset of the course, and after the eight-week fluency disorders coursework) for undergraduate SLP students. A significant positive change emerged between the first pre- and the post-test scores for 8% of the ratings and a favorable shift between the second pre-test of 6% of the ratings in contrast with the post-*POSHA–S* ratings. The third contributed data from 27 fourth-year undergraduate students majoring in speech-language pathology and audiology in Bosnia and Herzegovina. The students completed a Bosnian-Herzegovinian version of *POSHA–S* on three occasions: before the course (Pre), after a basic fluency disorders course (Post 1), and again at the end of an advanced fluency disorders course (Post 2). Significant changes in the desired direction occurred in 7% and 11% of the 60 potential *POSHA–S* ratings between the Pre versus Post 1 and Pre versus Post 2 ratings, respectively.

Interestingly, the investigations of these three programs (New York City, West Virginia, and Bosnia and Herzegovina) demonstrated robust evidence that attitudes of SLP students can be mitigated using fluency disorders coursework. The *POSHA–S* remained a consistent measure across these studies despite the wide variation in course content/duration, instructors, sampling procedures, and number and demographics of the participants. The authors point out the three groups of SLP students began with higher than average pre-*POSHA–S* scores, which could have contributed partially to the improved alteration in attitudes. An addition of a comparable group of control participants would have constituted a stronger design.

More recently, Hughes, Gabel, Roseman, and Daniels (Chapter 15) examined the effects of an interdisciplinary training program in raising awareness and changing attitudes of graduate students. Along with eight SLP students, they also involved eight school counseling students in the study. An Intensive Stuttering Clinic for Children and their Families (ISCCF) program run by the authors was used to provide both groups of students with information about stuttering in general and an opportunity to directly witness the social and emotional effects of stuttering for children who stutter and their families. Both groups of students completed a pre-clinic survey followed by short presentations about the other group's work. While the SLP students were involved in providing therapy, the counseling student group watched therapy and also engaged actively with children who stutter enrolled in the ISCCF program. After the eight-day clinic, both groups took a post-clinic survey and wrote a reflection paper. Although the data were primarily qualitative (open-ended questions), there were some quantitative questions in the post-clinic survey. Results indicated that, overall, school counseling and SLP graduate students felt more equipped to work with children who stutter after participating in the clinic. They also appeared to develop a better appreciation for each other's fields and a readiness to collaborate in future. The authors concluded that school counselors and SLPs can assist children who stutter to navigate the academic environment and advocated for a clear demarcation of roles for the two disciplines.

ALTERING ATTITUDES OF PRE-SERVICE AND IN-SERVICE TEACHERS TOWARD STUTTERING. In a pilot and follow-up study, Gottwald et al. (2011, 2014) selected a more varied sample consisting of 10 speech-language pathologists, 18 undergraduate students in a communication disorders program, 10 teachers, and 20 college professors from New Hampshire, U.S. The participants completed the *POSHA–S* before and after viewing an 11-minute DVD, purposely designed for the study, which featured facts about stuttering and the personal experiences of three stutterers. General findings showed that a brief exposure to life histories of people who stutter can improve feelings and attitudes toward stuttering. The most notable changes were observed in beliefs about people who stutter, knowledge about causes of stuttering, and how to interact with an individual who stutters. The teachers exhibited the greatest change (Overall Stuttering Scores on *POSHA–S* increased from 39 to 52), students displayed a considerable change (25 to 35), and SLP scores did not change (55 to 56), presumably because their pre-DVD attitudes were so positive. Professors did show a positive OSS change from 36 to 47.

Abdalla and St. Louis (2014) explored the effect of a 17-minute documentary video in ameliorating attitudes toward stuttering of 99 pre-service (48 controls, 51 experimental) and 103 in-service public school teachers (49 controls, 54 experimental) in Kuwait as measured by an Arabic adaptation of the *POSHA–S*. In a quasi-experimental design, both groups of participants were tested twice (pre- versus post-treatment) with a one-week interval. Only the experimental group viewed the video before completing the post-test survey. Pre-treatment comparisons showed that the control and experimental groups held similar attitudes toward stuttering. As predicted, the pre- and post-treatment ratings for both control groups remained unchanged since they did not view the video between the two treatment sessions. A significant shift in attitudes (mostly in a positive direction) was observed in the experimental pre-service teachers. Favorable changes were noted in various aspects of the disorder, notably traits, etiology, symptoms, and social distance, as well as strategies for dealing with students who stutter in the classroom. The findings were further reinforced by the fact that a control group of pre-service teachers failed to show such changes. Surprisingly, no changes in knowledge, beliefs, or attitudes toward people who stutter surfaced for the experimental in-service teachers after viewing the video. Two possible reasons for this discrepancy related to the fact that all the experimental pre-service teachers were females and younger while the experimental in-service teachers were all older males. Nevertheless, the authors hypothesize that the differences may have stemmed from variables related to teaching rather than sex or age for three reasons: (1) the two groups were similar in the pre-testing; (2) sex of the respondents did not affect *POSHA–S* results in two international studies (St. Louis, 2012a; St. Louis, LeMasters, & Poormohammad, Chapter 9); and (3) age has not yet been shown to be a strong predictor of *POSHA–S* attitudes after college (e.g., St. Louis, Chapter 1). In any case, the authors inferred that it is possible to positively modify certain listeners' perceptions of people who stutter using an educational documentary video that presented factual and emotional aspects of stuttering.

Potential Factors Contributing to Inconsistency in Results

Studies that have attempted to ameliorate negative stereotypes toward people who stutter have been inconclusive. Some have reported positive changes, while others have found either no shift in attitude or a change in the reverse direction (i.e., intervention allegedly reinforced the negative stereotypes). These varied results prompt us to ask whether the researchers considered the following foundational questions:

WERE THE RESEARCHERS REFERRING TO THE SAME PHENOMENA? When attempting to change attitudes, it is important to understand that an attitude can be explicit or implicit, each requiring a different type of measurement (Bohner & Dickel, 2011). On similar lines, stereotype can be simple or complex (see Boyle & Blood, Chapter 2, for more details). The two layers of stigma, namely, public stigma and self-stigma (Boyle, 2013a; Boyle & Blood, Chapter 2), need to be delineated too. For instance, are the participants from the public displaying stigma because they devalue the person who stutters due to her stuttering? On the other hand, could the members of the public be reacting to the self-stigma (i.e., negative internalized feelings stemming from public stereotypes, prejudice, and discrimination) exhibited by the individual who stutters?

DID THE RESEARCHERS CONSIDER CAUSES OF NEGATIVE STEREOTYPING OR STIGMA? Various explanations have been offered to explain the origin of stigma toward people who stutter. For example, the anchoring-adjustment theory explains that stereotypes about stuttering may be based on a fluent speaker's personal experience with typical disfluencies (MacKinnon, Hall, & MacIntyre, 2007) In other words, as postulated by White and Collins (1984), negative feelings (e.g., nervous or shy) may be associated with people who stutter because, superficially, stuttering simulates the typical disfluencies that fluent speakers experience when confronted with anxiety-provoking situations like public speaking. Goffman's (1963) explanation of stigma and Wright's (1983) idea of "spread phenomenon" would predict negative perceptions of a specific disability (in this case stuttering) to generalize or spread to views about the whole person, e.g., other characteristics such as the individual's capability, personality, and intelligence.

HOW DO NEGATIVE ATTITUDES FORM AND THEN BECOME ROOTED? This is another point worth bearing in mind when attempting to change attitudes. According to Bohner and Dickel (2011), "an attitude is an evaluation of an object of thought" (p. 392). These objects can be something in the person's mind and can range from abstract to mundane, including people, groups, ideas, and things. Two main theories address the question of how attitudes are formed and prevail (see Bohner & Dickel, 2011 for a review). One set of theories argue in favor of what they refer to as the "mental file-drawer" whereby attitudes are viewed as being already stored in long-term memory but tagged according to context and ready to be accessed and employed as warranted. Others postulate that we construct attitudes *on the go*. For example, Schwarz (2007) indicates that attitudes are "evaluative judgments, formed when needed, rather than enduring personal dispositions" (p. 639). Each of these views may influence changes in one's attitudes toward people who stutter given that there are various ways these attitudes were constructed and accessed.

WHAT WERE THE RESEARCHERS TRYING TO CHANGE EXACTLY? This is indeed a key question. While attitudes, stereotypes, and stigma are interconnected and have been studied, what matters most is how they affect the listeners' behavior toward the person who stutters. We need to be sure that once an attitude changes, its attendant behavior does too. For instance, the listener may no longer perceive the stutterer as introverted, but still be disinclined to offer her a job. The fluently speaking classmate may no longer hold a negative stereotype of low intelligence toward a peer who stutters, but may still bully the latter about his stuttering.

WHO NEEDS INTERVENTION TO CHANGE ATTITUDES AND IN WHAT CONTEXT? It is necessary to determine whether the self-stigma of the person who stutters or the public stigma displayed by the fluent listener should be targeted for intervention. It is likely that self- or public stigma would need to be modified through varying strategies.

Procedural Variables That May Affect Attitude Change

It could very well be that attitudes are notoriously difficult to change. Researchers have shown that listening to stuttered speech can cause fluent listeners cognitive, affective, and physical discomfort (Guntapalli, Everheart, Kalinowski, Nanjundeswaran, & Saltuklaroglu, 2007; Susca & Healey, 2002). This may be another reason for the difficulty in ameliorating negative attitudes toward stuttering and people who stutter in some participants like in-service teachers (Abdalla & St. Louis, 2014) and students (Leahy, 1994; McGee et al.,1996; Synder, 2001). Also, several challenges in altering attitudes could be related to variables associated with the effectiveness of the stimuli, accuracy of the measuring instruments, and selection criteria for participants (Delaney, 2001; Snyder, 2001).

PARTICIPANT SELECTION. When selecting participants for studies, it seems that researchers have not always considered pre-treatment knowledge of stuttering and exposure to people who stutter. This may have contributed to lack of consistency in the findings. Studies do not seem to have treated these groups of participants (i.e., those who had previous exposure versus those who did not) differently. McGee et al. (1996) observed that "exposure may provide the genesis and/or serve to enforce negative stereotypes as opposed to sensitize individuals and instill positive attitudes" (p. 245). We are not certain whether exposure to stuttering would have a negative or positive influence in changing attitudes. However, it may be worthwhile to take previous exposure into account and find or develop an alternative approach for those who already have exposure to people who stutter to ensure that the educational campaign has the desired effect.

Studies diverge in how the participants were recruited, with many lacking randomization, which may have contributed to selection bias. A number of studies recruited SLP students enrolled in university classes (e.g., Delaney, 2001; Leahy, 1994; Snyder, 2001). On the other hand, several studies were careful in avoiding SLP-related biases in participant selection (e.g., Abdalla & St. Louis, 2014; Flynn & St. Louis, 2011; McGee et al., 1996). In some reports, the reader is not provided with sufficient details about the participants, e.g., their background and ethnicity (e.g., Leahy, 1994; Snyder, 2001), in order to determine if these variables in participant selection might have contributed to lack of attitudinal change toward stuttering.

STIMULI TO EFFECT CHANGE. Researchers have adopted various creative approaches to effect changes in respondents' post-treatment attitudes toward people who stutter. Some have opted for coursework and exposure to stutterers while others have resorted to video or live presentations. An examination of these various methodologies does not provide a consistent picture. For example, reorganizing coursework for students enrolled in a fluency course was one type of stimuli. But the coursework used as stimuli differed in duration and content, as well as the inclusion of direct exposure to people who stutter as an integral component of the educational program. The kind of education and exposure could have influenced the program's outcome in changing stereotypes. Leahy (1994) provided SLP students with intensive coursework, as well as direct exposure to people who stutter through therapy. Her educational program for the students specifically addressed the stuttering stereotype. Yet at the end of a year, no substantial change in attitudes was found. Worrisome was the fact that attitudes seemed to worsen. Also, training graduate SLP students using various modules like emotional intelligence skills or multicultural training did not improve overall attitudes toward people who stutter substantially compared to regular coursework (Junuzović-Žunić et al., Chapter 14; Reichel & St. Louis 2004, 2007).

Video-based instruction is appealing because, when well-planned and carefully edited, the videos can provide both factual and emotional information. They provide the important scientific benefit of maintaining the same treatment in varying groups of viewers (e.g., Flynn & St. Louis, 2011). Hence, several studies that sought to alter attitudes of participants toward people who stutter have used videos. The content of these videos have attempted to integrate both factual and emotional aspects of stuttering even though they have differed in length of presentation. McGee et al. (1996), Snyder (2001), and Mayo et al. (2008) showed their participants video footage about people who stutter, i.e., *Speaking of Courage* and *Voices to Remember* (Bondarenko, 1992a, 1992b). These professionally recorded and carefully edited videos have a powerful impact on most audiences (St. Louis, 1994). However, McGee et al. and Snyder found the documentaries to have little to no effect in sensitizing their participants to people who stutter. In fact, McGee et al. noted that the film appeared to reinforce rather than change stereotypes among high school students. On the other hand, Mayo et al. reported a significant change using the same tool (i.e., a documentary video). Both Snyder and Mayo et al. edited and shortened the original documentary, *Speaking of Courage* (Bondarenko, 1992a). Mayo et al. specifically indicated how they ensured the parts of the video selected for their study had an overall positive tone whereby the personality of the main character was portrayed as determined and outgoing. It is unclear whether the components used by Snyder are comparable to Mayo et al. However, one could speculate that these differences may partially explain why Mayo et al. found a positive change using the same original documentary while Snyder did not. Another study also found improvement in attitudes using a professionally designed video (Flynn & St. Louis, 2011). Gottwald et al. (2011, 2014) and Abdalla and St. Louis (2014) reported that a specially designed video presentation was effective in altering attitudes of American teachers (and professors) and Arab teacher trainees.

The stimuli alone cannot fully explain why participants across studies differed in their attitudinal changes given that videos were found to be effective by some investigators (e.g., Flynn & St. Louis, 2011; Gottwald et al., 2011, 2014; Mayo et al., 2008). While the type of stimuli used to change attitudes may partially explain the lack of consensus in changing attitudes of fluent speakers toward stuttering, the stimuli adopted in a study must be meaningful for the targeted population. For example, Abdalla and St. Louis (2014) interviewed a fluent teacher and students who stutter in their documentary video, which was geared toward changing stuttering attitudes in teachers in Kuwait. Success in changing attitudes of high school students reported by Flynn and St. Louis (2011) may be partly due to the students' ability to relate in age and empathy to the youth who stutters featured in their presentations. In contrast, mismatch in age between the adult speakers who stutter in the documentary, *Voices to Remember*, and the adolescent participants in McGee et al. (1996) may have contributed to why a change in the desired direction was not observed.

It is also crucial to preview and carefully screen the content of the stimuli to ensure that it does not reinforce rather than dispel the participants' pre-treatment negative stereotypes of people who stutter (McGee et al., 1996). Vignettes from the *Voices to Remember*, according to McGee et al. (1996), may have reinforced their participants' preexisting unfavorable perceptions of people who stutter. McGee et al. (1996, p. 245) cited two examples from *Voices to Remember*; the first was a clinician who said, "When a child can't communicate fluently, they tend to withdraw and sometimes they just can't get anything out and when they can't communicate, they can't show people their personality." The second is when a husband who stutters reveals to his spouse, "If you want it in a few words, I'm hiding behind other people, and I have for an awfully long time."

The differences in results can partially be accounted for by variation in information. In other words, the content of the stimuli can influence which post-ratings change. For example, Flynn and St. Louis (2011) found differences in type of changes depending on what was addressed in the video versus the oral presentation. Specifically, greater positive change emerged for employment-related items (e.g., "People who stutter can do any job they want") after viewing the video that showcased a stutterer's success in being hired as a bartender. On the other hand, more positive changes occurred in items pertaining to causes when the stutterer specifically delineated the etiology of stuttering during the oral presentation. Therefore, the absence of demonstrable changes following intervention may be dependent upon the information presented in the educational program itself and not the type of stimuli per se.

INSTRUMENTS TO MEASURE CHANGE. A variety of measures have been used to study a shift in participants' attitudes toward people who stutter. Semantic differential scales (Woods & Williams, 1976) have been widely used with conflicting outcomes. McGee et al. (1996) and Leahy (1994) reported no significant differences in the ratings of their participants, while Mayo et al. (2008) and Reichel and St. Louis (2004) indicated that seven to eight items on the modified semantic differential scale displayed a positive change in their students. Some researchers have questioned whether the semantic differential method is sufficiently sensitive for accurately measuring attitudes toward people who stutter (Healey, Gabel, Daniels, & Kawai, 2007). Flynn and St. Louis (2011) opine that the semantic differential scale may foster changes related to other uncontrolled independent variables; hence, it may be too sensitive in tapping the numerous changes implicated in viewing an entire video or interacting with people who stutter. Later, St. Louis, Williams, Ware, Guendouzi, and Reichel (2014) explored the validity of the semantic differential scale (Woods & Williams, 1976) and *POSHA–S* in measuring attitudes of 321 university students toward stuttering. Ratings of *POSHA–S* correlated with 77% of the semantic differential scale items, while the reverse correlation was true for only 45% of the *POSHA–S* ratings. The authors suggested that the two measures seem to suit different types of research. For example, *POSHA–S* appears to be more sensitive in detecting changes in attitudes in multicomponent public education campaigns. These methodological observations could partly explain the conflicting findings of these studies. Snyder (2001), on the other hand, used the *CATS*, an instrument that did not use bipolar adjectives like the previous studies and yet found no substantive modification in the attitudes of graduate SLP students. As Snyder (2001) pointed out, the lack of consistent findings could have been due to the measures themselves. This suggestion prompted some researchers to consider *POSHA–S* (St. Louis, 2005, 2011a) a more standardized instrument that has been specifically designed to measure public opinion. Indeed, several studies have shown it to be an effective means for measuring changes in post-treatment attitudes toward stuttering. Flynn and St. Louis (2011) found *POSHA–S* scores improved in adolescents; Gottwald et al. (2011, 2014) in teachers, professors, and students; and Junuzović-Žunić et al. (Chapter 14) in SLP students. Discrepancy between questionnaires versus open-ended questions emerged in some of the studies. Although changes were not substantial, students in Reichel and St. Louis (2007) and Leahy (1994) commented on the benefits of the educational program and the positive impact it had on them.

EXPERIMENTAL DESIGN, ANALYSES, AND INTERPRETATION. The experimental designs adopted by studies attempting to change attitudes toward stuttering vary widely. The majority of studies (e.g., Flynn & St. Louis, 2011; Gottwald et al., 2011, 2014; Junuzović-Žunić et al., Chapter 14; Mayo et al., 2008; McGee et al., 1996; Snyder, 2001; Reichel & St. Louis, 2007) used a pre-test-post-test design, which involved comparing the pre-test scores of a group of experimental participants to their scores following completion of an educational program. A subset of these studies was interested in contrasting results for two or more conditions. For instance, Snyder (2001) explored variations in two types of films (emotional versus factual), while Flynn and St. Louis (2011) focused on measuring differences in a live oral presentation, video presentation, and combined video and live oral presentation. An alternative to the pre-test-post-test design was a quasi-experimental randomized design adopted by Abdalla and St. Louis (2014) and, to some extent, by Delaney (2001) and Reichel and St. Louis (2004). This design involved the inclusion of a control group that was statistically comparable to the experimental group; however, the control group did not receive treatment even though they completed both the pre- and post-treatment measures.

Research to date has focused on short-term change in stuttering attitudes where only one post-test was administered either immediately after the treatment (Mayo et al., 2008), 72 hours later (Snyder, 2001), or one week later (Abdalla & St. Louis, 2014). Although a few studies that mainly used coursework (e.g., Junuzović-Žunić et al., Chapter 14; Leahy, 1994; Reichel & St. Louis, 2004, 2007) measured ratings after one semester or one year, there are no specific studies that have attempted to explore long-term change where the same post-test was readministered twice (immediately after treatment and again after a certain amount of time lapse like six months).

When surveying respondents, some studies controlled for differences in rating a typically fluent person versus a person who stutters. Some asked the participants to rate a hypothetical fluent person and a stutterer of both sexes before and after an educational program (e.g., Delaney, 2001), others had hypothetical cases of only male speakers (Leahy, 1994; McGee et al., 1996), and yet the majority did not provide the respondents with a specific reference case (e.g., Flynn & St. Louis, 2011; Junuzović-Žunić et al., Chapter 14; Mayo et al., 2008; Snyder, 2001). Incorporating as many as five hypothetical cases (a female who stutters and two adult and two eight-year-old males who are fluent or stutter), Delaney (2001) made it rather difficult to draw conclusions regarding the study's main purpose, which was to measure effectiveness of a treatment program in altering attitudes toward stuttering in general. Terminology used to label the hypothetical cases may sometimes introduce biases. For instance, McGee et al. (1996, p. 242) refer to their hypothetical case who does not stutter as a "typical normal high school male speaker." The use of "normal" instead of "fluent" may have introduced a bias in the listeners, causing them to attribute negative stereotypes to the person who stutters who, by analogy, was not normal.

Another source of difference pertains to the type of analyses conducted to measure effectiveness of the treatment programs. Some researchers have resorted to descriptive analyses (e.g., Leahy, 1994; Reichel & St. Louis, 2007); others used parametrical statistics like t-tests (Flynn & St. Louis, 2011; Gottwald et al., 2011, 2014; McGee et al., 1996; Reichel & St. Louis, 2004) and analysis of variance (Mayo et al., 2008). Yet others have opted for non-parametric tests such as Wilcoxon signed-ranks test (Delaney, 2001; Snyder, 2001), Chi-Square test of independence (Reichel & St. Louis, 2004), or the McNemar test (Abdalla & St. Louis, 2014). Such differences add to the difficulties involved in drawing comparisons across studies.

A distinction in how the data are interpreted is another source of variation among researchers. Reichel and St. Louis (2004) described *POSHA–S* and *EIS* trends as being in a positive direction even though statistical comparisons between the pre- and post-test responses were not significant. On the other hand, several others (e.g., Abdalla & St. Louis, 2014; Flynn & St. Louis, 2011; Snyder, 2001) focus only on comparative ratings that were statistically significant.

Conclusion and Future Considerations

The purpose of this review was to critically evaluate the current state of research that has attempted to change the attitudes of fluent individuals toward people who stutter. As well, this review was intended to provide an evidence base for designing and evaluating future attempts to prevent and amend negative stereotyping of people who stutter. Leahy (1994) indicated that a "well-directed propaganda about the nature of the stutterer stereotype, the possible effects of this on therapy, as well as emphasizing the individuality of the client presentation would reduce students' negative attitudes to 'the stutterer'" (p. 42). Indeed, we are well aware that when designing an educational program intended to reduce negative attitudes toward people who stutter, it is crucial that goals and subgoals of the program be clearly delineated. It seems rather difficult to expect the anticipated outcome for each type of goal using a single type of measurement (e.g., multiple-choice test).

It would be fruitful to begin any education program by first considering the implications of the questions posed in the attitude change section of this chapter. We need to look at exactly what we wish to change and develop measurable goals, e.g., "By the end of the video intervention program, the participant(s) will label x." Furthermore, it is critical to consider the stimuli chosen to change attitude and its content. For example, how will selecting the movie *The King's Speech* (a 2010 film that portrays King George VI's struggle with stuttering and the positive impact Lionel Logue, an Australian speech therapist, had on him) help participants achieve the examiner's predetermined objectives? The investigator should take into account whether the selected measurement is consistent, reliable, and designed to capture the predetermined objectives. It also seems worth revisiting the four key processes Leahy (1994) cites, based on McDavid and Harari (1974, p. 90), for how an intervention campaign can alter persistent attitudes: "1) arousal of the interest and attention of the audience to the attitudinal issue in question; 2) exposure of the audience to new information and ideas; 3) selected guidance of the audience's attention towards a certain range of information or ideas; and 4) crystallization of action related to the attitude in question."

More rigorous methods of data collection using a mixed-method design (quantitative and qualitative) will provide us with better information about how participants construe stuttering and help us in generating more appropriate educational campaigns that can induce positive attitudinal changes. Further research employing different types of interventions (e.g., direct contact coupled with information) is warranted before it will be clear which interventions have a stronger influence on changing attitudes.

Appendix A: Changing Attitudes Toward Stuttering: Summary of Findings in Peer-reviewed Journals

	Leahy (1994)	Snyder (2001)	McGee et al. (1996)	Flynn and St. Louis (2011)	Langevin and Prasad (2012)	Abdalla and St. Louis (2014)
Findings	Negative/No change/ Positive; stuttering stereotype (3/11 = 27%)	Emotional film: Minimal change (1/50 = 2%); Altered auditory feedback video (3/50 = 6%)	Pre: Negative (11/25 = 44%); Post: Negative (14/25 = 56%); Pre/post: no difference	Oral OSS: Pre = 19, Post = 44; Film OSS: Pre = 18, Post = 33; Film + Oral OSS: Post = 43	*PATCS* and *Provictim* total scores: Positive changes from pre to post; changes higher for children unfamiliar with stutterer and non-perpetrators	*POSHA-S* + added items: Pre = 11, Post = 24 for experimental pre-trainees (44% shift), but no change for in-service teachers
Analysis/ Design	Descriptive: Pre vs. post (control and experimental groups)	Inferential: Wilcoxon signed-ranks test; pre vs. post (two conditions)	Inferential: Paired t-test; pre vs. post	Inferential: Paired t-test; pre vs. post (three conditions)	Inferential: Paired t-test, ANOVA, Wilcoxon signed-ranks test, Kruskal-Wallis test; pre vs. post	Inferential: McNemar test; pre vs. post for control and experimental groups
Measurement	SDS Student report	CATS	SDS	POSHA-S + added items Student report	PATCS and *Provictim* scales	POSHA-S + added items
Stimuli	Fluency disorder course + clinical exposure	Film (*Speaking of Courage*); Video (*Altered Auditory Feedback*)	Film (*Voices to Remember*)	Film (*True Life*: I Stutter*); Live Oral by person who stuttered Oral + Film	Instruction and video (stuttering education and bullying prevention [TAB]); program delivered by teachers	Video (specially-designed video featuring three people who stutter [17 minutes])

Key: *CATS = Clinician Attitude Toward Stuttering, OSS = Overall Stuttering Score, PATCS = Peer Attitudes Toward Children Who Stutter, POSHA-S = Public Opinion Survey of Human Attributes–Stuttering, SDS = Semantic Differential Scale, SLP = speech-language pathologist, TAB = Teasing and Bullying: Unacceptable Behaviour program*

CONTINUED

Changing Attitudes Toward Stuttering: Summary of Findings in Peer-reviewed Journals
CONTINUED

	Leahy (1994)	Snyder (2001)	McGee et al. (1996)	Flynn and St. Louis (2011)	Langevin and Prasad (2012)	Abdalla and St. Louis (2014)
Participants	13 SLP students (third- and fourth-year undergrad)	55 SLP students (first-year grad)	36 high school students	83 high school students (33 males, 50 females)	608 third- to sixth-grade students (mean age = 9.7 years; 330 males, 278 females)	103 practicing teachers; 99 teacher trainees
Location	Ireland	United States	Canada	United States	Canada	Kuwait

Key: CATS = Clinician Attitude Toward Stuttering, OSS = Overall Stuttering Score, PATCS = Peer Attitudes Toward Children Who Stutter, POSHA–S = Public Opinion Survey of Human Attributes–Stuttering, SDS = Semantic Differential Scale, SLP = speech-language pathologist, TAB = Teasing and Bullying: Unacceptable Behaviour program

Appendix B: Changing Attitudes Toward Stuttering: Summary of Findings in Conference Papers

	Delaney (2001)	Reichel and St. Louis (2004, 2007)	Mayo et al. (2008)	Gottwald et al. (2011, 2014)	Hughes et al. (Chapter 15)	Coleman et al. (2013)	Junuzović-Žunić et al. (Chapter 14)
Findings	Some positive change; one subcategory SDS = n.s.	Mixed, modest for tests; student reports very positive	Positive (fairly to quite or neutral shifts) (8/25 = 32%)	Teachers' OSS: Pre = 39, Post = 52; Students' OSS: Pre = 25, Post = 5; SLPs' OSS: No change (ceiling effect); Professors' OSS: Pre = 36, Post = 47	Positive interdisciplinary collaboration (student SLPs and school counselors); participants provided suggestions for progress (e.g., clarify roles)	Positive changes in perceptions after the story; increase in objective responses, knowledge; improved attitudes; less listener avoidance	B & H OSS: Pre = 25, Post 1 = 33, Post 2 = 37; NYC OSS: Pre = 9, Post = 20; WV OSS: Pre 1 = 31, Pre 2 = 32, Post = 46
Analysis/ Design	Inferential: Wilcoxon; pre vs. post (control/exp.)	Inferential: t-test; Qualitative: Student report	Inferential: ANOVA; pre vs. post	Inferential: Paired t-test; pre vs. post	Qualitative: Pre vs. post	Descriptive: Pre vs. post	Inferential: Paired t-test; pre vs. two posts (B & H); pre vs. post (NYC); two pre vs. post (WV)
Measurement	SDS; ATS	Emotional Intelligence Scale (EIS); POSHA-E; student report	SDS	POSHA-S	Open-ended; pre and post-clinic survey; questions; reflection papers	Responses to nine questions	POSHA-S

Key: ATS = Attitude Toward Stuttering scale; B & H = Bosnia and Herzegovina, NYC = New York City, n.s = not significant, OSS = Overall Stuttering Score, POSHA-S = Public Opinion Survey of Human Attributes–Stuttering, SDS = Semantic Differential Scale, WV = West Virginia

CONTINUED

Appendix B: Changing Attitudes Toward Stuttering: Summary of Findings in Conference Papers
CONTINUED

	Delaney (2001)	Reichel and St. Louis (2004, 2007)	Mayo et al. (2008)	Gottwald et al. (2011, 2014)	Hughes et al. (Chapter 15)	Coleman et al. (2013)	Junuzović-Žunić et al. (Chapter 14)
Stimuli	Clinical exposure	Emotional intelligence module; fluency disorder course; clinical exposure	Film (Speaking of Courage)	Video (Specially designed 11-minute)	Presentation; observations and services for stutterers in intensive stuttering clinic	Story about character who stutters; video of 6-year-old boy who stutters	Fluency disorders coursework
Participants	18 SLP students (second-year undergrad)	77 SLP students (grad) (2004); 20 SLP students (grad) (2007)	43 students (undergrad) (15 males, 29 females)	10 teachers; 10 SLP students; 10 SLPs; 20 professors	8 SLP students (grad, all female); 8 school counseling students (grad; 2 males, 6 females)	4 fluent children (4-6 years)	B & H: 27 SLP students (senior undergrad); NYC: 86 SLP students (grad); WV: 13 SLP students (senior undergrad)
Location	UK	U.S.	U.S.	U.S.	U.S.	U.S.	Bosnia and Herzegovina; U.S.

Key: ATS = Attitude Toward Stuttering scale; B & H = Bosnia and Herzegovina, NYC = New York City, n.s = not significant, OSS = Overall Stuttering Score, POSHA–S = Public Opinion Survey of Human Attributes–Stuttering, SDS = Semantic Differential Scale, WV = West Virginia

Part Two

RESEARCH: ATTITUDES OF THE NON-STUTTERING PUBLIC

Chapter 6

_____

American Indian Perceptions of Stuttering

Ann M. Beste-Guldborg, Kenneth O. St. Louis, Nichole Campanale

ABSTRACT

Negative attitudes toward stuttering are widespread across the world, yet little is known about American Indian attitudes toward the disorder. This study examines perceptions of stuttering in 1,572 American Indians from 95 tribal entities across four regions of the United States, using the *Public Opinion Survey of Human Attributes–Stuttering (POSHA–S)*, a valid and reliable instrument to measure stuttering attitudes. Results indicated moderately positive beliefs about stuttering and neutral to moderately negative reactions to the disorder. Overall Stuttering Scores parallel the *POSHA–S* database median value for samples, but with significant differences between groups on various subscores and component scores.

Introduction

Stuttering Attitudes and Stigma

Stuttering is known to exist across the world (Cooper & Cooper, 1996) with negative attitudes toward people who stutter well documented and widespread (Abdalla & St. Louis, 2012; Al-Khaledi, Lincoln, McCabe, Packman, & Alshatti, 2009; de Britto Pereira, Rossi, & Van Borsel, 2008; Doody, Kalinowski, Armson, & Stuart, 1993; Ip, St. Louis, Myers, & An Xue, 2012; Özdemir, St. Louis, & Topbaş, 2011b; St. Louis & Roberts, 2010). Traits associated with people who stutter include anxiousness, shyness, nervousness, emotional maladjustment, introversion, unassertiveness, and incompetency (Boyle, Blood, & Blood, 2009; Craig, Tran, & Craig, 2003; Gabel, 2006; Klassen, 2001; Woods & Williams, 1976; Yairi & Williams, 1970), and listeners commonly hold that stuttering is of psychological origin (Bloodstein & Berstein Ratner, 2008). Collectively these beliefs form the "stuttering stereotype," a common misconception among the populace (Blood, 1999; Boyle et al., 2009; Cooper & Cooper, 1985; Ham, 1990).

Family, Culture, and Stuttering Attitudes

Johnson (1961) advanced the belief that family views can impact one's stuttering. Though much of his early work was refuted, his perspectives regarding family attitudes toward stuttering are still widely accepted. Some attitudes are passed down generationally, without question (Bengston, Biblarz, & Roberts, 2002), and evidence suggests attitudes toward stuttering form similarly in early childhood, often without personal experience (Blood, 1999; Bloodstein, 1995; Guitar, 2005; Shapiro, 1999; Sheehan, 1970; Van Riper, 1971).

Johnson (1944) also theorized that cultural values influence stuttering. Twenty years ago, Bebout and Arthur (1992) reported significant differences in cross-cultural attitudes toward speech disorders, and today there is evidence that beliefs about the cause, nature, and treatment of stuttering may be culturally specific (Abdalla & St. Louis, 2012; de Britto Pereira et al., 2008; Özdemir et al., 2011b; Robinson & Crowe, 2002; Xing Ming, Jing, Yi Wen, & Van Borsel, 2001).

American Indians and Stuttering

Early reports suggested stuttering did not occur in American Indians (Johnson, 1944; Snidecor, 1947; Stewart, 1960). Since some evidence was advanced that Indian vernacular did not include a word for stuttering, Johnson (1944) premised that stuttering did not exist. He and others pointed to permissive child-rearing practices and tolerant attitudes toward language development as explanation for this reputed lack of stuttering (Snidecor, 1947; Stewart, 1960; Johnson, 1944). These ideas held until field evidence showed reference to stuttering in various American Indian tribal vernaculars (Lemert, 1953; Miller, 1972). In particular, evidence emerged of stuttering among the Bannock-Shoshoni people (Zimmerman, Liljeblad, Frank, & Cleeland, 1983), a tribe that Stewart (1960) considered "nonstuttering." Indications were that stuttering was not only present but also stigmatized and ridiculed (Zimmerman, Liljebald, Frank, & Cleeland, 1983).

American Indian Culture and Attitudes Toward Disability

Traditional American Indian culture is rooted in respect for the tribe and its people (Garrett & Garrett, 1996; Pewewardy, 2002) and is manifest in both commonalities and diversity among tribes (Garrett & Myers, 1996; Garrett & Pichette, 2000; Hodgkinson, 1990; Keltner, Crowell, & Taylor, 2005). Cultural distinctions occur because of tribal history and tradition, geographic location, familial influence, and level of acculturation to mainstream values and beliefs (Garrett & Garrett, 1994; LaFromboise, 1998; Turnbull, Brotherson, & Summers, 1985).

Evidence is conflicted about contemporary American Indian views toward disability (Joe & Miller, 1987; Keltner et al., 2005; Pengra & Godfrey, 2001). Cultural themes like collectivity and harmony suggest positive attitudes, adjustment, and inclusion of people regardless of ability (Keltner et al., 2005). Similarly, Clay (1992) indicates the value of relationships and cultural precepts of respect, dignity, and reciprocity overshadow the idea that a disability needs to be fixed and instead promote acceptance as is. Others (Joe & Miller, 1987; Pengra & Godfrey, 2001) suggest American Indians are reluctant to define and perceive a person as disabled.

In contrast, there are indications that some American Indians define disability from a mainstream medical model or as something to be fixed or reduced, as well as from a functional perspective placing emphasis on performance within society (Keltner et al., 2005; Lomay & Hinkebien, 2006; National Council on Disability, 2003). The reality is many American Indians are bicultural and have learned to combine traditional with mainstream views. Nonetheless, traditional culture remains important in the perception of individuals with disabilities (Garrett & Pichette, 2000; Joe & Miller, 1987; LaFromboise, 1998).

Culturally Appropriate Services

Speech-language pathologists are encouraged to provide culturally relevant services, responding to people within the context of their cultural backgrounds (American Speech-Language-Hearing Association, 2014a). The American mainstream interpretation of disability is that something is wrong and should be fixed (Murugami, 2009), whereas some American Indians accept disability as a part of "what is" and not as something "broken" (Joe & Miller, 1987; Pengra & Godfrey, 2001). Culturally appropriate service delivery to American Indians requires an understanding of not only individual views but also traditional cultural values, including attitudes and beliefs toward stuttering (Murugami, 2009; National Council on Disability, 2003; O'Connell, 1985).

Need for Study

There is an emergence of literature examining the beliefs of Indigenous peoples across the world toward stuttering (Bebout & Arthur, 1992; de Britto et al., 2008; St. Louis, 2008; St. Louis, Filatova, Coşkun, Topbaş, Özdemir,

Georgieva, McCaffrey, & George, 2011). Evidence suggests that negative attitudes exist across cultures and geographic locations; however, perceptions may be culturally specific (Abdalla & St. Louis, 2012; Özdemir et al., 2011b; Tellis, Blood, Blood, Lubker, St. Louis, Yaruss, Pill et al., 2000). There are few published studies examining American Indian perceptions of stuttering (e.g., St. Louis, Przepiórka, Beste-Guldborg, Williams, Błachnio, Guendouzi, Reichel, & Ware, 2014). The purpose of this study was to examine the perceptions of American Indians toward stuttering and to determine differences among tribal groupings.

Method

Survey Instrument

The *Public Opinion Survey on Human Attributes–Stuttering (POSHA–S)* is an established, internally consistent, reliable, and valid measure used to examine perceptions of stuttering worldwide (St. Louis, 2005, 2008, 2009, 2011a, 2012c; St. Louis, Lubker, Yaruss, Adkins, & Pill 2008; Özdemir, St. Louis, & Topbaş, 2011a; St. Louis, Reichel, Yaruss, & Lubker; 2009). For this study it was adapted minimally according to instrument guidelines by a group of American Indian professionals familiar with disability.

PARTICIPANTS, DATA COLLECTION, AND ANALYSIS. Participants were self-proclaimed American Indians with tribal affiliations recognized as Northern Plains, Eastern, Southwest, and Northwest as determined by the *Tribal Directory of Indians* at the Web site, indians.org. After approval was obtained, respondents were recruited from published e-mail addresses of various tribal organizations in each region and sent an e-mail link to the survey. Participation was voluntary and respondents were asked to pass the survey link on to others as desired. A total of 1,572 self-identified American Indian adults, representing people from 95 tribal entities across 36 states, took part in the study.

Data were converted to a -100 to +100 scale (0 = neutral) and analyzed using standard *POSHA–S* scoring guidelines (St. Louis, 2011a). Responses were calculated, clustered, and averaged into component scores and subscores, two reflecting stuttering and one relating to other negative human attributes (i.e., mental illness and obesity). Both stuttering subscores were combined to determine an Overall Stuttering Score. In addition, t-test comparisons with Bonferroni correction $p \leq .00417$ were calculated to determine significant pairwise differences.

Results

Respondent Characteristics

Table 6.1 summarizes *POSHA–S* demographic information for the sample and by tribal grouping. The mean age of respondents was 38 years with a range of 18 to 75 years. The majority were females (70%), married (70%), parents (76%), and working or attending college as students (94%). The mean number of years of education was 13.3. Very few of the participants reported themselves as a person who stutters or who is mentally ill, but one-quarter of the sample reported themselves as obese. Most described incomes (-27) were well below the *POSHA–S* average for samples, which was close to 0. Nearly a third (31%) did not know a person who stutters, a higher percentage than for the other four human attributes measured.

Stuttering Attitudes in American Indians

Figure 6.1 represents converted mean *POSHA–S* component scores, subscores, and Overall Stuttering Scores (OSS) for the sample and the tribal groupings. Points closer to the periphery imply positive attitudes, while those closer to the center are negative (St. Louis, 2011a). American Indian perceptions of stuttering and people who stutter, as evidenced by an Overall Stuttering Score of 20, were similar to people across the world as the median Overall Stuttering Score i.e., 17, from 222 *POSHA–S* database samples obtained from 36 countries around the world. Beliefs about people who stutter were positive (BEL = +42) while reactions to stuttering were more negative (SR = -3), a profile seen in nearly all *POSHA–S* archive studies (St. Louis, 2011a). Respondents showed strong belief in the potential of people who stutter (+70), as well as sound understanding of who could/should help (+50) and how to help (+35). There was solid conviction that an SLP should be involved in treatment (+94). When asked if a traditional spiritual leader should assist in the treatment of stuttering, a question specific to this study, respondents were neutral (-8). A belief in the stuttering stereotype was evidenced by negative scores on variables representing people who stutter as "nervous/excitable" (-12) and "shy/fearful" (-8). Respondents reacted strongly when asked if they would want to be a person who stutters (-82), and reported a lack of knowledge (-25) and little personal experience with stuttering (+10). Respondents were unclear of knowledge sources for stuttering (-3), but reported receiving information most often from specialists (+26), visual media (+6), and school (0). Table 6.2 specifies numerical values for the sample as a whole and the various tribal groupings.

Table 6.1. Demographic Characteristics of Four Tribal Regions

Demographic Variable	All American Indians	Northern Plains	Eastern	Southwest	Northwest
Number	1,572	639	205	395	333
Age: Mean (year)	38.3	34.1	40.8	47.3	33.8
Total schooling: Mean (year)	13.3	13.1	13.4	13.8	12.8
Sex: Males (% total)	30%	34%	30%	26%	26%
Sex: Females (% total)	70%	66%	70%	74%	74%
Married (% of total)	70%	63%	66%	86%	68%
Parent (% of total)	76%	72%	69%	84%	77%
Student (% of total)	21%	26%	11%	9%	29%
Working (% of total)	73%	65%	85%	87%	67%
Relative income (-100 to +100)	-27	-27	-6	-43	-21
Self-identification (% total)					
Stuttering	1%	1%	2%	<1%	<1%
Mentally ill	1%	1%	<1%	1%	1%
Obese	25%	16%	13%	20%	56%
Left-handed	9%	10%	12%	9%	8%
Intelligent	72%	68%	77%	71%	77%
No persons known who (are) (% total)					
Stuttering	31%	37%	33%	25%	27%
Mentally ill	20%	19%	23%	22%	16%
Obese	7%	5%	4%	6%	11%
Left-handed	13%	11%	17%	12%	15%
Intelligent	1%	1%	1%	<1%	0%
Self-rating of health and abilities (-100 to +100)					
Physical health	40	34	67	34	44
Mental health	51	48	69	44	51
Ability to learn	62	62	71	60	59
Speaking ability	52	52	66	51	44
Self-rating of life priorities (-100 to +100)					
Be safe/secure	75	74	81	77	71
Be free	59	63	70	64	38
Spend time alone	23	18	56	16	17
Attend social events	-6	-6	25	-25	-2
Imagine new things	27	25	63	12	28
Help less fortunate	52	50	71	44	53

CONTINUED

Table 6.1. Demographic Characteristics of Four Tribal Regions *CONTINUED*

Demographic Variable	All American Indians	Northern Plains	Eastern	Southwest	Northwest
Have exciting experiences	-45	-52	-24	-58	-32
Practice my religion	16	8	37	11	22
Earn money	58	62	67	52	53
Do job/duty	72	74	78	68	68
Get things done	73	78	78	71	65
Solve big problems	58	61	71	57	48
Completion time: Mean (minutes)	8.0	7.5	8.9	8.0	8.3

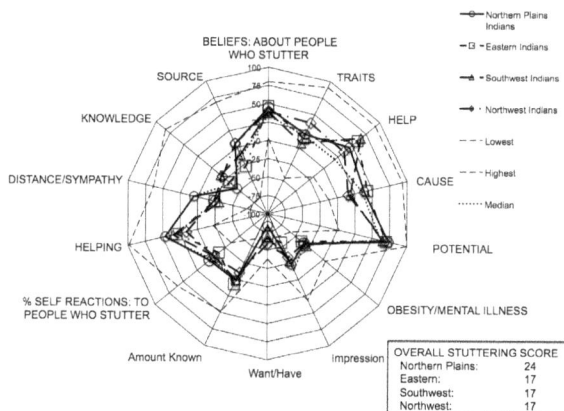

Figure 6.1: Summary *POSHA–S* graph for Native American tribal groupings showing component scores, subscores, and Overall Stuttering Scores in relation to the highest, lowest, and median sample means from the *POSHA–S* database.

Stuttering Attitudes Among Groups

Although Overall Stuttering Scores, Belief subscores, and Self Reaction subscores were reasonably similar, pair-wise *t*-test comparisons using the Bonferroni correction (p ≤ .00417) revealed significant differences among the tribal groups with percentages significant ranging from 43% between the Northern Plains and Eastern groups to 67% between the Northern Plains and Southwest and Northern Plains and Northwest groups. Cohen's *d* effect size was calculated

Table 6.2. Mean Ratings for All Respondents and Four Tribal Regions for *POSHA–S Overall Stuttering Scores*, Subscores, Components, and Items. Pair-Wise Statistically Significant Differences (p ≤ .00417) are Shown at the Right by Asterisks (*)

POSHA–S Variable	All Amer. Indians	Northern Plains	Eastern	Southwest	Northwest	Plains vs. Eastern	Plains vs. SW	Plains vs. NW	Eastern vs. SW	Eastern vs. NW	SW vs. NW
OVERALL STUTTERING SCORE	*20*	*24*	*17*	*17*	*17*	*	*	*			
Beliefs About People Who Stutter	*42*	*44*	*47*	*39*	*39*		*	*	*	*	
Traits/Personality	20	20	14	7	37		*	*		*	*
Have themselves to blame[a]	79	83	82	61	89		*		*		*
Nervous or excitable[a]	-12	-9	-10	-28	1	*					*
Shy or fearful[a]	-8	-14	-30	-13	22			*		*	*
Stuttering Should Be Helped by:	50	45	60	66	35	*	*	*		*	*
Speech and language therapist	94	89	94	99	98		*	*	*		
Other people who stutter	30	22	33	49	22		*				*
Medical doctor[a]	26	25	51	49	-13	*	*	*		*	*
Spiritual leader[b]	-8	-2	-15	-10	-12						
Stuttering Is Caused by:	29	38	43	18	15	*	*	*	*		
Genetic inheritance	10	17	18	5	-2		*				
Learning or habits[a]	-7	-8	7	-6	-15						
A very frightening event[a]	15	23	34	-11	17	*			*		*
An act of God[a]	60	75	84	67	8		*	*	*	*	
A virus or disease[a]	23	40	25	9	4	*	*				
Ghosts, demons, spirits[a]	73	81	90	45	81	*			*		*
Potential	70	74	70	65	69	*					
Can make friends	92	93	90	92	94						
Can lead normal lives	79	83	79	79	70			*			
Can do any job they want	59	64	44	58	60	*					
Should have jobs requiring good judgment	50	56	67	31	51		*		*		*
Self Reactions to People Who Stutter	*-3*	*3*	*-13*	*-6*	*-5*	*	*	*	*	*	
Accommodating/Helping	35	46	30	35	16	*	*	*		*	*
Try to act like the person was talking normally	59	77	59	37	51	*	*	*	*		
Person like me	-37	-25	-71	-2	-83	*	*	*	*		*
Fill in the person's words[a]	33	56	36	50	-36	*		*		*	*
Tell the person to "slow down" or "relax"[a]	-3	17	-5	-27	-10	*	*	*	*		
Make joke about stuttering[a]	81	76	93	73	97	*		*	*		*
Should try to hide their stuttering[a]	78	62	74	98	74		*		*		*

CONTINUED

Table 6.2 *continued*: Mean Ratings for All Respondents and Four Tribal Regions for *POSHA–S Overall Stuttering Scores*, Subscores, Components, and Items. Pair-Wise Statistically Significant Differences (p ≤ .00417) are Shown at the Right by Asterisks (*).

POSHA–S Variable	All Amer. Indians	Northern Plains	Eastern	Southwest	Northwest	Plains vs. Eastern	Plains vs. SW	Plains vs. NW	Eastern vs. SW	Eastern vs. NW	SW vs. NW
Social Distance/Sympathy	-14	5	-24	-31	-23	*	*	*			*
Feel comfortable or relaxed	12	27	-3	12	-9	*		*			*
Feel pity[a]	26	46	22	5	17	*	*	*			
Feel impatient (not want to wait while the person stutters)[a]	36	65	-1	27	12	*	*	*	*		
Concern about my doctor[a]	14	21	9	-2	21		*				*
Concern about my neighbor[a]	13	43	-19	-25	23	*	*	*		*	*
Concern about my brother or sister[a]	-54	-15	-62	-93	-78	*	*	*	*	*	*
Concern about me[a]	-78	-54	-79	-99	-98	*	*	*	*	*	
Impression of person with stuttering	-10	-9	-13	-8	-11						
Want to have stuttering	-82	-76	-71	-96	-84		*	*	*	*	*
Knowledge/Experience	-30	-45	-31	-16	-19	*	*	*	*	*	
Amount known about stuttering	-25	-30	-31	-18	-22		*				
People with stuttering known	-76	-82	-72	-75	-71	*	*	*			
Personal experience (me, my family, friends)	10	-25	9	44	35	*	*	*	*	*	
Knowledge Source	-3	6	-28	-11	6	*	*		*	*	*
Television, radio, films	6	32	-19	-33	16	*	*			*	*
Magazines, newspapers, books	-19	-10	-48	-29	-8	*	*			*	
Internet	-25	-31	-45	-33	6			*		*	*
School	0	-14	2	15	9			*	*		
Doctors, nurses, other specialists	26	54	-32	26	8	*	*	*	*	*	
Obesity/Mental Illness	-34	-35	-39	-32	-34				*		
Overall Impression	-31	-23	-56	-28	-34	*		*	*	*	
Obesity	-23	-22	-51	-15	-17	*			*	*	
Mental illness	-39	-24	-60	-41	-50	*	*	*	*		
Want to Have	-72	-83	-69	-68	-58	*	*	*			*
Obesity	-65	-79	-66	-55	-50	*	*	*		*	
Mental illness	-79	-87	-71	-81	-67	*		*			*
Amount Known about	0	2	7	1	-10		*		*	*	
Obesity	4	6	8	11	-9		*		*	*	
Mental illness	-5	-2	6	-9	-11				*		

[a] The signs of the mean ratings for this item are reversed so that higher scores reflect "better" attitudes and lower scores "worse" attitudes.
[b] Added item not included in a component or subscore of the *POSHA–S*.

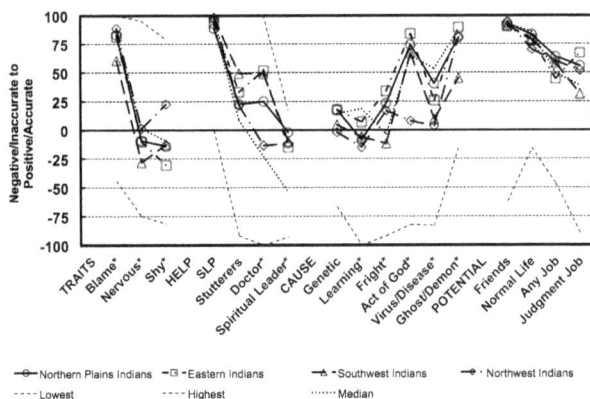

Figure 6.2: Mean item and component scores contributing to the *POSHA–S* Beliefs subscore for American Indian tribal groupings in relation to the highest, lowest, and median sample means from the *POSHA–S* database.

for those comparisons with significant findings. The mean *d* for this sample was .478 indicating a moderate average effect size (range .044 = 1.191). (It should be noted that the large percentages of significant differences were heavily influenced by the large sample sizes.) Northern Plains Indians had a significantly higher Overall Stuttering Score (+24) followed by all three other tribal groupings (+17).

Figure 6.2 lists items and components contributing to the Belief subscore. Although all groups showed positive beliefs about stuttering, Eastern (+47) and Northern Plains (+44) Indians reported significantly higher scores. All groups believed strongly in the potential of people who stutter with little significant difference among them. There was robust belief that people who stutter could make friends and lead normal lives and moderate to strong certainty that they could hold any job, including those requiring good judgment.

Southwest Indians understood most accurately who could help (+66) with solid consensus among all groups that a speech-language pathologist should be consulted. While all groups showed general neutrality or slight negativity in not rejecting the use of a spiritual leader in treatment, respondents were much more likely to reject the idea that a higher power or spirit may influence the presence or absence of stuttering. Southwest and Northwest Indians rated these variables siginifcantly different than the other groups. Eastern respondents reported the most accurate understanding of cause (+43) and were least likely to consult a spiritual leader (-15).

Evidence of the stuttering stereotype, as noted by negative scores on trait

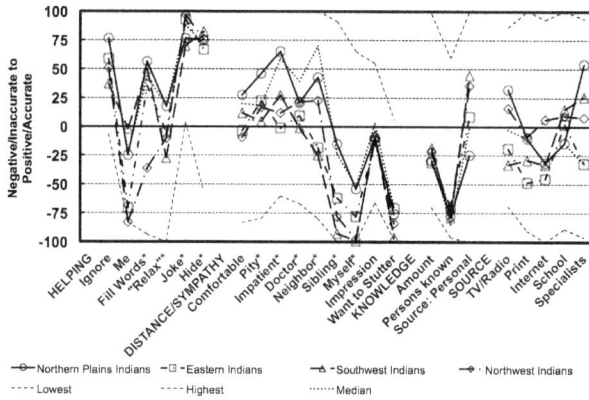

Figure 6.3: Mean item and component scores contributing to the *POSHA–S* Self Reactions subscore for American Indian tribal groupings in relation to the highest, lowest, and median sample means from the *POSHA–S* database.

variables related to nervousness/excitability and shyness/fearfulness, emerged in all groups and was significantly strongest in Southwest (nervous/excitable = -28) and Eastern Indians (shy/fearful = -30). Trait and personality scores were generally positive for all groups, with Northwest and Northern Plains Indians rating personality significantly higher than the others.

Figure 6.3 lists variables combined to derive the Self Reactions subscore. All groups showed slightly negative to neutral reactions to stuttering with significant differences between all but Northwest and Southwest Indians. Help scores were moderate to strong, indicating a general knowledge of appropriate interactions and assistance among all groups; however, significant differences were evident in many of the variables.

Northern Plains Indians understood best how to help (+46), and felt most at ease with the disorder (+5). All other groups had significantly lower social distance/sympathy scores. A robust sense of discomfort was revealed among all groups when asked if they would want to stutter, with Southwest Indians showing the strongest reaction (-96). General impressions of people who stutter were neutral to slightly negative in all groups with no significant differences evident.

All groups reported little knowledge or experience with stuttering, with Northern Plains Indians indicating the least knowledge (-45) and experience (-25). Interestingly, this group was most likely to gain information about the disorder from a specialist (+54). Southwest Indians reported significantly more personal experience with stuttering and were likely to gain information from specialists (+26) and school (+15). Both Northern Plains (+77) and Southwest Indians (+70) were somewhat but significantly more likely than others to make a joke about stuttering.

Discussion

Negative attitudes toward stuttering are widespread (Cooper & Cooper, 1996; de Britto Pereira et al., 2008; Ip et al., 2012; Özdemir et al., 2011b; St. Louis & Roberts, 2010), although much of the research has focused on people from Westernized cultures (Abdalla & St. Louis, 2012; Allard & Williams, 2008). There is an international movement to understand attitudes toward stuttering from a worldwide perspective (St. Louis, 2005, 2011b) with the goal to diminish the social stigma associated with stuttering and improve treatment practices. This study provides insight into American Indian perceptions of stuttering both as a whole and from a regional perspective.

The evidence that traditional American Indians are more accepting of disability and view it as something that "is" rather than something to be "fixed" is mixed (Clay, 1992; Joe & Miller, 1987; Keltner et al., 2005; Lomay & Hinkebein, 2006; Pengra & Godfrey, 2001). This study did not support the traditional premise. Results revealed that perceptions toward stuttering of American Indians from four regions and more than 95 tribal entities, though different from each other among the variables, were not remarkably different from the worldwide population database median (St. Louis, 2011a). Like most samples, American Indians in this study held moderately positive beliefs about people who stutter, neutral to slightly negative self reactions toward stuttering, and somewhat positive overall perceptions about the disorder. Findings may represent an acculturated rather than traditional view of disability as postulated in Garrett and Pichette (2000) and Turnbull et al. (1985).

Selected findings bear discussion. It was interesting that three of the four groups had very similar overall stuttering scores, yet very mixed subscores and component scores, many of which were significantly different. This finding could suggest subtle tribal or regional influence and should be explored further. Two of the tribal groups reported, with greater propensity than the median value for 222 *POSHA–S* sample means analyzed, that they would joke about stuttering. Humor is a generally acceptable part of daily life in Indian culture (Garrett, 1996). The use of jokes and "teasing" is common, and laughter is used to relieve stress and create an atmosphere of sharing and connectedness (Garrett & Garrett, 1994; Herring, 1994). It has been shown that Indians use humor to dissipate tension in difficult situations (Deloria, 1988). Finally, it is interesting that while the use of spiritual leaders to treat stuttering was neutral, findings suggested a belief that other powers play a causal role. This is not surprising as, while there is heterogeneity of American Indian cultures, spirituality is considered an essential dimension (Brant, 1990).

Several cautions are in order. First, because of the convenience/snowball sampling procedures, a representative sample of American Indians may not have been secured for this study. Also, the sampling technique may have influenced results in another way by attracting individuals compelled to respond based on their interest in or closeness to the topic of stuttering. Finally, knowledge of one culture does not necessarily generalize to an understanding of closely related cultures (Pengra & Godfrey, 2001), and one tribal culture is no more or less representative of all American Indian cultures (Kramer, 1996). Complete understanding of another culture is never possible because perceptions are always filtered through one's own cultural perspectives and experiences (Fish, 2000; Selig, 1998). Bearing this, findings should be interpreted carefully.

Chapter 7

Sudanese Perceptions, Attitudes, and Knowledge of Stuttering

Yomna Elsiddig, Charles Haynes, Julie Atwood, Kenneth O. St. Louis

ABSTRACT

Sudan is a large nation in eastern North Africa with a rich Afro-Arab tradition. Due to many factors, speech and language services are limited in scope and resources. Although social environments do not cause stuttering, they influence how stuttering is experienced, how it develops, and how it affects people's lives. This project employed an adapted version of the *Public Opinion Survey of Human Attributes–Stuttering (POSHA–S)* with 108 native respondents to explore Sudanese public beliefs, attitudes, and knowledge of stuttering. Public opinion results indicated a marginally positive view of stuttering relative to other attributes, but also the presence of negative personality stereotypes in over half of respondents. The study suggests the need for the dissemination of current scientific knowledge and education about stuttering in Sudan.

Introduction

Stuttering has been identified universally in people of all cultural backgrounds and referenced throughout history (Guitar, 2013). Though social environments do not cause stuttering, they impact the way it develops and how it affects people's lives. The attitudes of clients, their families, and communities are critical to the therapeutic process (Bebout & Arthur, 1992). Several studies have explored perceptions and beliefs regarding stuttering within the United States as well as within other countries and have revealed stigmatizing perceptions and negative stereotypes that are present across cultures (Doody, Kalinowski, Armson, Stuart, 1993; Gabel, 2006; St. Louis, 2005, Chapter 1).

Sudan, a large nation in the eastern part of North Africa, is home to 30 million people, five million of whom live in the capital city of Khartoum (Central Intelligence Agency, 2014). The cultural fabric is composed of both Arab and African traditions, creating an Islamically faith-based, yet superstitious, society. Sudan has attempted to address issues of disability since the government passed the Act on Welfare and Rehabilitation of Disabled Persons in 1984. However, the law's full-scale implementation has yet to be established due to many problems, including "emotional, social, and financial difficulties" (World Health Organization, 2012).

The field of speech-language pathology is relatively new in Sudan, with most developments happening within the past 10 years. In 2013, there were no undergraduate or graduate programs in speech-language pathology in Sudan and in order to study in this area or pursue licensure or certification, students had to leave the country. Therefore, most clinicians who offer speech and language services in Sudan have degrees in early childhood development and/or clinical psychology. Currently, there are 28 public and private clinics that offer speech and language services, and only one, the Sudanese Stuttering Organization, is dedicated solely to the support and services of people who stutter (Government of Sudan, Ministry of Social Development, 2013).

The International Project on Attitudes Toward Human Attributes (IPATHA) was launched in 1999 as an initiative to explore public attitudes toward stuttering in different nations. The *Public Opinion Survey of Human Attributes—Stuttering* (*POSHA–S*) was created and by September, 2013, had been used in over 30 countries (St. Louis, 2005). Two recent studies conducted in the Middle Eastern country of Kuwait using the *POSHA–S* determined that Arab parents and teachers showed limited knowledge regarding the prevalence of stuttering and the extent to which it occurs across races. Many respondents believed that stuttering could be cured, but also judged that a speech-language pathologist (SLP) would be the professional to treat stuttering. However, over 80% of respondents believed that stuttering is caused by psychological or emotional factors, and 66% believed that stuttering is an act of God (Allah). These were among the first findings regarding perceptions and attitudes toward stuttering among Arab and Muslim nations and set up a basis for studying other cultures with a similar religious and cultural fabric, like Sudan (Abdalla & St. Louis, 2012; Al-Khaledi, Lincoln, McCabe, Packman, & Alshatti, 2009).

Purpose

While recent studies have begun to expand and analyze other cultures' beliefs about stuttering, nothing is known about the Sudanese population regarding these views. The general question driving the research was: What are Sudanese knowledge, beliefs, and attitudes toward stuttering? Additional specific hypotheses accorded special focus in this study were (1) that Sudanese will perceive negative personality stereotypes of people who stutter as being "nervous, shy, or fearful"; (2) that the societal belief will be that stuttering is caused by "an act of God (Allah)" and by "ghosts, spirits, and demons"; and (3) that an imam (religious leader) and a medical doctor will more often be seen as sources of help for people who stutter than will the SLP.

Methods

The *POSHA–S* was translated into Modern Standard Arabic for the two studies conducted in Kuwait, making it also applicable for the Arabic-speaking majority of Sudan. The first page of this survey collects demographic information, including age, gender, birthplace, income, education, religion, and marital status. The remaining pages contain the questionnaire. Questions on the *POSHA–S* pertain to (1) the overall impression of a person with a specific attribute, (2) how the respondent would feel if he/she had the attribute, (3) the amount of knowledge the respondent has about the attribute, and (4) the type of action taken if the respondent were talking to a person with the attribute.

The *POSHA–S* survey participants were recruited over a four-week period through convenience sampling from four different locales. After obtaining official human subjects clearance, the first author approached potential participants and described the questionnaire as an anonymous public opinion survey on human attributes. The location distribution was as follows: 75 respondents from Khartoum's main public park (Al-Saha Al-Khadra), 25 respondents from residents of the first author's family's neighborhood (Arkaweet neighborhood), 10 respondents from the University of Khartoum, and five respondents from local shop owners (Al-Balabil and Al-Taif neighborhoods). The researcher provided adequate time (~25 minutes) for survey completion and clarification, as well as gave additional time when needed. A total of 115 questionnaires were distributed, with a total return of 108 (94% response rate). Table 7.1 provides characteristics of the survey respondents.

POSHA–S survey data were analyzed with general descriptive statistics, including frequency distribution cross-tabulations. Chi-Square ($X2$) tests were

Table 7.1. Demographic Data for *POSHA–S* Respondents

VARIABLE	
Number in sample	108
Mean age in years	30.0 (range 12–63 years)
Gender, *n* (%)	
Males	57 (54.3%)
Females	48 (45.7%)
Education, *n* (%)	
High school diploma or less	27 (26.0%)
Bachelor's degree	63 (60.6%)
Postgraduate degree	14 (13.5%)
Marital Status (married), *n* (%)	38 (40.9%)
Work Situation, *n* (%)	
Student	31 (31.0%)
Working	56 (55.0%)
Not working	15 (14.7%)
Know friend/relative who stutters (yes), *n* (%)	27 (25.0%)

used to explore relationships between education and attitudes, knowledge, and beliefs about stuttering. For the current study, only questions and items related to the specific hypotheses were analyzed.

Results

It was hypothesized that Sudanese people would perceive negative personality stereotypes of people who stutter as nervous, shy, or fearful. These stereotypes about people who stutter were reported by slightly over half of participants. More than half agreed that people who stutter are shy and fearful (no = 32.7%, plus not sure = 10.6%), and 53.4% agreed that the people who stutter are nervous and excitable (no = 34%, not sure = 12.6%). At the same time, participants conveyed many positive perceptions of stuttering people: All respondents believed people who stutter can make friends, 89.3% believed they can do any job they want, and almost all respondents, 97.0%, agreed that people who stutter can lead normal lives. Moreover, 90.4% of participants did not believe that people who stutter have themselves to blame for their stuttering.

In some sections of the *POSHA–S*, stuttering is placed among four other attributes for comparative purposes and to control for response bias. Figure

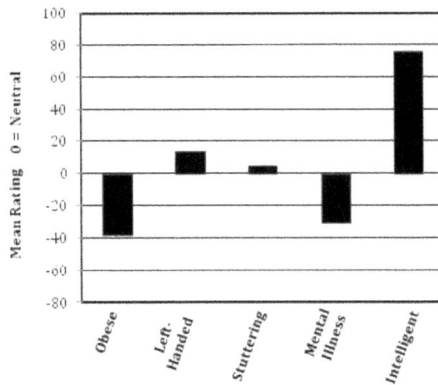

Figure 7.1: Mean rating scores of respondents' overall impressions of five attributes converted to a -100 to 100 scale, 0 = neutral.

7.1 demonstrates the mean scores (converted to a scale of -100 to +100, 0 being neutral) of all respondents to the statement "My overall impression of a person who is . . ." Of the five attributes, "Intelligent" received the most positive impression at 76 and "Obese" received the most negative score at -38. "Stuttering" received a marginally positive score of 5, higher than "Mentally ill" (M = -31), but lower than "Left-Handed" (M = 14).

Mean scores and converted ratings for "The amount I know about people who are . . ." indicate that "Stuttering" was the attribute respondents knew the least about, receiving a mean rating of -21. Respondents knew the most about people who are "Intelligent," with a mean rating of 46. Knowledge of people who are "Left-Handed" showed a mean score of 7, or higher than "Mentally ill" but lower than "Obese." Figure 7.2 presents all of the attributes and respondents' mean reported level of knowledge.

It was hypothesized that the Sudanese societal beliefs about the cause of stuttering would be associated with "an act of God (Allah)" and by "ghosts, spirits, and demons." Most respondents, 83.0%, indeed attributed the cause of stuttering to "an act of God (Allah)," while only 3.0% of respondents attributed it to "ghosts, demons, and spirits." Genetic inheritance as a cause for stuttering was the second highest response at 66.0%.

A follow-up Chi-Square test revealed no relationship between level of education and "an act of God (Allah)" as a perceived cause for stuttering. However, significant results were found between level of education and the attribution of stuttering to "genetic inheritance": participants with a bachelor's degree or

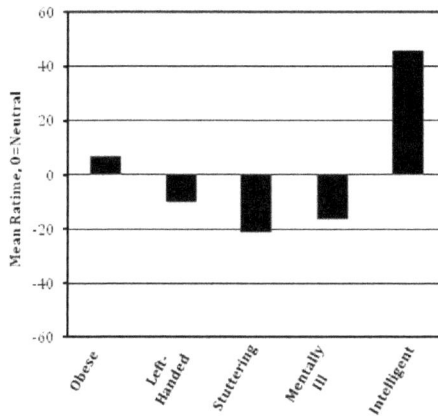

Figure 7.2: Mean rating scores of respondents' level of knowledge of five attributes converted to a -100 to 100 scale, 0 = neutral.

higher were more likely than those with less education to attribute the cause of stuttering to genetic inheritance ($X2 = 14.07$, p = .03).

The specific hypothesis that an imam and a medical doctor will more often be seen as sources of help for people who stutter was investigated through responses to the statement "I believe stuttering should be helped by . . ." The vast majority of respondents, 90.0%, chose "a speech-language pathologist" in response to this statement. Table 7.2 presents respondents' choices to this and the other sources for intervention for people who stutter.

Table 7.2: Sources of Help for People Who Stutter

Statement	Yes (%)	No (%)	Unsure (%)
I believe stuttering should be helped by			
A speech-language pathologist	90.0	6.0	4.0
A religious leader or imam	37.5	46.8	15.6
A medical doctor	66.6	23.0	10.4

Discussion

Selective data from the *POSHA–S* showed that Sudanese ratings of the overall impression of stuttering were relatively positive compared to the negative human attributes of obesity and mental illness. Neutral and positive human attributes,

151

left-handedness and intelligence, were rated higher on the scale than stuttering. Negative stereotypes about stuttering people did exist in slightly over half the participants, as was anticipated. In terms of knowledge about stuttering, respondents self-reported low levels of knowledge, yet 90.0% correctly indicated an SLP as a source of help for people who stutter, and 66.0% attributed genetic inheritance as a cause. Additional analysis of the *POSHA–S* revealed that participants received most of their knowledge about stuttering from personal experience, and the least from doctors, nurses, and specialists. This suggests the need for the dissemination of scientific knowledge and general information about stuttering in clinics, hospitals, and other specialized centers.

While negative stereotypes and some lack of knowledge about stuttering were evident, general attitudes toward people who stutter were largely positive as all respondents believed that people who stutter can make friends, and 97.0% believed they could lead normal lives. Additionally, 89.3% believed stuttering individuals can do any job they want, and 90.4% of participants did not believe that people who stutter have themselves to blame for their stuttering. These results are highly encouraging and may speak to increased acceptance of people who stutter and more positive societal attitudes toward disability.

One of the demographic items added to the *POSHA–S* was a 1–5 rating scale of respondents' priority value placed on "practicing my religion." The average rating was 4.75 out of 5, one of the highest valued items on that section. A strong explanatory preference for monotheism over superstition was evident in the responses to the statement, "I believe stuttering is caused by . . ." wherein 83.0% attributed it to "an act of God (Allah)," and only 3.0% to "ghosts, demons, and spirits." Given the historical mix of Islam and animism in Sudan's history, it was hypothesized that both would be seen as causes. This response suggests a clear distinction between faith in one God versus superstition as a cause for the disorder. There was no relationship between level of education and choosing "an act of God (Allah)" as a perceived cause for stuttering. However, participants with a bachelor's degree or higher were more likely to attribute the cause of stuttering to genetic inheritance than were those with less than that degree.

As Cheng (1989) notes, cultural background can have enormous impact upon people's attitudes toward the perceived source of a speech-language disorder and the efficacy or desirability of intervention. Overall, findings of generally positive attitudes toward stuttering within Sudanese society are encouraging, but still indicate the need for educational campaigns by health care professionals and educators to increase knowledge levels and understanding of stuttering among the general public. Future research should collect data on the incidence and prevalence rates of stuttering and other speech and language disorders in

Sudan. Additionally, *POSHA–S* results should be further analyzed to see how various demographic variables, such as age, sex, and income, affected perceptions, attitudes, and beliefs on stuttering. The results of this study should be incorporated into follow-up comparative studies with other *POSHA–S* results from other Muslim and non-Muslim nations. Findings may be useful to SLPs working throughout the Middle East and East Africa, as well as clinicians in Western countries working with stuttering individuals and families of people who stutter from Sudan.

Chapter 8

Public Attitudes Toward Mild Versus Severe Stuttering in the United States and Kuwait

Kenneth O. St. Louis, Fauzia Abdalla, Megan E. Burgess, Chelsea D. Kuhn

ABSTRACT

Research has been mixed regarding whether or not public attitudes toward stuttering are affected by severity of stuttering. This study sought to compare attitudes toward hypothetical stuttering described as either mild or severe in two widely different cultures and languages. Two hundred student respondents were recruited in the United States and Kuwait to fill out modified versions of the *Public Opinion Survey of Human Attributes–Stuttering (POSHA–S)* in English and Arabic, respectively. One version described any reference to stuttering and other human attributes (e.g., obesity and mental illness) as "mild"; another version, handed out alternatively, described them as "severe." Respondents rating "severe stuttering" had modestly less positive attitudes overall than those rating "mild stuttering" in both countries, although the differences were not uniformly in that direction. Eight to 13% of ratings were significantly different statistically. Combining both versions for each country yielded more positive attitudes from American respondents in general than Kuwaiti respondents, but again, exceptions for individual ratings did occur. Severity of hypothetical stuttering is a weak predictor of public attitudes toward stuttering.

Introduction

As made abundantly clear in this book's annotated bibliography (Hughes, Chapter 21) and summary chapters (e.g., Boyle & Blood, Chapter 2; Langevin, Chapter 3), numerous and burgeoning research projects exploring public attitudes and/or behavior toward stuttering as a condition and those who stutter have clearly documented negative bias, stereotypes, stigma, and discrimination. A number of studies have focused specifically on the effects of stuttering severity on attitudes toward stuttering, and results have been mixed. Some investigations reported more positive public attitudes toward people with mild stuttering than with severe stuttering (e.g., Collins & Blood, 1990; Turnbaugh, Guitar, & Hoffman, 1979). Other studies have shown no difference as a function of severity (e.g., Gabel, Hughes, & Daniels, 2008). These studies used different procedures and measures. For example, Collins and Blood (1990) showed 84 female college students a video recording of people speaking with severe stuttering or mild stuttering, with order counterbalanced. They measured the attitudes of the participants with a 14-item 7-point bipolar adjective (semantic differential) scale. For 13 of 14 items, those with severe stuttering were rated lower than those with mild stuttering. Gabel (2006) and Gabel et al. (2008) respectively asked 260 college students to rate attitudes on the 25-item Woods and Williams (1976) bipolar adjective (semantic differential) scale and on the appropriateness of 43 careers for hypothetical people who stutter severely versus mildly (as well as whether or not they had sought speech therapy). The investigators found more positive attitudes in mild stutterers than severe stutterers for only two of 25 adjective pairs (i.e., tense and self-derogatory), but no difference as a function of severity for any of the 43 careers.

Due to these and other mixed findings, the primary purpose of this study was to determine the extent of differences in attitudes toward people who stutter described as mild versus severe on a standard measure of public attitudes, and if there would be differences in such attitudes in two widely different cultures, the United States and Kuwait. A secondary purpose was to compare overall attitudes toward stuttering between the two countries, regardless of severity.

Method

The *Public Opinion Survey of Human Attributes–Stuttering* (*POSHA–S*) was developed as a standard measure of public attitudes for a wide variety of settings, groups, languages, and geographic areas (e.g., Abdalla & St. Louis, 2012; Ip, St. Louis, Myers, & An Xue, 2012; Özdemir, St. Louis, & Topbaş, 2011b; Przepiórka, Błachnio,

St. Louis, & Wozniak, 2013; St. Louis, 2011a, 2012c). Its components, scoring, and sociometric characteristics have been widely reported (e.g., Przepiórka et al., 2013; St. Louis, 2011a, 2012c; St. Louis, Williams, Ware, Guendouzi, & Reichel, 2014). The *POSHA–S* database, to which numerous samples have been compared, has also been documented in all recent publications, and at the time of the analyses of the data herein (circa April 2013) contained 169 different samples representing 7,197 respondents from 26 countries and 18 languages.

On the *POSHA–S*, respondents rate a hypothetical person who stutters with no exemplars, definitions, or explanations, except for using a "stuttering disorder" instead of "stuttering" in order to rule out any vernacular usages or connotations that refer to normal disfluency. Severity of stuttering is unspecified in the standard *POSHA–S*. For this study, we created two versions of the *POSHA–S*, one relating to a hypothetical person with mild stuttering (Re: Mild) and another relating to a hypothetical person with severe stuttering (Re: Severe). For example in the standard *POSHA–S*, one item is "People who stutter are shy and reserved." The Re: Mild version changed the item to "People with mild stuttering are shy and reserved," and the Re: Severe version changed it to "People with severe stuttering are shy and reserved."

The Re: Mild and Re: Severe versions also contained changes in the four other attributes in the general section to which stuttering can be compared. Each of the attributes had a mild or slight version and a severe or strong version. Mentally ill became either "mildly mentally ill" or "severely mentally ill," obese became "somewhat obese (overweight)" or "morbidly obese," left-handed became "mostly left-handed" or "completely left-handed," and intelligent became "fairly intelligent" or "extremely intelligent."

Both mild and severe versions were translated to Arabic for use in Kuwait by the second author and back-translated to English as recommended by St. Louis and Roberts (2010). In the United States and Kuwait, paper-and-pencil version of the English and Arabic versions, respectively, were collated alternately and distributed in that way to ensure random assignment of either version to respondents. Authors recruited convenience samples of individuals in their classes or others known to them. Most of those taking the English version were college students in the United States, and all those taking the Arabic version were students in Kuwait. Speech-language pathology (SLP) students or practitioners were excluded from participation since their attitudes have been shown to be more positive than non-SLP respondents (St. Louis, Przepiórka, Beste-Guldborg, Williams, Błachnio, Guendouzi, Reichel, & Ware, 2014).

As has been explained in numerous studies (e.g., Ip et al., 2012; Özdemir et al., 2011b; Przepiórka et al., 2013; St. Louis, 2011a, 2012c), *POSHA–S* mean ratings were converted to scaled ratings from -100 to +100, with 0 being neutral.

Some items are inverted so that higher scores reflect more positive or accurate attitudes and lower scores, less accurate or positive attitudes. Pair-wise *t*-test comparisons between standard attitude ratings were run for individual items, components or clusters of related items, subscores or clusters of related components, and an Overall Stuttering Score or mean of two stuttering subscores (Beliefs and Self Reactions). The Bonferroni correction was applied such that p ≤ .00417 (.05/12) was taken as significant for pair-wise comparisons. Cohen's *d* effect sizes were calculated for significant differences (Cohen, 1988). Finally, comparisons of the means for this study could be compared with the highest, lowest, and median sample means observed to date (circa April 2013) in the *POSHA–S* database.

Results

Demographic characteristics of the respondents are shown in Table 8.1. One hundred respondents filled out the *POSHA–S* in the United States, 50 responding to the Re: Mild version and 50 to the Re: Severe version. In Kuwait, 111 filled it out, 56, the Re: Mild version and 55, the Re: Severe version. Respective return rates in the United States and Kuwait were 69% and 74%. More females than males filled out the *POSHA–S* in Kuwait; thus, the sample was reduced at random to match the 50 in each group as in the United States and to equalize the number of male and female respondents.

Relatively few respondents were married or had children in either country, but the Kuwaitis rated their incomes relative to family and friends as well as others in their country higher than the Americans did. Race and religion were essentially as expected. Sixteen percent and 22% of the Americans and Kuwaitis, respectively, regarded themselves as "somewhat overweight," with 0% and 2% regarding themselves as "morbidly obese." Two percent to 6% identified themselves with "mild stuttering" or "mild mental illness" compared to 0% to 4% with "severe" variants.

Table 8.2 shows the results for the Overall Stuttering Scores, subscores, and components for Re: Mild and Re: Severe in each country. It also shows all the statistically significant pair-wise comparisons for these variables and any items for which a difference existed. Figures 8.1 and 8.2 show the respective U.S. and Kuwait results graphically.

In the United States samples, 4/60 (7%) of the non-independent (paired) *t*-test pair-wise comparisons were significantly different (p ≤ .00417). The mean Cohen's *d* effect size of the four significant differences was .70 or "moderate-large" (Cohen, 1988), all favoring Re: Mild over Re: Severe. They were: personal knowledge source for stuttering (item), knowledge of stuttering

Table 8.1: Demographic Summary of American and Kuwaiti Respondents in Re: Mild Versus Re: Severe Samples

Demographic Variable	U.S. Re: Mild	U.S. Re: Severe	Kuwait Re: Mild	Kuwait Re: Severe
Number	50	50	50	50
Age (year)	23.9	25.3	20.8	21.1
Education (year)	13.3	13.1	13.1	12.7
Male/Female (%)	44 / 56	34 / 66	50 / 50	50 / 50
Student/Working (%)	86 / 24	84 / 30	98 / 0	100 / 0
Married/Parent (%)	8 / 8	12 / 12	20 / 14	6 / 4
Income Score (-100 to +100)	1	15	22	32
Race (Caucasian /Arab + Kuwaiti/ Other) (%)	90 / 0 / 10	98 / 0 / 2	0 / 89 / 11	0 / 100 / 0
Religion (Christian/Muslim/Other) (%)	95 / 0 / 5	93 / 2 / 5	0 / 100 / 0	0 / 100 / 0
Self Identification (%)				
Obese	16	0	22	2
Mentally Ill	4	0	2	0
Stuttering	6	0	4	4
No People Known (%)				
Obese	2	12	6	12
Mentally Ill	32	38	40	58
Stuttering	26	52	20	40

(component), impression of obesity (item), and the obesity/mental illness subscore. The Overall Stuttering Scores differed only by 3 points, 24 for Re: Mild and 21 for Re: Severe. Both of these were above the *POSHA–S* database median of 15 for stuttering, *without reference to severity*, as can be seen also for the Beliefs and Self Reactions subscores and components in Figure 8.1. American Re: Mild ratings for Obesity ("somewhat overweight")/Mental Illness ("mildly mentally ill") were about average, compared to database averages without reference to severity, whereas Re: Severe ratings ("morbidly obese" and "severely mentally ill") were below average.

The Re: Mild versus Re: Severe samples from Kuwait differed significantly on nearly twice as many comparisons, i.e., 8/60 (13%), again all favoring Re: Mild. The mean Cohen's *d* was .60 or "moderate." Significantly different ratings were: school source for stuttering knowledge (item), impression of stuttering (item), want overweight/obesity (item), impression of obesity/mental illness (component), want to have obesity/mental illness (component), social distance/sympathy

Table 8.2: Mean Ratings for Re: Mild Versus Re: Severe for *POSHA–S* Overall Stuttering Scores, Subscores, Components, and Items (Pair-wise Statistically Significant Differences [p ≤ .00417] Are Highlighted with Shading)

POSHA–S Variable	U.S. Re: Mild	U.S. Re: Severe	Kuwait Re: Mild	Kuwait Re: Severe
OVERALL STUTTERING SCORE	24	21	19	9
Beliefs About People with Mild/Severe Stuttering	40	41	23	18
Traits/Personality	13	25	13	-1
Have themselves to blame[a]	90	82	92	66
Nervous or excitable[a]	-20	-6	-14	-27
Shy or fearful[a]	-30	0	-38	-43
Mild/Severe Stuttering Should Be Helped by:	30	37	-2	3
Speech and language therapist	96	96	76	82
Other people who stutter	2	31	-20	-30
Medical doctor[a]	-8	-16	-62	-42
Mild/Severe Stuttering Is Caused by:	40	37	7	-3
Genetic inheritance	20	49	16	26
Learning or habits[a]	-14	14	14	-16
A very frightening event[a]	6	-4	-36	-54
An act of God[a]	62	39	-74	-74
A virus or disease[a]	72	35	39	26
Ghosts, demons, spirits[a]	92	90	86	74
Potential	78	67	72	75
Can make friends	100	90	90	90
Can lead normal lives	96	86	88	80
Can do any job they want	64	54	76	80
Should have jobs requiring good judgment	50	36	36	48
Self Reactions to People with Mild/Severe Stuttering	8	1	15	-1
Accommodating/Helping	44	54	45	24
Try to act like the person was talking normally	74	96	98	100
Person like me	-42	-22	0	10
Fill in the person's words[a]	42	36	26	-16
Tell the person to "slow down" or "relax"[a]	26	42	17	-10
Make joke about mild/severe stuttering[a]	82	94	70	56
Should try to hide their mild/severe stuttering[a]	84	76	58	6

CONTINUED

159

Table 8.2 *continued*: Mean Ratings for Re: Mild Versus Re: Severe for *POSHA–S* Overall Stuttering Scores, Subscores, Components, and Items (Pair-wise Statistically Significant Differences [p ≤ .00417] Are Highlighted with Shading)

POSHA–S Variable	U.S. Re: Mild	U.S. Re: Severe	Kuwait Re: Mild	Kuwait Re: Severe
Social Distance/Sympathy	33	21	27	4
Feel comfortable or relaxed	54	26	80	70
Feel pity[a]	34	2	22	-20
Feel impatient (not want to wait while the person stutters)[a]	64	60	78	63
Concern about my doctor[a]	60	40	24	0
Concern about my neighbor[a]	90	88	74	43
Concern about my brother or sister[a]	46	46	18	-6
Concern about me[a]	12	2	-2	-26
Impression of person with mild/severe stuttering	2	3	1	-12
Want to have mild/severe stuttering	-68	-74	-50	-80
Knowledge/Experience	-20	-50	-21	-30
Amount known about mild/severe stuttering	-30	-47	-23	-28
People with mild/severe stuttering known	-78	-92	-79	-84
Personal experience (me, my family, friends)	48	-10	40	22
Knowledge Source	-24	-21	8	-3
Television, radio, films	4	22	26	12
Magazines, newspapers, books	-52	-35	-2	-6
Internet	-50	-39	2	8
School	20	0	42	-22
Doctors, nurses, other specialists	-44	-53	-26	-8
Mild/Severe Obesity/Mental Illness Subscore	-28	-44	-27	-44
Overall Impression	0	-22	-8	-37
Mild/Severe Obesity	-7	-36	-10	-37
Mild/Severe Mental Illness	6	-7	-6	-36
Want to have	-85	-93	-51	-81
Mild/Severe Obesity	-83	-95	-44	-83
Mild/Severe Mental Illness	-87	-91	-57	-79
Amount Known about	1	-17	-24	-16
Mild/Severe Obesity	20	-4	-3	4
Mild/Severe Mental Illness	-18	-31	-45	-35

[a] The signs of the mean ratings for this item are reversed so that higher scores reflect "better" attitudes and lower scores "worse" attitudes.

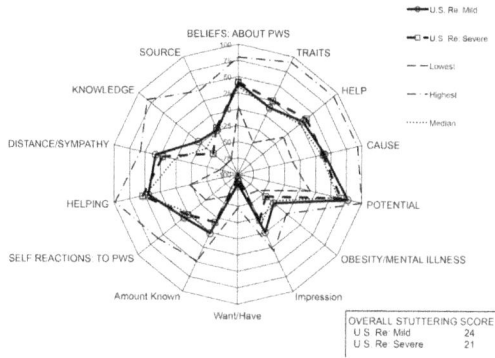

Figure 8.1: Summary graph of American respondents' ratings of Re: Mild versus Re: Severe.

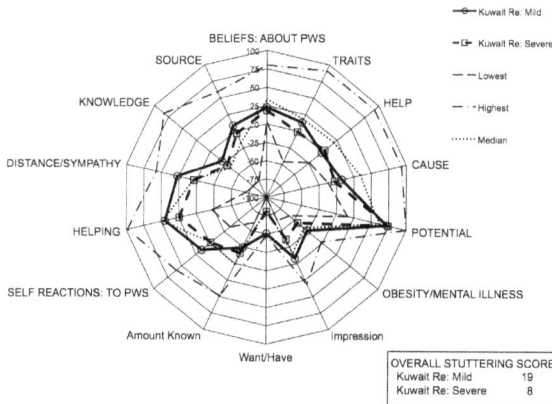

Figure 8.2: Summary graph of Kuwaiti respondents' ratings of Re: Mild versus Re: Severe.

(component), and Self Reaction to people who stutter (subscore). Figure 8.2 shows that the Kuwaiti Overall Stuttering Scores more strongly favored the Re: Mild over Re: Severe than was the case in the American samples, i.e., 19 and 8, respectively, or a 10-point difference. Whereas both American respondents were generally above average on both Belief and Self Reactions, Figure 8.2 reveals that the Kuwaiti samples for both Re: Mild and Re: Severe were below average for all Belief components except for potential of a stutterer. By contrast, their Self

Reaction ratings for Re: Severe were close to or slightly below average, and their Self Reaction ratings for Re: Mild were generally above average.

Inspecting Table 8.2 further indicates that, although not significantly different, for 12/60 (20%) of the American comparisons, the means were actually higher (better) for Re: Severe than Re: Mild. Higher Kuwaiti means for Re: Severe over Re: Mild ratings also occurred for 13/60 (22%) of the comparisons. Aside from one example each for source of knowledge of the mild or severe stuttering person, which might not be considered less positive attitudes, these still suggest that severe stuttering (or obesity and mental illness) are not uniformly rated less positively than mild attributes. Examples of trends favoring Re: Severe include correctly identifying a genetic cause for stuttering or trying to ignore stuttering in the United States and advisability of having a job requiring good judgment or being helped by "people like me" in Kuwait. Not included in the *POSHA–S* score was another puzzling result, i.e., non-significantly better overall impressions of and wanting to be "fairly intelligent" compared to "extremely intelligent" in Kuwaiti respondents.

The ratings were combined for Re: Mild and Re: Severe for both American and Kuwaiti samples and then compared between the two countries. Combined Overall Stuttering Scores were 23 for the United States and 14 for Kuwait. American attitudes were significantly different from Kuwaiti attitudes for 20/60 (33%) of the ratings (mean Cohen's d = .62 ["moderate"]). Of these, 13/60 or 22% favored the United States over Kuwait, while 7/60 or 11% favored Kuwait over the United States. Three examples of the latter were sources of knowledge (component), comfort around a stuttering person (item), and wanting/having obesity or mental illness (component).

Additionally, the two countries were compared on the Re: Mild ratings only, yielding Overall Stuttering Scores of 24 versus 19 for the United States and Kuwait, respectively, and 9/60 (15%) of the differences significant with the mean d = .93 or "large." Five of 60 (8%) favored the United States, while 4/60 (7%) favored Kuwait. Differences between the United States and Kuwait, compared for Re: Severe only, were somewhat larger, with OSSs of 21 versus 9. In this case, 10/60 (17%) were statistically significant, with the mean d = .88 or "large," and all favored the United States. These results indicate that American attitudes toward severe stuttering are more favorable than those for Kuwait. For mild stuttering, however, Kuwaiti attitudes were nearly as likely as American attitudes to be more positive.

Discussion

The results of this investigation of attitudes toward mild versus severe stuttering in widely different cultures add needed information to a growing body of epidemiological evidence on public attitudes toward stuttering. Severity of stuttering, however interpreted by the two populations sampled, did have an expected effect on *POSHA–S* measured attitudes. That this result occurred for both predominantly American and exclusively Kuwaiti students suggests that severity of stuttering as a predictor of public attitudes is a robust finding in two widely different cultures speaking very different languages. Yet although significant differences between Re: Mild and Re: Severe in both countries all favored the Re: Mild version of the *POSHA–S*, the results were far from uniform in that direction. A substantial minority of ratings reflected more accurate, informed, or positive attitudes toward severe stuttering, obesity, or mental illness.

Our overall finding of better attitudes toward mild than severe stuttering is in slight agreement with Gabel's (2006) findings for better attitudes on only two of 25 bipolar adjective ratings. By contrast, they are not in agreement with Gabel et al.'s (2008) finding that perceived severity of stuttering "mild" versus "severe" did not affect university students' judgments of role entrapment, or what occupations a person who stutters should or should not hold. The two *POSHA–S* items related to vocation, i.e., people who stutter can do any job they want or should have jobs where they have to correctly understand and decide important things (have good judgment), were different for the two countries. In the United States, hypothetically mild stuttering was associated with better attitudes than severe stuttering, 50 and 64 versus 36 and 54, but in Kuwait, the results were reversed, 36 and 76 versus 48 and 80.

When attitudes of hypothetical mild versus severe stuttering were rated on our modified *POSHA–Ss*, severity had a modest but not uniform negative effect. We conclude that severity of a hypothetical stutterer, though present, is only a weak predictor of public attitudes toward stuttering in general. The term "hypothetical" is important. Without confirming research, these results cannot be generalized to beliefs about and reactions to a real person who stutters, whose actual stuttering might be rated mild or severe by listeners. We cannot know if our results would be the same as those of respondents rating, for example, a presumably mild stutterer with two to three repetitive iterations on initial syllables or short one- to two-second blocks or pauses, all without obvious accessory behaviors versus a presumably severe stuttering with complex combinations of 10–15 repetitions, 10–30-second prolongations or blocks, and accompanying signs of struggle, tension, lack of eye contact, and so on. The study by Collins and Blood

(1990) addressed this issue with exemplars of mild versus severe stuttering and did show that attitudes toward severe stuttering were more negative on a bipolar adjective scale than toward mild stuttering. It is difficult to compare our results to theirs because they used a bipolar adjective scale, and a recent study by St. Louis et al. (2014) indicates that the *POSHA–S* has quite low correlations with the widely used Woods and Williams (1976) bipolar adjective scale.

Comparisons between the United States and Kuwait using combined Re: Mild and Re: Severe data revealed larger differences with fully one-third of the *POSHA–S* ratings being statistically significant. In general, attitudes toward stuttering of the U.S. respondents were better than those from Kuwait, but with a 1:2 ratio of Kuwaiti attitudes being more positive. Analyzing country comparisons for Re: Mild and Re: Severe separately, fewer differences reached significance, due in part to less statistical power related to one-half the sample size. Yet, inspecting both comparisons, it was apparent that significant ratings of severe stuttering all favored the United States while, for mild stuttering ratings, about half favored the United States and half Kuwait.

We caution that the data presented were generated mostly from college students, whose attitudes might not be representative of the general populations in each country. Also, we caution that attitudes toward hypothetically mild versus severe stuttering might well not correspond to attitudes toward specific individuals manifesting such variability in stuttering symptoms. One potential area of future research would be to compare the effects of hypothetical versus real stuttering on the *POSHA–S*.

Chapter 9

_____

Public Attitudes Toward Males Versus Females Who Stutter: United States and Iran

Kenneth O. St. Louis, Staci N. LeMasters,
Ahmad Poormohammad

ABSTRACT

Research has been mixed regarding the effect of sex on attitudes toward stuttering, whether considering the sex of the respondents or the sex of the people who stutter. This study compared attitudes toward hypothetical males versus females who stutter, as well as the effect of the sex of respondents on such attitudes in two widely different cultures and languages. Adult respondents were recruited in the United States and Iran to fill out modified versions of the *Public Opinion Survey of Human Attributes–Stuttering* (*POSHA–S*) in English and Farsi, respectively. One version described any reference to people who stutter as "males who stutter"; another version, handed out alternatively, described them as "females who stutter." Other *POSHA–S* attributes were similarly modified. American or Iranian attitudes toward hypothetical males versus females who stutter were very similar with no significant differences. There were also virtually no differences in either country between male and female respondents. Combining male and female versions for each country yielded more positive stuttering attitudes from American respondents in general than Iranian respondents. Together with other research using the *POSHA–S* showing no differences in attitudes of males versus female respondents, this study demonstrated that sex of a hypothetically stuttering person is not a predictor of public attitudes toward stuttering.

Introduction

All the chapters in this volume document the large and rapidly growing area of research confirming that non-stuttering members of the public hold negative or stigmatizing attitudes toward stuttering (e.g., Boyle & Blood, Chapter 2; Gabel, Chapter 4). Most of this research has involved asking respondents to rate hypothetical people who stutter (e.g., Abdalla & St. Louis, 2012; Flynn & St. Louis, 2011; Gabel, Blood, Tellis, & Althouse, 2004; Hughes, Gabel, Irani, & Schlagheck, 2010a; Özdemir, St. Louis, & Topbaş, 2011b; St. Louis & Roberts, 2010). In her comprehensive review of the literature, Hughes (2008) summarized research on attitudes toward stuttering for males versus females, both from the perspective of the sex[1] of the respondent and the sex of the person who stutters. The results have been mixed. In one frequently cited study with only 20 respondents, Burley and Rinaldi (1986) reported no differences in attitudes toward males versus females who stuttered, regardless of the sex of the respondents, but more negative attitudes from their male respondents compared to their female respondents. Using a similar design with the same measure, but with a control group and more respondents, Patterson and Pring (1991) found no differences in stuttering attitudes of males versus females. Yet, Weisel and Spektor (1998) found that adult males had more negative attitudes than females. Among young children, Hartford and Leahy (2007) reported no differences for boys and girls. Similarly, Langevin (2009) reported no significant differences from school-aged children's attitudes toward stuttering with respect to their sex, but in another investigation, a few comparisons resulted in more positive attitudes for girls than for boys (Langevin, Kleitman, Packman, & Onslow, 2009). Evans, Healey, Kawai, and Rowland (2008) found that the sex of middle-school students did not make a difference in their stuttering attitudes.

Cross-cultural comparisons have also been considered to be important. In a few items from similar oral questionnaires from three widely divergent cultures (Belgium, China, and Brazil), Van Borsel and colleagues found that males had more positive or accurate perceptions of those who stutter than females on some items, but for other items, the reverse was observed (de Britto Pereira, Rossi, & Van Borsel, 2008; Van Borsel, Verniers, & Bouvry, 1999; Xing Ming, Jing, Yi Wen, & Van Borsel, 2001). de Britto et al. (2008), for example, reported that female respondents were more likely to believe that the prevalence of stuttering was less than 1% of the population and that those who stutter had no differences in intelligence than male respondents. Regarding intelligence, 41% of males accorded those who stutter higher than average IQs, compared to 8% of females.

As explained in detail elsewhere (St. Louis, 2011a, 2012c, 2014) the *Public Opinion Survey of Human Attributes–Stuttering* (*POSHA–S*) was developed as a standard measure of public attitudes in widely variant settings, groups, languages, and geographic areas (e.g., Abdalla & St. Louis, 2012; Ip, St. Louis, Myers, & An Xue, 2012; Özdemir, St. Louis, & Topbaş, 2011a, 2011b; Przepiórka, Błachnio, St. Louis, & Wozniak, 2013; St. Louis, 2011a, 2012c). Its components, scoring, and sociometric characteristics have been widely reported (e.g., Przepiórka et al., 2013; St. Louis, 2011a, 2012c; St. Louis, Williams, Ware, Guendouzi, & Reichel, 2014). The *POSHA–S* does not define stuttering and does not mention the sex of the hypothetical person who stutters. To determine whether or not respondents' sex affected results on the *POSHA–S*, St. Louis (2012a) randomly selected one male and one female respondent from each of 50 different worldwide samples. None of the 60 *POSHA–S* ratings between male and female raters was statistically significant. Nevertheless, based on impressions from earlier work (e.g., Burley & Rinaldi, 1986), authors continue to consider respondents' sex as a potentially important factor in stuttering attitudes (e.g., Abdalla & St. Louis, 2014; Ip et al., 2012).

In addition to mixed findings from previous research on stuttering attitudes of males versus females, the question remains: Is there a difference in public attitudes *toward* males versus females who stutter? Also, the need exists to further consider cross-cultural comparisons; we chose to compare Iran and the United States. To our knowledge, public attitudes toward stuttering have not been reported in the scientific literature for Iran. Also, Iran was a logical choice for comparison with the United States because a generation of Islamic law in Iran imposed after the revolution of 1979 resulted in discrepancies in certain legal issues between men and women, e.g., a person's legal value or weight of legal testimony (IHRD, 2014). It is plausible, therefore, that greater differences in attitudes toward stuttering males versus females might exist in Iran versus the United States. The primary purpose of this study, then, was to determine the extent of differences in attitudes toward stuttering individuals described either as males or females on a standard measure of public attitudes in two widely different cultures, the United States and Iran. A secondary purpose of the study was to compare overall attitudes toward stuttering between the two countries, regardless of sex of the hypothetical stuttering individual.

Method

As noted, the *Public Opinion Survey of Human Attributes–Stuttering* (*POSHA–S*) was developed as a standard measure of public attitudes for a wide variety of groups, settings, geographic areas, and languages. For this study, the authors created two versions of the *POSHA–S*, one relating to a hypothetical male who stutters (Re: Male) and another to a hypothetical female who stutters (Re: Female). For example, in the standard *POSHA–S*, one item is "People who stutter are nervous and excitable." The Re: Male version was modified to "Males who stutter are nervous and excitable," and the Re: Female version was changed to "Females who stutter are nervous and excitable." The Re: Male and Re: Female versions also changed the four other attributes in the general section (intelligence, left-handedness, obesity, and mental illness) similarly.

The male and female versions were translated to Farsi (Persian) for use in Iran by the third author and back-translated to English by a Farsi- and English-speaking colleague as recommended by St. Louis and Roberts (2010). Printed paper-and-pencil versions of the modified English and Farsi *POSHA–S*s were collated alternately and handed out in order so that random assignment of either version to respondents was ensured. Authors recruited convenience samples of colleagues, family members, friends, and others known to them, but excluding speech-language pathologists (SLPs) or SLP students because their attitudes have been shown to be more positive than non-SLP respondents (St. Louis, Przepiórka, Beste-Guldborg, Williams, Błachnio, Guendouzi, Reichel, & Ware, 2014).

Both male and female versions of *POSHA–S* mean ratings were converted to a conventional -100 to +100 scale, with 0 being neutral (St. Louis, 2012c). Some items are inverted so that higher scores reflect more positive or accurate attitudes, and lower scores less accurate or positive attitudes. Independent *t*-tests were also run between individual items, components or clusters of related items, subscores or clusters of related components, and an Overall Stuttering Score (OSS) or mean of two stuttering subscores (Beliefs and Self Reactions). The Bonferroni correction was applied such that $p \leq .00417$ (.05/12) was taken as significant for pair-wise comparisons. Cohen's *d* effect sizes were then calculated for significant differences (Cohen, 1988). Finally, comparisons of the means for this study could be compared with the highest, lowest, and median sample means observed to date. The *POSHA–S* database, to which numerous samples have been compared, has also been documented in all recent publications (e.g., St. Louis, 2012c). At the time of this research (circa April 2013), it contained 167 different samples representing 7,197 respondents from 26 countries and 18 languages.

Results

Demographic characteristics of the respondents are shown in Table 9.1. In the United States 117 adults responded to the *POSHA–S*, 55 (15 men and 40 women) to the Re: Male version and 62 (20 men, 41 women, and one not specified) to the

168

Table 9.1: Demographic Summary of American and Iranian Respondents for Re: Male Versus Re: Female Samples

Demographic Variable	U.S. Re: Male	U.S. Re: Female	Iran Re: Male	Iran Re: Female
Number	55	62	50	51
Age (year)	38.4	39.9	32.3	30.9
Education (year)	13.4	14.4	14.6	14.1
Male/Female (%)	27 / 73	33 / 67	62 / 38	24 / 76
Student/Working (%)	35 / 69	35 / 58	36 / 56	39 / 37
Married/Parent (%)	64 / 56	60 / 53	48 / 40	47 / 35
Income Score (-100 to +100)	1	5	-3	-8
Race (Caucasian/Iranian, Aryan, Fars/Other, NR [%])	94 / 0 / 6	96 / 0 / 4	4 / 58 / 38	0 / 59 / 41
Religion (Christian/Muslim/Other, NR [%])	84 / 2 / 14	72 / 2 / 26	0 / 72 / 28	0 / 75 / 25
Self Identification (%)				
Obese	5	16	14	8
Mentally Ill	2	2	50	33
Stuttering	0	0	36	37
No People Known (%)				
Obese	3	0	2	0
Mentally Ill	36	35	24	24
Stuttering	42	48	28	18

Re: Female version. In Iran, 101 completed it, 50 (31 men and 19 women) and 51 (12 men, 38 women, and one not specified) to the Re: Male and Re: Female versions, respectively. Respective return rates in the United States and Iran were 84% and 92%.

Students comprised 35% to 39% of the respondents in the four groups, and 37% to 69% reported they were working. Income scores, relative to respondents' family or friends and to all the people in their countries, were average to slightly above average for the Americans and slightly to somewhat below average for the Iranians. Race and religion percentages were what would be expected. Unexpected, however, were the one-third to one-half of the Iranians who identified themselves as mentally ill and more than one-third self-identifying as stuttering. Presumably related to this, fewer Iranians than Americans reported knowing no one with these attributes.

Overall Stuttering Scores (OSSs), subscores, and components for Re: Male and Re: Female in each country are shown in Table 9.2. With shaded cells, it also shows all of the statistically significant pair-wise comparisons for independent *t*-tests on any rating in which a significant difference existed (p ≤ .00417). In columns 1 and 2, the means for all the male and female respondents in the United States are shown for Re: Male and Re: Female, and in columns 3 and 4, parallel data are shown for Iran. None of the differences between Re: Male or Re: Female were significant for either country. Figures 9.1 and 9.2 show these respective U.S. and Iranian results graphically where it can be seen that the Re: Male and Re: Female profiles for each country were essentially parallel and overlapping. OSS values were also very similar, 20 versus 22, respectively for the United States and 11 versus 12 for Iran.

Columns 5 to 8 of Table 9.2 show the *POSHA–S* means for male and female respondents in the United States, and columns 9 to 12 show the means for the Iranian male and female respondents. In each case men's reactions to hypothetical males versus hypothetical females who stutter is shown, as well as women's reactions to male stuttering versus female stuttering. American men had 10 points worse OSSs for males who stutter versus females, i.e., 15 versus 25. American women's OSS values were closer to equal yet slightly favoring stuttering males over females (22 versus 20). The same pattern was observed for the Beliefs subscore (i.e., composite for those items external to the respondents). By contrast, the Self Reactions subscore (i.e., reflecting ratings internal to the respondents) for stuttering females was more positive than such ratings of stuttering males by both American men and women.

The men versus women respondent results in Iran were somewhat different. For the OSS and Belief subscore, both Iranian men and women had slightly better attitudes toward Re: Female than Re: Male, while with the Self Reactions subscore, Re: Male and Re: Females were about even. Nevertheless, for these three measures, the mean ratings of Iranian men were more positive than for Iranian females by 5–7 points.

In spite of these apparent trends, only three *POSHA–S* items were significantly different in the two country samples: American men being more likely to report filling in a stuttering male's words than a stuttering female's words, American women reporting knowing more about female obesity than male obesity, and Iranian men more strongly believing that males should *not* hide their stuttering than females should. None of the differences were significant for Iranian females. These rare significant differences, accounting for 1/60 or 2% of each of the three groups, nonetheless had "large" to "very large" effect sizes, with Cohen's *d* values of 1.24, 0.75, and 1.17, respectively.

Since so many of the Iranians identified themselves as stuttering, whether or not they meant normal disfluency or the fluency disorder of stuttering, we sorted

Table 9.2. Mean Ratings for Re: Male Versus Re: Female for *POSHA–S* Overall Stuttering Scores, Subscores, Components, and Items (Pair-wise Statistically Significant Differences [p ≤ .00417] Are Highlighted with Shading)

POSHA–S Variable	U.S. Total Re: Male	U.S. Total Re: Female	Iran Total Re: Male	Iran Total Re: Female	U.S. Males Re: Males	U.S. Males Re: Females	U.S. Females Re: Males	U.S. Females Re: Females	Iran Males Re: Males	Iran Males Re: Females	Iran Females Re: Males	Iran Females Re: Females
Column	1	2	3	4	5	6	7	8	9	10	11	12
Number	55	62	50	51	15	20	40	41	31	12	19	38
OVERALL STUTTERING SCORE	20	22	11	12	15	25	22	20	14	16	7	10
Beliefs About Males/Females Who Stutter	43	43	16	18	37	50	46	40	18	22	12	7
Traits/Personality	30	33	12	22	27	40	32	28	17	28	4	19
Have themselves to blame[a]	85	85	83	96	80	90	88	83	90	83	74	100
Nervous or excitable[a]	6	15	-10	-2	7	25	5	7	-3	25	-21	-13
Shy or fearful[a]	0	0	-38	-27	-7	5	3	-5	-34	-25	-42	-29
Males/Females Who Stutter Should Be Helped by:	14	13	7	9	5	27	18	6	9	14	4	8
Speech and language therapist	91	93	96	92	93	90	90	98	93	92	100	92
Other people who stutter	-22	-31	-4	-2	-21	10	-23	-53	6	17	-22	-8
Medical doctor[a]	-26	-25	-71	-62	-57	-20	-15	-28	-73	-67	-67	-59
Stuttering in Males/Females Is Caused by:	51	49	-1	-5	44	53	53	48	0	-1	-3	-6
Genetic inheritance	30	16	19	37	50	20	23	18	23	58	11	29
Learning or habits[a]	39	30	35	37	0	30	53	28	37	42	33	37
A very frightening event[a]	40	48	-79	-84	40	65	40	38	-87	-75	-67	-87
An act of God[a]	43	56	-37	-49	43	50	43	58	-39	-17	-33	-58
A virus or disease[a]	63	57	17	-8	43	65	70	53	17	-42	17	5
Ghosts, demons, spirits[a]	91	90	38	35	86	85	93	93	47	25	22	39
Potential	78	78	46	47	72	80	81	76	48	46	42	47
Can make friends	96	98	80	84	100	100	95	98	83	75	74	86
Can lead normal lives	98	100	84	82	93	100	100	100	87	92	79	78
Can do any job they want	76	74	20	16	47	80	88	71	19	17	21	14
Should have jobs requiring good judgment	42	39	0	6	47	40	40	37	3	0	-5	8

CONTINUED

171

Table 9.2 *continued*: Mean Ratings for Re: Male Versus Re: Female for *POSHA–S* Overall Stuttering Scores, Subscores, Components, and Items (Pair-wise Statistically Significant Differences [p ≤ .00417] Are Highlighted with Shading)

POSHA–S Variable	U.S. Total Re: Male	U.S. Total Re: Female	Iran Total Re: Male	Iran Total Re: Female	U.S. Males Re: Males	U.S. Males Re: Females	U.S. Females Re: Males	U.S. Females Re: Females	Iran Males Re: Males	Iran Males Re: Females	Iran Females Re: Males	Iran Females Re: Females
Self Reactions to Males/Females Who Stutter	*-3*	*1*	*7*	*5*	*-6*	*0*	*-2*	*1*	*9*	*10*	*3*	*3*
Accommodating/Helping	45	50	42	32	30	50	50	50	40	17	45	37
Try to act like the person was talking normally	85	79	72	80	100	70	80	83	61	58	89	86
Person like me	-43	-61	-27	-33	-50	-45	-40	-70	-30	-17	-22	-36
Fill in the person's words[a]	37	59	10	-4	-21	75	58	50	7	-33	16	8
Tell the person to "slow down" or "relax"[a]	19	41	21	-14	14	30	20	45	24	-25	16	-13
Make joke about the person's stuttering[a]	94	97	96	100	79	90	100	100	93	100	100	100
Should try to hide their stuttering[a]	75	87	78	63	60	80	80	90	83	17	68	76
Social Distance/Sympathy	32	40	-5	-7	27	48	33	36	-3	1	-8	-9
Feel comfortable or relaxed	44	52	10	16	47	85	43	35	10	25	11	13
Feel pity[a]	37	31	9	8	43	40	35	25	14	-8	0	16
Feel impatient (not want to wait while the person stutters)[a]	57	67	46	45	29	65	68	68	55	33	32	50
Concern about my doctor[a]	47	71	33	27	13	65	60	73	57	25	-5	32
Concern about my neighbor[a]	87	95	65	63	80	95	90	95	53	67	84	61
Concern about my brother or sister[a]	67	71	-45	-55	80	85	63	63	-50	-33	-37	-61
Concern about me[a]	0	29	-68	-58	27	55	-10	15	-74	-17	-58	-70
Impression of male/female who stutters	-4	2	-21	-29	-13	-3	0	4	-14	-25	-33	-31
Want to be like a male/female who stutters	-51	-56	-74	-80	-60	-56	-48	-57	-80	-58	-64	-86
Knowledge/Experience	-40	-50	-14	-7	-35	-50	-41	-50	-4	6	-30	-11
Amount known about males/females who stutter	-47	-59	-49	-44	-47	-78	-47	-50	-40	-21	-65	-51

CONTINUED

172

Table 9.2 *continued*: Mean Ratings for Re: Male Versus Re: Female for *POSHA–S* Overall Stuttering Scores, Subscores, Components, and Items (Pair-wise Statistically Significant Differences [p ≤ .00417] Are Highlighted with Shading)

POSHA–S Variable	U.S. Total Re: Male	U.S. Total Re: Female	Iran Total Re: Male	Iran Total Re: Female	U.S. Males Re: Males	U.S. Males Re: Females	U.S. Females Re: Males	U.S. Females Re: Females	Iran Males Re: Males	Iran Males Re: Females	Iran Females Re: Males	Iran Females Re: Females
Males/females who stutter known	-90	-88	-48	-46	-91	-87	-89	-89	-43	-35	-56	-49
Personal experience (me, my family, friends)	18	-2	55	71	33	15	13	-10	70	75	32	68
Knowledge Source	-50	-37	4	1	-49	-47	-51	-33	2	17	6	-5
Television, radio, films	2	-11	38	16	-50	5	20	-20	37	8	39	21
Magazines, newspapers, books	-61	-23	31	-2	-79	-45	-55	-13	28	42	37	-16
Internet	-65	-52	-27	-22	-14	-55	-83	-53	-30	-8	-22	-29
School	-48	-30	-17	-6	-29	-55	-55	-18	-7	-8	-33	-8
Doctors, nurses, other specialists	-78	-69	-6	20	-71	-85	-80	-63	-17	50	11	8
Male/Female Obesity/Mental Illness Subscore	*-40*	*-34*	*-46*	*-51*	*-41*	*-42*	*-40*	*-31*	*-40*	*-44*	*-56*	*-53*
Overall Impression	-18	-12	-42	-48	-27	-17	-15	-10	-33	-50	-57	-48
Males/females who are obese	-26	-20	-16	-31	-27	-23	-26	-20	-2	-42	-39	-29
Males/females who are mentally ill	-10	-4	-68	-64	-27	-11	-4	-1	-64	-58	-75	-67
Want to be	-69	-75	-79	-86	-60	-75	-72	-77	-78	-73	-82	-89
Like a male/female who is obese	-69	-77	-67	-78	-50	-75	-76	-79	-67	-71	-67	-80
Like a male/female who is mentally ill	-68	-74	-92	-93	-70	-75	-68	-76	-88	-75	-97	-99
Amount Known about	-33	-15	-17	-19	-35	-36	-33	-6	-10	-9	-29	-23
Male/female obesity	-19	11	-15	-21	-17	-13	-19	20	-9	-13	-26	-23
Male/female mental illness	-48	-40	-19	-16	-53	-59	-46	-33	-12	-5	-31	-23

[a]The signs of the mean ratings for this item are reversed so that higher scores reflect "better" attitudes and lower scores "worse" attitudes.

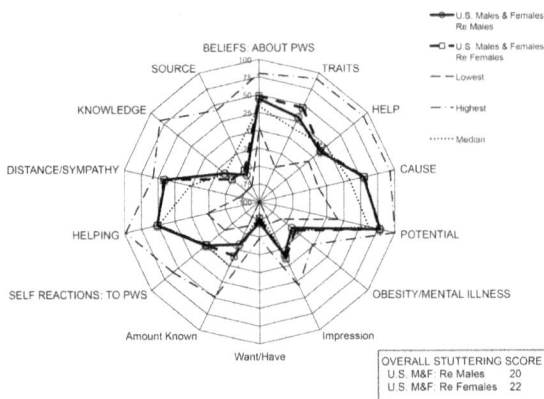

Figure 9.1: Summary graph of American respondents' ratings of Re: Male versus Re: Female.

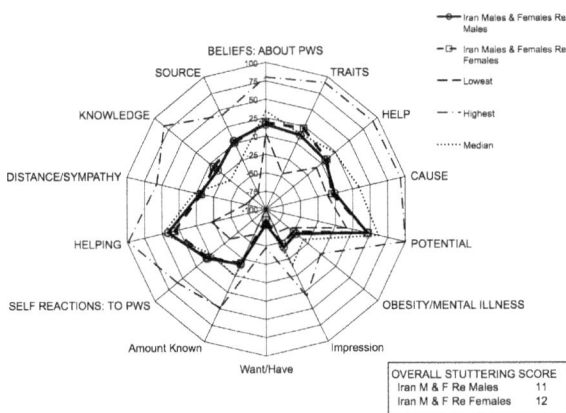

Figure 9.2: Summary graph of Iranian respondents' ratings of Re: Male versus Re: Female.

both the Re: Male and Re: Severe groups from Iran according to respondents who either self-identified as stuttering themselves or not. Of the 50 Re: Male group, 18 regarded themselves as stuttering (12 men and six women), and of the 51 Re: Female group, 19 self-identified as stuttering (13 men and six women). This left 32 in each group who did not self-identify as stuttering. OSS values for Re: Male and Re: Female calculated for the self-identified stuttering respondents were, respectively, 23 and 12, favoring the hypothetical stuttering males. For those who did not regard themselves as stuttering, the OSSs were 4 for Re: Male and 11 for Re: Female, favoring the hypothetically stuttering females. Given the 2:1 male-to-female sex ratio, it is likely that these individuals were stutterers, no doubt because the third author is an SLP who gave the modified *POSHA–Ss* to individuals who probably stuttered either then or in the past. Since the possibility of confounding of the results might have occurred, we ran all pair-wise *t*-tests between Re: Male versus Re: Female both for the self-identified stuttering respondents and those who did not self-identify as stuttering. None of the 60 *t*-tests was significant for either pair of analyses; thus, we determined that if any confounding did occur because one-third of the Iranian respondents may have stuttered, (1) the confounding was almost exactly balanced between the two groups by number and respondent sex ratio, and (2) the confounding factor had no effect on differences in attitudes toward hypothetical males versus females who stutter.

Re: Male and Re: Female ratings were combined to address the secondary purpose of the study, i.e., to compare overall public attitudes toward stuttering in the United States versus Iran. The combined OSS value for the United States was 21 versus 11 for Iran, and the percentage of significant differences was dramatically different from the male-female comparisons. Fifty-five percent (33/60) of the combined *POSHA–S* comparisons were statistically significant, with a mean effect size of $d = 0.828$ or "large" (range = 0.40 to 1.87). Of the 33 differences, 26 or 79% favored the United States, while seven or 21% favored Iran. The three largest differences favoring the Americans were: rejecting that stuttering is caused either by an emotionally traumatic experience (44 versus -82) or an Act of God (Allah) (50 versus -43), or concern if a sibling stuttered (69 versus -50). The three largest differences favoring the Iranians were knowledge of stuttering from specialists (7 versus -73), or from magazines, newspapers, and books (14 versus -41), and source of knowledge from personal experience.

Discussion

The results presented here provide quite unambiguous support for the proposition that sex of a hypothetical stutterer does not affect adults' attitudes toward stuttering in two countries that speak different languages and hold widely different cultural, religious, and political traditions. Moreover, the sex of the respondents themselves made only slight differences in their attitudes in either country. Together with the study by St. Louis (2012a) showing that the sex of respondents had no effect on measured *POSHA–S* attitudes, it is reasonable to conclude that the much-debated effect of sex on attitudes can be partly put to rest. No doubt, there have been—and will continue to be—reported instances from the literature wherein sex makes a difference, especially if all the items of various measures are considered (e.g., de Britto Pereira et al., 2008; Langevin et al., 2009; Xing Ming et al., 2001). However, these data are quite clear with respect to *POSHA–S* summary results that neither the sex of respondents nor the sex of a stuttering person has a significant effect on attitudes.

The combined Re: Male and Re: Female data comparisons between the American versus Iranian respondents generated large differences. St. Louis (2012c) concluded that ≥ 30% of the 60 *POSHA–S* comparisons can be interpreted as a large difference. In this case 55% of the ratings were significant. These results confirm other studies that have shown that stuttering attitudes in Middle Eastern countries are not as positive as those in North America (Abdalla & St. Louis, 2012; Al-Khaledi, Lincoln, McCabe, Packman, & Alshatti, 2009; Özdemir et al., 2011a, 2011b; St. Louis, Chapter 1). Returning to the *POSHA–S* graphs in figures 9.1 and 9.2, aside from the differences in pairs of OSSs between the two countries, the profiles in each of the figures were visibly different, suggesting not only a difference in magnitude of the measured attitudes, but also unique differences from item to item. Özdemir et al. (2011a) reported another finding of profile differences between two samples from Turkey, one that was obtained via convenience sampling and the other via probability sampling.

Other differences between the two samples are noteworthy. Unlike the American sample, more than one-third of the Iranians self-identified themselves as people who stutter. Whether this meant in Farsi, as it sometimes does in English, that one stumbles over words is not clear. Nevertheless, it is likely that a substantial number of the Iranians did, in fact, stutter, based on their 2:1 male-to-female sex ratio (Bloodstein & Bernstein Ratner, 2008). The analyses carried out between the 12 and 13 self-identified stutterers in the Re: Male and Re: Female groups and between the two parallel groups of 32 non-stuttering identified respondents indicates that, whether or not one-third of them stuttered, it had very little measured effect on the overall results. Moreover, even though the Iranian sample included stuttering people, whose attitudes have been shown to be more positive than non-stutterers (e.g., St. Louis, Kuhn, & Lytwak, Chapter 16), the fact that the Iranian attitudes were less positive than those for the United States argues further that the results were not seriously confounded.

Overall, this study adds strong evidence that sex does not affect stuttering attitudes, either in respondents or in people responded to. One implication is that the female- or male-dominated samples seen in the literature on public attitudes (e.g., Abdalla & St. Louis, 2014) very likely do reflect the attitudes of both the female and male population.

Note

[1] In many recent articles, including some in this volume, the term "gender" is used to refer to whether a person is male or female (e.g., Hughes, 2008). The term "sex" is used in the paper rather than "gender" because, in epidemiology, there are important differences between the terms (Kreiger, 2003). The *POSHA–S* asks respondents to identify their "sex" either "male" or "female."

Chapter 10

Recognizing Positive Aspects of Stuttering: A Survey of the General Public

Stephanie Hughes, Edward A. Strugalla

ABSTRACT

In this study, fluent speakers from the general public responded to open-ended questions about the effects of stuttering on the lives of people who stutter. The development of traits such as compassion, motivation, and perseverance were associated with stuttering people only after participants were asked to think about positive aspects of stuttering. Fluent speakers appear to emphasize disabling aspects of stuttering unless prompted to do otherwise. In addition, some of the seemingly positive aspects of stuttering described by participants could prove problematic for people who stutter. For example, many fluent speakers believed that stuttering is positive because stuttering individuals work hard to compensate for their stuttering, and often excel in careers that do not require strong verbal communication skills. The findings of the study indicate that more research on positive stuttering stereotypes is warranted in order to better understand fluent speakers' attitudes toward people who stutter.

Introduction

Social Perspectives on Disability

Theories of disability are often proposed in the context of a medical or a social model. In the medical model, health care providers presume that an individual who has some degree of bodily impairment will suffer because of the functional

178

limitations they experience (Giddens, 2006). From this perspective, the goal of medical and other professionals is to reduce the presumed suffering of their patients by fixing or otherwise curing their bodily ailments (Silvers, 1998). The social model of disability, on the other hand, proposes that in many cases it is the discriminatory practices of society that causes people with impairments to be disabled (Giddens, 2006).

With respect to stuttering, pioneering researchers came to the realization long ago that the medical model of disability does not suit stuttering particularly well. Van Riper (1982) noted that typically fluent listeners can heavily influence the success of communicative interactions with people who stutter. Stuttering is, in great part, an impairment in which the reactions of fluent speakers are often more disabling than speech disfluencies. Furthermore, the development of the World Health Organization's International Classification of Impairments, Disabilities, and Handicaps and its subsequent adaptation for stuttering (Yaruss, 1998; Yaruss & Quesal, 2004b) encouraged speech-language pathologists (SLPs) to address stuttering from a social disability perspective. Specifically, SLPs should recognize that fluent speakers may limit or restrict the ability of people who stutter to engage in the same occupational, educational, and social opportunities afforded to fluent speakers.

The general trend toward considering stuttering from a social disability perspective highlights the importance of societal attitudes toward stuttering when providing fluency therapy to stuttering clients. It is often supposed that both people who stutter and fluent speakers have specific roles that they are to play when communicating with each other. People who stutter, for example, feel responsible for the emotional comfort of their listeners (Plexico, Manning, & Levitt, 2009a). The same holds true for fluent speakers, as it has long been held that fluent speakers should make stuttering speakers feel as comfortable as possible by "acting and speaking [so] that the stutterer will feel secure in one's presence, will feel that he is being accepted as an individual, and will feel that he has nothing to lose by stuttering" (Johnson, 1934, p. 44). Johnson fell short of providing specific advice on how fluent speakers can achieve these objectives, and research suggests that, nearly 80 years later, fluent speakers are still unsure of how they can be of most help to stuttering individuals (Hughes, Gabel, Irani, & Shlagheck, 2010b). Thus, despite a desire to be helpful communicative partners, people who stutter and fluent speakers tend to be uneasy when conversing with each other.

Positive Stereotypes

Several decades of research have highlighted the negative attitudes of fluent speakers toward stuttering (e.g., Crowe & Walton, 1981; Hulit & Wirtz, 1994;

Woods & Williams, 1971; Gabel, Blood, Tellis, & Althouse, 2004). Some improvements in these attitudes have been measured (e.g., Cooper & Cooper, 1996), but people who stutter continue to be stereotyped as shy, quiet individuals who are poor communicators. The social model of disability suggests that these stereotypes prevent stuttering people from participating fully in social and occupational opportunities (Yaruss & Quesal, 2004b).

It is important to note that fluent speakers rarely take an entirely negative view of stuttering. In most studies, people who stutter are perceived as anxious, shy, and less employable individuals who are nonetheless also intelligent, friendly, and cooperative (Hughes, Gabel, Irani, & Schlagheck, 2010a). Personal narratives of individuals who stutter have also revealed that stuttering is not viewed as an entirely positive or negative phenomenon by people who stutter, and that personal opinions toward one's stuttering may shift as a product of time, therapy, and/or life experiences (Daniels, Gabel, & Hughes, 2012; Klompas & Ross, 2004; Plexico, Manning, & DiLollo, 2005; Plexico, Manning, & Levitt, 2009a, 2009b).

The nature and nuances of fluent speakers' positive attitudes toward stuttering and people who stutter have not been analyzed in the literature on stuttering with any great depth. The extent to which fluent speakers believe all people who stutter have positive traits or experience positive outcomes because of stuttering is not known. Positive traits ascribed to groups of marginalized people may have negative effects, as positive stereotypes often have negative correlates. In his review of the literature, Czopp (2008) described how women are often viewed as nurturing but weak, and people of Asian descent as highly competent in mathematical abilities but emotionally cold. This dichotomy seems to apply to people who stutter, as Hughes and colleagues (2010a) reported that stuttering people may be perceived as friendly and warm people who are nonetheless poor communicators. In general, positive stereotypes may be as restricting and limiting as negative stereotypes (Czopp, 2008).

Purpose

Given the scarcity of research related to positive perceptions of stuttering, the purpose of this study was to gather and analyze data related to fluent speakers' impressions of the effects of stuttering, including any positive effects that stuttering might have on the lives of people who stutter. The following research questions guided the study: (1) To what extent do fluent speakers believe that stuttering can have positive consequences for people who stutter? and (2) What is the nature of fluent speakers' beliefs regarding the positive effects of stuttering?

Methods

Participants

A total of 510 members of the general public (62% female, 38% male) served as participants in this study. The total did not include 12 participants who reported that they stuttered and were thereby not included in the data set. Seventy-five percent of participants knew at least one person who stutters. Most participants (74.5%) were White/Caucasian and had at least a four-year college degree. Participants were recruited by speech-language pathology graduate students in fluency disorders and research methods classes. These students were told not to recruit from university students, practicing speech-language pathologists, or people younger than age 18. Participants were invited to take part in the study by an e-mail that contained a link to an online questionnaire; thus, those who decided to complete the survey were anonymous.

Survey Instrument

The electronic questionnaire was adapted from a version developed by Hughes et al. (2010b). The Hughes et al. survey asked university students to answer such questions as, "How do you think people who stutter are affected by their stuttering?" and "If you were a person who stutters, how would your life be different?" In addition to these open-ended questions, this study's questionnaire asked the close-ended ("yes" or "no" response) question, "Do you think that people who stutter can be positively affected by their stuttering? In other words, do you think anything good can come from stuttering?" Participants who indicated that stuttering is associated with positive outcomes were asked to elaborate on their answer, i.e., "If you have not already done so in your previous survey answers, please elaborate on how people who stutter may be positively affected by their stuttering." The questionnaire was administered electronically via Survey Monkey.

Data Analysis

Data analysis focused on questionnaire items that corresponded to whether participants believed that stuttering can have positive effects (e.g., close-ended question analyzed with descriptive statistics) and what, specifically, these positive effects are (e.g., open-ended question analyzed for themes among participants' responses). Thematic analysis and classification of positive versus negative effects of stuttering were conducted in a manner described in a previous study by the first author (Hughes et al., 2010b). To reduce bias, the qualitative data analysis was completed by the second author, who had experience with qualitative data analysis but did not have an interest in the outcome of the study. The first author agreed that the themes extrapolated from the data by the first author were valid. She subsequently analyzed a subset of the data to determine the extent to which the authors were in agreement on how individual statements should be coded (i.e., aligned with themes). Reliability was satisfactory as the authors were in agreement for more than 90% of responses.

Results

The question "How do you think people who stutter are affected by their stuttering?" elicited responses from 509 of the 510 participants. Only 4.3% (n = 22) provided at least one trait, quality, or effect of stuttering that was judged to be positive, such as becoming a better listener, overcoming stuttering, or being a more compassionate person. The close-ended survey item, "Do you think that people who stutter can be positively affected by their stuttering?" elicited responses from 504 participants. Of these participants, 67.9% (n = 343) selected the "yes" option and the remaining 31.9% (n = 161) selected "no."

As noted, participants who believed that people who stutter could be positively affected by stuttering were asked to elaborate on these positive effects in an open-ended questionnaire item. Of the 343 participants who were eligible to answer this question, 91.3% (n = 313) did so. The four major themes derived from the analysis of this data set are presented in the sections below.

Theme 1: People Who Stutter Develop Empathy and Compassion for Others

Participants reported that stuttering individuals tend to be more understanding of differences and disabilities in the general population as compared to fluent speakers. One participant wrote, "I think that [people who stutter] would learn to better accept people for who they are on the inside instead of looking at people for their imperfections." Similarly, a participant stated that people who stutter "have the potential to be more understanding of other's differences and shortcomings." Only a few participants discussed in any detail why stuttering should necessarily lead people to be more compassionate, empathetic, or nicer to others.

Theme 2: Stuttering Can Result in Personal Growth or Character Strength

Similar to Theme 1, participants indicated that stuttering can engender positive outcomes by helping people who stutter to be stronger or have greater strength of character. One participant, noting that there are successful people who stutter, wrote that "the struggle to communicate makes people much better human beings." Other participants reported that stuttering could build self-confidence "if you don't let it bother you," or if people who stutter "overcome their stuttering." Indeed, overcoming stuttering was a concept noted by many participants, including one who wrote: "To overcome this problem would give that person a feeling of being able to accomplish anything they wanted after conquering the speech problem." Similarly, another participant wrote: "I feel that people who stutter and overcome that speech impediment could feel an astounding sense of accomplishment and confidence." The specifics of what it means to "overcome" stuttering were not explained by any of the participants.

Theme 3: People Who Stutter Tend to Focus on Helping Others

Several participants indicated that people who stutter could be quite successful in careers where they work with people who stutter, people who have other types of speaking difficulties, or people who have disabilities in general. One participant wrote that stuttering individuals could be successful in helping others who stutter because people who stutter "will have more motivation to find a cure" for stuttering. In this same vein, a participant stated, "[people who stutter] may want to help others who are in the same situation. They may also want to participate in new tests or experiments." Other participants believed that people who stutter can be advocates, educators, or role models. "I think people who stutter can help others know more about [stuttering] and understand that it is something that won't necessarily be a negative quality to have," wrote one participant. "Perhaps they could be an inspiration to others with verbal difficulties, helping them to feel more confident," wrote another. One the most representative statements related to this theme came from the participant who wrote:

> I think that a person who has the ability/skill to accept their own shortcomings also has the ability to transmit that self-confidence to others. This could very well lead to a life not affected as much by the condition. This person may also be a positive role model for others in the same situation.

Theme 4: People Who Stutter Can Work Hard to Develop Skills in Areas Other Than Speaking

Participants indicated that people who stutter often develop strengths in other areas to "compensate for a perceived weakness." Stuttering may, stated one participant, "motivate [people who stutter] to excel at other things. Instead of speech, they may concentrate on sports or other types of art." "They will be forced to work on themselves to develop new skills to overcome stuttering," wrote another participant. People who stutter were advised to "explore new avenues for careers." For example, participants cited singer Mel Tillis as someone who has a suitable career for a person who stutters: "Mel Tillis can sing, but stutters when he talks!" wrote one participant. In some cases, participants appeared to believe that people who stutter may be able to overcome their stuttering specifically because they develop strengths in areas other than speech: "If they are able to excel and overcome their stuttering because of other gifts they may have they will be extremely proud," noted one participant.

Conclusions and Discussion

The results of this study indicated that most fluent speakers who are members of the general public view stuttering from a deficit perspective. That only 4% of participants reported positive aspects of stuttering when asked to describe the effects of stuttering for people who stutter is striking, especially because nearly 70% of participants indicated that stuttering can have positive effects when asked this question in a yes/no format. Therefore, unless they are asked to consider otherwise, many fluent speakers focus on what stuttering people are not able to do. When prompted to consider positive effects of stuttering, however, many members of the general public readily associated stuttering with seemingly positive outcomes or traits. This finding suggests that fluent speakers have contradictory impressions of stuttering and people who stutter that are complex and highly nuanced.

An argument can be made, from a historical perspective, that many researchers have concentrated their efforts on measuring and changing negative attitudes toward people who stutter instead of measuring and fostering positive attitudes. Consider that in their groundbreaking studies, Yairi and Williams (1970) and Woods and Williams (1971) asked SLPs to list traits that described boys and men who stutter. One-third of traits were considered positive, yet Woods and Williams concluded that stereotypes of people who stutter were strongly negative and pervasive. They did not call for researchers to examine the basis and consequences of positive stereotypes of stuttering people, such as intelligence, cooperativeness, and friendliness. The rather one-sided findings in these influential early stereotyping studies may have set in motion a way of thinking that has fostered undue attention to stigma of stuttering to the exclusion of a more accurate, holistic view of public attitudes.

Another consideration is that the literature on disabilities and stereotyping suggests that even positive stereotypes may be harmful to minorities and those with disabilities. The results from this study suggest that fluent speakers view stuttering as an affliction that severely limits one's ability to be a good communicator. Any inherent strengths that people who stutter possess are viewed as resulting from overcoming stuttering or searching for its cure as an inspiration to others who are equally afflicted. The idea of overcoming stuttering is a curious one and was not readily explained by participants. Does overcoming stuttering mean achieving fluent speech, effectively "curing" one's own stuttering? Or does it mean accepting one's stuttering and living a "normal" life? Such questions may be an area of future research that can provide additional insights into fluent speakers' perceptions of optimal management of stuttering by people who stutter.

In addition, the nature of participants' responses seemed to indicate that individuals who stutter must work hard to be successful in spite of their stuttering. This finding suggests that people who stutter are not viewed as skilled communicators, and that fluent speakers believe that stuttering speakers should develop skills in other (ostensibly non-speech) areas to be successful in life. Only a few participants discussed specifically which skills, talents, or "gifts" should be developed to help one "overcome" stuttering, and these had to do with singing, art, or sports. These results are consistent with occupational stereotyping studies in which people who stutter are often encouraged by fluent speakers to pursue careers which do not seem to require high levels of communicative competence (e.g., Gabel et al., 2004).

It is also potentially problematic that some participants tended to view people who stutter who "overcome" their stuttering as role models for others who stutter and people with disabilities in general. Such occurrences may very well be positive for both people who stutter and others, but one cannot help but think of "model minorities"—those people who because of their race or ethnicity are expected to perform better in certain areas as compared to others, and "super crips"—people who perform heroic feats or accomplish tremendous tasks despite their disabilities (see Davis, 2010, for a review of the disability literature and further explanation of these terms). What pressures might people who stutter face if to be successful by fluent speakers' standards is to either speak fluently or become enormously successful at some non-speaking career, such as music or visual arts?

The results of this study may raise more questions than they answer with respect to fluent speakers' positive perceptions of people who stutter. Future studies could seek input from stuttering people in order to obtain a more holistic view of stuttering that encompasses not only the impairments and social restrictions associated with stuttering, but the personal strengths that stuttering can engender (e.g., Corcoran & Stewart, 1998). It may also be helpful for researchers who study attitudes toward stuttering to triangulate their findings with researchers who have investigated attitudes toward disabilities in general. In so doing, we may begin to develop a firmer foundation from which to hypothesize about the nature of attitudes toward stuttering and how we may change fluent speakers' attitudes toward people who stutter.

Part Three

RESEARCH: ATTITUDES OF PROFESSIONALS

Chapter 11

Attitudes Toward Stuttering: A Look at Selected Helping Professions

Ann M. Beste-Guldborg, Kenneth O. St. Louis, Nichole Campanale

ABSTRACT

Negative perceptions of stuttering are known to exist in some helping professions, but the picture is incomplete. This study examines perceptions of stuttering in 509 members of the mental health, education, health care, and law enforcement professions. It uses the *Public Opinion Survey of Human Attributes–Stuttering* (*POSHA–S*), a valid and reliable instrument to measure stuttering attitudes. Results indicate parallel perceptions about the disorder among the professions with some notable exceptions. Findings of particular interest are the presence of the stuttering stereotype and anxiety related to interactions with people who stutter among all the professional groups.

Introduction

Listener Attitudes, Stereotype, and Stigmatization

Listeners often hold negative views of stuttering and people who stutter; consequently, misconceptions, stereotypes, and stigmatization are prevalent (Allard & Williams, 2008; Blood, 1999; Boyle & Blood, Chapter 2; Woods & Williams, 1976; Yairi & Williams, 1970). People who stutter are depicted, as anxious, shy, nervous, sensitive, reactionary, weak, emotionally maladjusted, incompetent, unsociable, and unheroic (Boyle, Blood, & Blood, 2009; Craig, Tran, & Craig,

189

2003; Hulit & Wirtz, 1994; Klassen, 2001). Likewise listeners classify stuttering as a "psychological" condition, and these beliefs together form the *stuttering stereotype*, an idea without empirical support (Blood, 1999; Bloodstein & Bernstein Ratner, 2008; Boyle et al., 2009; White & Collins, 1984).

Stereotypes surrounding stuttering have wide-ranging effects in the lives of people who stutter (Blood, 1999; Craig, 2010; Gabel, Chapter 4; Hughes, Gabel, & Palasik, 2011). Many exhibit anxiety-related conditions and low self-esteem, in part, as a result of their own and others' perceptions, stereotypes, and stigmatization (Boyle, 2013b; Craig & Tran, 2006; Tran, Blumgart, & Craig, 2011). Often stuttering individuals internalize negative stereotypes and accept them as the truth (Irani & Gabel, 2008). The consequences limit social, educational, occupational, and other life experiences (Gabel, Blood, Tellis, & Althouse, 2004; Koedoot, Bouwmans, Franken, & Stolk, 2011; Klompass & Ross, 2004; Yaruss & Quesal, 2004b).

Research has found that professionals who interact with, support, and have influence over people who stutter are among those with negative and stereotypical attitudes. These include teachers (Crowe & Walton, 1981; Yeakle & Cooper, 1986), school administrators (Lass, Ruscello, Pannbacker, Schmitt, Kiser, Mussa, & Lockhart, 1994), special educators (Ruscello, Lass, Schmitt, & Pannbacker, 1994), health care workers (Silverman & Bongey, 1997; Yairi & Carrico, 1992), law enforcement professionals (Johnson, 2006), vocational rehabilitation counselors (Hurst & Cooper, 1983b), social workers (Altholz, 1991), and speech-language pathologists (SLPs) (Cooper & Cooper, 1996; Silverman, 1982).

Negative Attitudes in Selected Helping Professions

EDUCATIONAL PERSONNEL. Children spend significant portions of their formative years in school and educational personnel have great influence over their development, attitudes, thoughts, and behavior (Dewey, 1933; Nisbett & Ross, 1980; Turner & Helms, 1995). The beliefs and attitudes of school staff affect their perceptions and judgments, which, in turn, can affect the emotional, educational, and social development of students (Bingham, Haubrich, White, & Zipp, 1990; Eisenhart, Shrum, Harding, & Cuthbert, 1988; Langevin, Chapter 3; Lewis, 1990; Nespor, 1987).

In the 1980s and 1990s, researchers examined teacher perceptions of people who stutter and found the majority to hold negative personality stereotypes (Crowe & Walton, 1981; Lass, Ruscello, Schmitt, Pannbacker, Orlando, Dean, Ruziska, & Bradshaw, 1992; Yeakle & Cooper, 1986). This was disturbing given the influence teachers have in the classroom. More recent studies have noted a positive shift in teacher attitudes toward stuttering, finding more tolerance, acceptance, and a small but greater understanding of strategies to help stuttering people (Abdalla & St. Louis, 2014; Cooper & Cooper, 1996; Irani & Gabel, 2008; Plexico, Plumb, & Beacham, 2013).

The attitudes of SLPs toward stuttering have also been studied. Early investigations revealed a plethora of negative attitudes toward both the disorder and stuttering individuals, including a belief in the stuttering stereotype (Cooper & Rustin, 1985; Lass, Ruscello, Pannbacker, Schmitt, & Everly-Myers, 1989; Ragsdale & Ashby, 1982; Silverman, 1982; Turnbaugh, Guitar, & Hoffman, 1979; Woods & Williams, 1971; Yairi & Williams, 1970). This was troubling given that attitudes SLPs hold influence not only interactions with clients but also therapeutic outcomes (Andrews & Cutler, 1974; De Nil & Brutten, 1991). In 1996, Cooper and Cooper reviewed attitudinal changes of SLPs during the period from 1973 to 1991 and found they were less likely to perceive people who stutter as possessing psychological disorders but still prone to hold unsubstantiated beliefs regarding personalities. A 2003 review of SLP attitudes indicated a continued reduction in negative attitudes toward people who stutter, especially with regard to the stuttering stereotype (Crichton-Smith, Wright, & Stackhouse, 2003).

There are several other educational personnel who are integral parts of the school and whose influences are important in the lives of children. Little is known about their attitudes toward stuttering. Only two studies exist: one examining school administrators' perceptions of stuttering people (Lass et al., 1994) and one exploring special educator beliefs (Ruscello et al., 1994). Both found a preponderance of stereotype regarding people who stutter, including a belief in the stuttering personality.

MENTAL HEALTH PROFESSIONALS. People seek or are forced into counseling, often reluctantly, usually during a vulnerable period of life (Hinson & Swanson, 1993; Kahn & Hessling, 2001; Richwood & Braithwaite, 1994). This includes stuttering individuals who engage in psychological counseling or psychotherapy to improve their interpersonal and social relationships (Altholz & Golensky, 2004; Ginsberg, 2000). A mental health practitioner's job is to help alleviate the mental anguish of their clients and assist them to achieve their full potential (Altholz & Golensky, 2004). For people who stutter, this is difficult unless counselors have accurate and current knowledge about stuttering (Ginsberg & Wexler, 2000).

Though formal studies regarding mental health professionals' attitudes toward stuttering are few (Altholz, 1991; Hurst & Cooper, 1983b), some references to stereotyping exist in the literature. Ginsberg and Wexler (2000) claimed that it was not uncommon for people who stutter to have had experiences with counselors who possessed little knowledge about stuttering and had outdated and stereotypic assumptions about the disorder. This included a labeling of stuttering people as nervous, uptight, unintelligent, socially inept, and maladjusted. In a 2004 call to action, Altholz and Golensky (2004) asserted that people who stutter faced stigmatization and discrimination as a result of misconceptions and misinformation about stuttering, including those contributed by mental health professionals. They alleged the key issues were lack of awareness and sensitivity.

HEALTH CARE PROFESSIONALS. Regular health care visits help people live long, healthy lives. Results of the National Health Interview Study (U.S. Department of Health and Human Services, Centers for Disease Control and Prevention, 2014a, 2014b) revealed that 82% of adults and 93% of children in the United States visited a health care provider in 2011. Among those visitors are numerous stuttering individuals. Doctors, public health nurses, and other health providers are often the first to see people who stutter. They are the "gatekeepers" to further intervention, and willingness to refer often depends on their knowledge and attitudes about the disorder (Lees, Stark, Baird, & Birse, 2000; Yairi & Carrico, 1992). Very little has been published with regard to health care worker attitudes toward stuttering (Lees et al., 2000; Rosenfield, 1981; Yairi & Carrico, 1992).

Inaccurate beliefs have been found among nurses. In a 1997 study, nurses were asked to rate physicians who stuttered on a semantic differential scale and classified them, most commonly, as afraid, tense, and nervous (Silverman & Bongey, 1997). In addition, these doctors were seen as less mature, intelligent, secure, and competent than physicians who did not stutter. In 1992, Yairi and Carrico studied pediatricians' practices relating to early childhood stuttering and found a significant percentage held outdated and erroneous beliefs about the disorder and its etiology. In addition, physicians were noted to associate stuttering with stereotypical personality characteristics (Yairi & Carrico, 1992). These doctors reported a lack of information about stuttering during formal medical training. A study by Lees et al. (2000) also found antiquated beliefs, a lack of knowledge, and stereotypical assumptions among primary care practitioners.

A review of the literature advising physicians and other medical personnel about stuttering revealed a mixture of appropriate and stereotypical information. One article included references to broken teeth and locking jaws as common consequences of severe stuttering (Rafuse, 1994). That same article went on to infer that "backtracking and relearning" were important constructs of treatment, as well as the need to build confidence, social skills, and self-control to address the emotional and psychological aspects of the disorder. Another account, written about the same time, referred to psychological and emotional issues with stuttering that precluded full participation in schools, inhibited development of personal relationships, and limited choice of careers (Lawrence & Barclay, 1998). This article went on to assert that people who stutter have poor self-image, a sense of failure, and a passive approach to life. Several unsubstantiated treatment options were suggested, including: use of a metronome, the "shadow" method, "syllabic" speaking, fluency initiating gestures (FIGs), and the Edinburgh Masker, a small apparatus strapped across the larynx that prevented a person who stutters from hearing his or her own voice through a voice-activated masking system.

An article published in 2000 for physicians presented more accurate than erroneous information from medical providers, but disturbingly asserted that some people who stutter were viewed to exhibit social anxieties so serious that speech therapy was not warranted. It also cautioned physicians that the experience of "one or two" dysfluencies after discharge could lead to complete regression of therapeutic gains (Costa & Kroll, 2000).

More recent literature about stuttering advised medical personnel appropriately with regard to etiology, presentation of the disorder, and therapy (Ashurst & Wasson, 2011; Prausse & Kikano, 2008). To our knowledge, no recent studies have investigated attitudes toward stuttering in health care professionals.

LAW ENFORCEMENT PROFESSIONALS. Police must quickly access emergencies using all possible cues (Fletcher, 1990). Social psychological literature shows wide acceptance by police officers of specific indicators of deceptive behavior, including: involuntary speech disruptions, gaze aversion, emotional agitation, mouth movements, and hand gestures (Akehurst, Kohnken, Bull, & Vrij, 1996; Johnson, 2006). In particular, officers believe that when people lie, they stutter or take long pauses while speaking. Studies have shown that these attitudes are common, not just among police officers, but among other law enforcement personnel, including institutional corrections officers (Lakhani & Taylor, 2003; Vrij & Semin, 1996), parole officers (Porter, Woodworth, & Birt, 2000), prosecutors (Stromwall & Granhag, 2003), and judges (Stromwall & Granhag, 2003).

Current law enforcement training reinforces these beliefs (Johnson, 2006). The most widely offered education in the United States for interviewing and interrogation is the Reid Method (Brown, 2001; Remsberg, 1997). It teaches officers to observe suspects for nonverbal indicators of stress or deception, including: fidgeting, shifting body posture, frequent leg/foot movements or hand gestures, touching the face or head, avoiding eye contact, fast or stuttered speech with frequent pauses, and profuse sweating (Blair & Kooi, 2004; Inbau, Reid, Buckley, & Jayne, 2001). Many of these behaviors are common among people who stutter, especially during periods of stress. In a recent article on community policing, McCullough (2014) called for officers to consider the presence of bona fide stuttering rather than deception when encountering speech disruptions and unusual facial or body movements as part of a policing situation.

Law enforcement personnel are concerned with stabilizing chaotic situations while keeping themselves and others safe (Chevigny, 1995). They must take in all available information and act quickly. They are taught to rely, in part, on their "gut" (Chevigny, 1995). But what informs their attitudes and perceptions? It is understood that officers of the law often view people with mental illness as dangerous, violent, and unpredictable (Modell, 2003; Watson, Corrigan, & Ottati, 2004). They commonly stigmatize these individuals on the spot, especially if the officers have had little experience with—or training about—mental illness (Watson et al., 2004). It would stand to reason that these attitudes and perceptions may carry over to individuals with other stigmatizing conditions like stuttering (Lamb, Weinberger, & DeCuir, 2002; Modell & Copp, 2007). Little is known about law enforcement attitudes and perceptions of people who stutter.

Need for the Study

Negative attitudes toward stuttering and people who stutter are widespread and unfounded. This leads to misinformation, stigmatization, and stereotyping (Blood, 1999; Bloodstein & Bernstein Ratner, 2008; Craig, 2010; Hughes, Gabel, & Palasik, 2011). Erroneous beliefs and lack of knowledge about stuttering expose people who stutter to a myraid of negative experiences, sometimes from trusted professionals and often at vulnerable points in life (Altholz, 1991; Cooper & Cooper, 1996; Crowe & Walton, 1981; Lass et al., 1994; McCullough, 2014; Ruscello et al., 1994; Silverman & Bongey, 1997; Yairi & Carrico, 1992).

Much is known about teacher and SLP attitudes toward stuttering and a positive shift has been noted (Cooper & Cooper, 1996; Crichton-Smith et al., 2003), but the picture is incomplete. These are the only helping professionals whose attitudes have been investigated with some thoroughness. Attitudes of other helping professionals have not been well studied, even amidst gross misunderstandings of the disorder (Blair & Kooi, 2004; Brown, 2001; Costa & Kroll, 2000; Ginsberg & Wexler, 2000; Johnson, 2006; Lees et al., 2000; Silverman & Bongey, 1997). A current awareness of attitudes toward stuttering in the helping professions is important as members play critical roles of support, assistance, and opportunity, and their actions have significant impacts on the self-perception, health, and quality of life of people who stutter (Ezrati-Vinacour & Levin, 2004).

In addition, there are calls for public education to reduce stigma associated with stuttering (Abdalla, Chapter 5; Blood, 1999; Klompas & Ross, 2004; St. Louis, Filatova, Coşkun, Topbaş, Özdemir, Georgieva, McCaffrey, & George,

2011). To do this well, a reliable understanding of attitudes and perceptions is needed. Likewise, it is helpful to understand attitudes as stuttering people might experience them within a particular setting. For example, a visit to the doctor may require not only contact with the physician but also with the medical secretary, nurse's aide, medical technician, nurse, and X-ray technician, each with his or her own attitude toward stuttering but together they define the experience. This study looks at attitudes toward stuttering in the helping professions from this broad experience perspective.

Method

Participants

Participants in this study were 509 employees within health care, mental health, education, and law enforcement settings. They were recruited from 2,072 published e-mail addresses of various professional and work organizations across all 50 states. Participants were sent an e-mail link to the survey, which included a cover letter, statement of informed consent, and the survey. In an effort to get as large a response rate as possible, participants were asked to pass the link on to other helping professionals as they saw fit. Involvement in the study was voluntary and only fully completed surveys were included in the data analysis.

Survey Instrument and Data Analysis

The *Public Opinion Survey on Human Attributes–Stuttering* (*POSHA–S*), a well-developed instrument to measure stuttering attitudes, was used with the addition of one question specifying employment setting (St. Louis, 2011a, 2012c). Data were converted to a -100 to +100 scale (0 = neutral) then analyzed according to *POSHA–S* guidelines (St. Louis, 2011a). Responses were clustered and averaged into component and subscores, two reflecting stuttering and one measuring two additional human attributes (mental illness and obesity). Both the Beliefs about People Who Stutter (BEL) and Self Reactions to Stuttering (SR) subscores were averaged to determine an Overall Stuttering Score (OSS).

Results

Respondent Characteristics

Table 11.1 summarizes *POSHA–S* demographic information for the sample and the professional groups. The mean age of respondent was 39 years with a range of 20 to 71 years. Mental health participants were oldest ($\overline{X}$ =49.1 years), and edu-

Table 11.1: Demographic Comparisons for All Helping Professions (HP) Followed Separately by Mental Health (MH), Health Care (HC), Education (ED), and Law Enforcement (LE)

Demographic Variable	All Professions	Mental Health	Health Care	Education	Law Enforcement
Number	509	119	133	141	116
Age: Mean (year)	39.3	49.1	36.2	33.8	39.7
Total schooling: Mean (year)	16.5	18.2	16.8	16.0	15.1
Sex: Males (% total)	41%	34%	47%	18%	71%
Sex: Females (% total)	59%	66%	53%	82%	29%
Married (% of total)	61%	44%	73%	69%	55%
Parent (% of total)	66%	76%	47%	74%	67%
Student (% of total)	7%	4%	6%	5%	15%
Working (% of total)	99%	100%	98%	99%	99%
Relative income (-100 to +100)	30	51	65	26	-26
Self identification (% total)					
Stuttering	1%	2%	1%	1%	1%
Mentally ill	1%	1%	1%	1%	1%
Obese	1%	1%	1%	1%	1%
Left-handed	11%	15%	12%	11%	5%
Intelligent	92%	97%	92%	91%	87%
No people known who (are) (% total)					
Stuttering	32%	18%	41%	23%	46%
Mentally ill	12%	0%	8%	26%	11%
Obese	6%	3%	0%	4%	20%
Left-handed	29%	25%	32%	23%	38%
Intelligent	0%	0%	0%	0%	0%
Self-rating of health and abilities (-100 to +100)					
Physical health	52	48	53	50	58
Mental health	55	46	59	56	61
Ability to learn	65	68	66	61	67
Speaking ability	56	66	58	45	56
Self-rating of life priorities (-100 to +100)					
Be safe/secure	83	89	82	79	82
Be free	63	75	65	53	59
Spend time alone	38	58	45	25	23
Attend social events	0	-1	15	-7	-7
Imagine new things	36	62	33	25	26
Help less fortunate	52	68	53	41	48
Have exciting experiences	-26	-5	-38	-50	-5
Practice my religion	32	58	28	21	24
Earn money	56	61	54	51	59
Do job/duty	72	84	71	66	70
Get things done	75	87	73	67	75

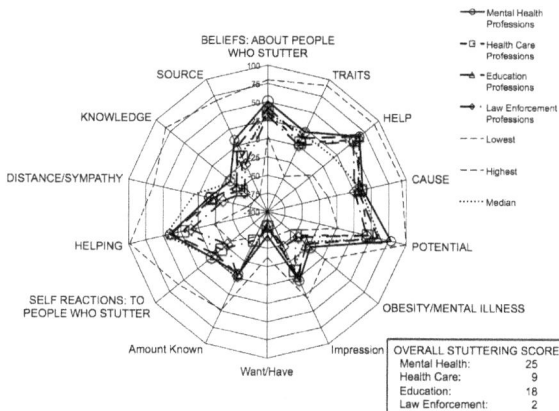

Figure 11.1: Summary POSHA–S graph for the Helping Professions, showing component scores, subscores, and Overall Stuttering Scores.

cation participants youngest ($\overline{X}$ = 33.8 years). The majority were females (59%), with the exception of law enforcement, where the percentage of female/male respondents was 29%/71%. More than half were married (61%), parents (66%), and most were working or retired (99%). The mean number of years of education was 16.5 with mental health professionals reporting the highest amount of schooling ($\overline{X}$=18.2 years), and law enforcement the lowest ($\overline{X}$=15.1 years). Described income levels in relation to others in the country varied from health care professionals as highest (+65) to law enforcement as lowest (-26). Most respondents knew or knew of a stuttering individual (68%) and considered themselves intelligent (92%), but virtually none reported as a person who stutters (<1%), mentally ill (<1%), or obese (<1%). Counselors and social workers made up the majority of mental health respondents (56%); nurses were the bulk of health care professionals (74%), teachers made up the majority of educational professionals (62%), and law enforcement participants were largely patrol officers or detectives/investigators (76%). An appendix lists all respondent occupations represented in each helping profession.

Stuttering Attitudes in All Helping Professions

Figure 11.1 shows graphically the mean ratings for the *POSHA–S* component scores and subscores. Points closer to the periphery indicate more positive and accurate perceptions while those closer to the center reflect more negative and inaccurate views (St. Louis, 2011a). Overall Stuttering Scores are shown at the lower right.

The sample OSS was slightly positive (+14), and much more so than the Obesity/Mental Illness subscore (O/MI -36). This score was similar to the median worldwide OSS (+17) as calculated from 222 *POSHA–S* database samples circa September 2014, though the point spread between groups was large (24 points). Consistent with all *POSHA-S* studies to date, BEL of +40 was more positive than SR of -13 for the sample and all groups.

Although visually, the profiles followed similar patterns, pair-wise *t*-test comparisons using the Bonferroni correction (p ≤ .00417) revealed significant differences among the groups with percentages significant ranging from 23% between the health care and education groups to 55% between mental health and law enforcement professionals (shown in Table 11.2 below). Cohen's *d* effect sizes were calculated for those comparisons with significant findings. The mean *d* for this sample was .685 indicating a moderate to large effect size (range = .08 to 1.08).

Table 11.2 provides converted mean values for *POSHA–S* variables; components; subscores for Beliefs (BEL), Self Reactions (RS), and Obesity/Mental Illness (O/MI); and Overall Stuttering Scores (OSS) for the total sample and each helping profession. Significant findings are noted by shading.

Stuttering Attitudes in Mental Health Professionals

Table 11.2 and Figure 11.1 indicate that mental health professionals consistently presented the most positive/accurate perceptions and had the highest OSS (+25), BEL (+51), and RS (0) of all groups. As with all groups in this study, perceptions of stuttering were much higher than perceptions of mental illness and obesity (O/MI -23).

This sample strongly believed in the potential of people who stutter (+78), knew who could assist (+65), and had the clearest understanding of a genetic basis for the disorder (+40). Still, there was a general unease with stuttering (Social Distance/Sympathy Score -15) and some evidence of the stuttering stereotype (Trait Score +21). This group reported little experience with the disorder (-33), and uncertainty about information sources related to stuttering (+9).

Stuttering Attitudes in Education Professionals

Education professionals demonstrated somewhat positive perceptions of stuttering with an OSS second highest in the sample (+18). As common in almost all *POSHA–S* studies, beliefs about people who stutter (+42) were far more positive than reactions to stuttering (-7). This group believed strongly in the potential of people who stutter (+60), felt they should be open about stuttering (+98), and knew who could help (+65). There was a sense of discomfort with stuttering (-20), uncertainty over information sources (-1), and lack of experience with

Table 11.2: Mean Ratings for All Respondents and Four Professional Categories for *POSHA–S* Overall Stuttering Scores, Subscores, Components, and Items (Pair-wise Statistically Significant Differences [p ≤ .00417] Are Shown at the Right by Asterisks [*])

POSHA–S Variable	All Professions	Mental Health (MH)	Health Care (HC)	Education (ED)	Law Enforcement (LE)	MH vs. HC	MH vs. ED	MH vs. LE	HC vs. ED	HC vs. LE	ED vs. LE
OVERALL STUTTERING SCORE	14	25	9	18	2	*	*	*	*	*	*
Beliefs About People Who Stutter	40	51	36	42	31	*	*	*			*
Traits/Personality	10	21	5	12	1			*			
Have themselves to blame[a]	80	92	73	87	70	*		*			
Nervous or excitable[a]	-29	-6	-32	-24	-54			*			*
Shy or fearful[a]	-23	-23	-26	-28	-13						
Stuttering Should Be Helped by:	61	65	57	65	54						
Speech and language therapist	96	97	95	98	96						
Other people who stutter	61	70	59	65	49						
Medical doctor[a]	25	29	17	33	18						
Stuttering Is Caused by:	32	37	35	31	26		*	*			
Genetic inheritance	17	40	18	9	1						
Learning or habits[a]	10	18	3	18	-3						
A very frightening event[a]	3	16	-7	6	-4						
An act of God[a]	69	54	79	72	68	*					
A virus or disease[a]	8	10	27	-15	10				*		
Ghosts, demons, spirits[a]	89	87	92	94	83						
Potential	56	78	45	60	44	*	*	*	*		*
Can make friends	81	94	74	84	71	*		*			
Can lead normal lives	60	84	49	64	44	*		*			
Can do any job they want	34	56	18	49	13	*		*	*		*
Should have jobs requiring good judgment	51	79	38	42	47	*	*	*			
Self Reactions to People Who Stutter	-13	0	-17	-7	-28	*	*	*	*	*	*
Accommodating/Helping	28	40	21	39	10	*		*	*	*	*
Try to act like the person was talking normally	72	77	57	75	82					*	
Person like me	-31	-12	-26	-24	-63		*			*	*
Fill in the person's words[a]	-1	23	-23	25	-32	*		*	*		*
Tell the person to "slow down" or "relax"[a]	-41	-4	-46	-28	-91	*		*		*	*
Make joke about stuttering[a]	92	97	92	89	92						
Should try to hide their stuttering[a]	78	62	74	98	74		*		*		*

CONTINUED

199

Table 11.2 *continued*: Mean Ratings for All Respondents and Four Professional Categories for *POSHA–S* Overall Stuttering Scores, Subscores, Components, and Items (Pair-wise Statistically Significant Differences [p ≤ .00417] Are Shown at the Right by Asterisks [*])

POSHA–S Variable	All Professions	Mental Health (MH)	Health Care (HC)	Education (ED)	Law Enforcement (LE)	MH vs. HC	MH vs. ED	MH vs. LE	HC vs. ED	HC vs. LE	ED vs. LE
Feel comfortable or relaxed	16	17	20	40	-21			*		*	*
Feel pity[a]	26	75	16	21	-5	*	*	*			
Feel impatient (not want to wait while the person stutters)[a]	49	40	56	71	25		*				*
Concern about my doctor[a]	-10	-12	-17	-15	6						
Concern about my neighbor[a]	-14	-7	-6	-38	-2		*		*		
Concern about my brother or sister[a]	-74	-74	-75	-74	-74						
Concern about me[a]	-92	-88	-83	-97	-97				*	*	
Impression of person with stuttering	-18	-5	3	-9	-66			*		*	*
Want to have stuttering	-85	-82	-86	-83	-88						
Knowledge/Experience	-47	-33	-54	-44	-58	*		*			
Amount known about stuttering	-51	-33	-58	-45	-67	*		*			*
People with stuttering known	-71	-71	-75	-70	-72						
Personal experience (me, my family, friends)	-19	6	-28	-18	-36			*			
Knowledge Source	-9	9	-16	-1	-28	*		*			*
Television, radio, films	-31	-12	-49	-26	-37	*					
Magazines, newspapers, books	-29	14	-38	-39	-50	*	*	*			
Internet	-1	9	-11	17	-21						*
School	7	17	5	21	-17						*
Doctors, nurses, other specialists	9	14	13	20	-14						
Obesity/Mental Illness	-36	-23	-49	-29	-44	*		*	*		*
Overall Impression	-13	4	-11	-2	-47	*		*		*	*
Obesity	-12	-3	-9	4	-44			*		*	*
Mental illness	-14	12	-13	-8	-50	*	*	*		*	*
Want to have	-78	-67	-80	-81	-83	*	*	*			
Obesity	-80	-65	-89	-88	-76	*	*			*	*
Mental illness	-75	-70	-70	-74	-89			*		*	
Amount Known about	-18	-6	-56	-5	-3	*			*	*	
Obesity	-16	-36	-28	4	-4		*	*	*	*	
Mental illness	-20	25	-85	-14	-1	*	*	*	*	*	

[a]The signs of the mean ratings for this item are reversed so that higher scores reflect "better" attitudes and lower scores "worse" attitudes.

stuttering (-44). As with mental health professionals, the education group identified traits associated with the stuttering stereotype (+12).

Stuttering Attitudes in Health Care Professionals

Health care professionals presented a similar yet less positive profile. The OSS was +9 with a higher BEL (+36) and somewhat negative RS (-17), a common delineation across *POSHA–S* studies. The O/MI was remarkably lower (-49). Like others, this group believed in the potential of people who stutter (+45) and understood where to seek assistance (+57). Comparably, they were unclear of cause (+35), did not know where to seek information (-16), and reported a lack of experience with stuttering (-54). Additionally there was discomfort (-19) and signs of the stuttering stereotype (+5).

Stuttering Attitudes in Law Enforcement Professionals

Law enforcement professionals reported the least experience with people who stutter (-58), yet showed a parallel but lower profile as compared to other groups. The OSS (+2) was below average (BEL = 31 and SR = -28) still much higher than the O/MI (-44). Like other groups, this sample believed in the potential of stuttering people (+44) and knew who could help (+54). They reported the greatest unease with people who stutter (-36) and stronger evidence of the stuttering stereotype (+1). Uncertainty of how to help (+10) and lack of knowledge about where to seek information (-28) were evident.

Discussion

Negative attitudes toward stuttering exist among individuals important in the lives of people who stutter (Irani, Gabel, Hughes, Swartz, & Palasik, 2009; Lass et al., 1994; Yairi & Carrico, 1992). This study examined stuttering attitudes in mental health, education, health care, and law enforcement professions from a perspective that included a variety of workers an individual who stutters may encounter within a particular setting. Understanding perceptions in this way may help to clarify the stigma that people who stutter could face in the experience of daily life and help to inform educational campaigns to reduce this stigma.

Similar attitudinal patterns were noted in all of the helping professions. The presence of the stuttering stereotype was evident in all groups to some degree as was a sense of unease in interaction with people who stutter. In addition, all groups were unclear about etiology and uncertain of where to turn for accurate information about the disorder. Consistent with the *POSHA–S* database median values, in all cases beliefs about stuttering people were more positive than reactions to stuttering, and all groups understood that SLPs could help in the treatment of stuttering as could people who stutter. Mental health professionals had the most positive and accurate beliefs regarding all human attributes studied, including stuttering. Further analysis of this trend may reveal important lessons for the training of helping professionals regarding both disabilities and stigmatizing conditions.

Surprisingly, the majority of respondents described little knowledge and experience with stuttering and reported specialists as a minimal source of information regarding the disorder.

It was predictable that law enforcement officials expressed the least positive beliefs/reactions toward stuttering (Modell & Copp, 2007). They typically interact with people who stutter in time-sensitive, stressful, and emotional situations where stuttering may be at its peak. They are trained to interpret signs of deception, including those related to altered speech patterns and excessive hand and body movements (Brown, 2001; Johnson, 2006; Remsberg, 1997). It is crucial, however, for both the fair treatment of stuttering individuals and the safety of officers, that the information officers use to interpret situations be filtered through an accurate knowledge base regarding the disorder of stuttering. Law enforcement agencies may want to reconsider the training of officers to detect suspicious behavior through speech disruptions, avoidance of eye contact, and hand gestures (Johnson, 2006). As long as the risk exists that police officers may unintentionally be taught to interpret the typical behaviors of people who stutter as suspicious, the risk of stigmatization remains, and since the literature suggests that a large number of police officers, corrections officers, prosecutors, and judges rely on these cues, efforts should be made to educate these professionals about stuttering.

The high degree of negative reaction by health care professionals was somewhat unanticipated, given the fact that practitioners are receiving more accurate information about stuttering through their professional journals (Ashurst & Wasson, 2011; Prausse & Kikano, 2008). Perhaps inaccurate information from earlier times continues to influence the profession in negative ways. Another possibility is that interactions in health care settings mirror those of law enforcement in some ways. If contacts are brief, time-bound, and pressured, stuttering may be increased, causing health care workers to form and act upon negative beliefs.

This study is possibly the first to examine beliefs about stuttering from the experience perspective. It gives a look at attitudes that people who stutter may encounter in daily life situations such as attending school, visiting the doctor, getting shots at public health, attending counseling, or getting pulled over by the police. Without a doubt, negative and inaccurate perceptions exist in the helping professions, more so in some than others. Clearly there is a need for education about stuttering in all of the professions. This study offers an understanding of how stuttering attitudes manifest and points to areas of strength and challenge in each group. Accordingly, it can be used to formulate setting specific educational programs to reduce stigma in each of the professional settings.

Limitations

Certain cautions are in order. First, because of the convenience/snowball sampling procedures used in this study, the sample may not be representative of the helping professions as a whole or individually. Second, the sampling technique may have influenced results by attracting individuals compelled to respond based on their interest in or closeness to the topic of stuttering, therefore skewing the results. Third, the respondents were heavily weighted as elementary teachers, nurses, police officers, and counselors, thereby reducing generalizability to additional members of the helping professions.

Future Directions

Educational and awareness campaigns should be undertaken with each of the helping professions to further educate them on the disorder of stuttering as well as common stereotypes associated with the disorder. These should involve both pre-service and in-service trainings that address perceptions through education and positive interaction with people who stutter. In addition, research should be carried out examining the efficacy of these educational campaigns in altering negative attitudes toward stuttering.

Appendix

MENTAL HEALTH PROFESSIONALS: secretary, mental health aide, licensed clinical social worker, addiction counselor, licensed clinical professional counselor, medical social worker, psychologist, and psychiatrist.

HEALTH CARE PROFESSIONALS: doctor, nurse, physical therapist, occupational therapist, phlebotomist, X-ray technician, laboratory technician, nurse's aide, licensed practical nurse (LPN), medical secretary, public health worker, intake specialist, physician assistant, nurse practitioner, dental assistant, and receptionist.

EDUCATION PROFESSIONALS: secretary, custodian, lunch room personnel, para-educator, secondary teacher, athletic director, special educator, school principal, superintendent, speech-language pathologist, school counselor, school psychologist, reading specialist, math tutor, attendance officer, school clerk, special education director, special education coordinator, elementary teacher, behavior specialist, cook, bus driver, home/school coordinator.

LAW ENFORCEMENT PROFESSIONALS: police officer, probation officer, sheriff, detective, highway patrol officer, judge, probation officer, parole officer, jailer, correction facility worker, juvenile detention officer, secretary, clerk of court, victim advocate, public defender, prosecutor, guard, intake specialist, private detective, police chief, patrolman, school resource officer, and community liaison.

Chapter 12

_____

Knowledge and Attitudes of Primary School Teachers about Stuttering Children in Sri Lanka

Saminda Kuruppu, Chantha K. Jayawardena

ABSTRACT

Knowledge and attitudes about stuttering and children who stutter was investigated among 84 primary school teachers of a leading international school in Colombo, Sri Lanka. Results showed that (1) a majority of teachers believed that a child with stuttering has the potential to overcome the stuttering problem, and (2) the child's everyday environment is an important factor in reinforcing or reducing his or her stuttering. Nearly half of the sample believed that many students who stutter are shy and quiet. Teachers who had previous experience in teaching three or more students with stuttering had more desirable answers than those who had very limited exposure to students with stuttering. It is recommended that creating awareness about stuttering among teachers would be important in fostering a classroom environment with healthy attitudes and actions toward children who stutter.

Introduction

People's knowledge and attitudes about health problems is important for several reasons. Increased knowledge about a specific health problem has the potential to eliminate myths and misconceptions and to change people's attitudes and behaviors toward individuals living with the health problem. Although stuttering (also known in various groups and geographical areas as dysfluency or stammering) cannot be completely cured only by therapeutic procedures, early identification and appropriate intervention ensure better outcomes, leading to improved quality of life of the affected individuals (British Stammering Association, 2014). Therefore, creating a more positive public environment around the condition would be a great relief for people who stutter and their loved ones.

Stereotyping is making generalizations about a particular group of people whereby the society attributes a defined set of characteristics to the group (White & Collins, 1984). One attaches a particular idea or image to a person who belongs to that particular group and makes a value judgment about the person, all without making an individual assessment about the person. The stereotypes can be positive or negative, but negative racial remarks, gender remarks, and sexual remarks are prime examples of stereotyping. Studies have indicated that the public often negatively stereotypes those who stutter, using descriptors such as shy, anxious, withdrawn, nervous, tense, hesitant, self-conscious, less competent, introverted, and insecure (Craig, Tran, & Craig, 2003). According to Smart (2001), people with disabilities often internalize negative stereotypes and accept them as the truth about themselves. This, in turn, can seriously contribute to a negative self-concept, or "self-stigma" among the affected individuals. Smart also pointed out that such internalization may be exacerbated if those stereotypes are repeated often and from people with authority (c.f. Boyle & Blood, Chapter 2).

School-age children spend a considerable amount of time at school, and teachers are typically regarded as authority figures who can have a significant influence on their lives during these formative years (Ministry of Education, Sri Lanka, 2014; Irani & Gabel, 2008). Accordingly, exploring teachers' knowledge and attitudes about stuttering would provide insight into not only the level of their awareness of the disorder but, more importantly, on how they deal with students who stutter in the classroom. Thus, such exploration becomes a prerequisite for dispelling misconceptions and eventually increasing sensitivity to the problem and promoting positive attitudes toward affected individuals.

School teachers have become the subjects in a growing number of studies of stuttering attitudes worldwide (e.g., Arnold & Goltl, 2013). Using a self-administered questionnaire and semi-structured interviews, Pachigar, Stansfield, and Goldbart (2011) investigated beliefs and attitudes of primary school teachers in Mumbai, India, toward children who stutter. Fifty-eight teachers responded to the questionnaire, and four of them were interviewed. Questionnaire results revealed the teachers believed that a child's environment influenced the occurrence of stuttering and that children who stuttered had the potential to overcome the condition. There was a strong agreement that punishment would not increase fluent speech. Sixty-two percent believed stuttering does not affect a child's IQ. Few (19%) teachers believed that children who stuttered were quiet and shy. A majority (69%) of teachers believed that ridicule is a common human reaction to stuttering; however, 62% did not believe that children should be taught to accept or expect ridicule. A significant correlation was not observed between teachers' work experience and overall attitudes toward stutterers. Two global themes emerged from the interviews. These related to (1) teachers' philosophies about stuttering, and (2) their perceived roles in supporting children who stutter. All teachers reported limited experience in teaching children who stutter, but their responses indicated a desire to do their best to support such children in the classroom.

In another study, Abdalla and St. Louis (2012) reported school teachers' knowledge, beliefs, and reactions regarding stuttering and toward people who stutter in Kuwait using an adapted version of the *Public Opinion Survey of Human Attributes–Stuttering* (*POSHA–S*). The results of this study suggested that the respondents had considerable awareness and exposure to stuttering: about 49% of the teachers indicated knowing a friend or a relative who stutters, and 69% of the in-service teachers had direct contact with a student who stutters in their classrooms. Approximately three-quarters of the teachers held positive attitudes given that they felt that people who stutter "can lead normal lives" and about four-fifths believed they "can make friends." Nevertheless and despite the fact that over 70% of the teachers deemed that people who stutter do not have a "lower level of academic performance in school," only 42% believed that people who stutter "can do any job they want." Nearly all teachers would "try to act like the person was talking normally" and would "not make a joke about stuttering." They reportedly never punish a child for stuttering. Very few differences were noted between opinions of teachers who were still in training and those who were practicing for an average of 11 years. Some of the most consistent findings with regard to people who stutter were that they were "nervous or excitable" and "shy or fearful." A follow-up study was conducted by the same authors to explore the effect of educational documentary video on changing attitudes among Kuwaiti school teachers toward stuttering (Abdalla & St. Louis, 2014). The student teachers demonstrated a positive change of attitudes after video presentation while practicing teachers did not.

Stuttering is a poorly attended health problem in the Sri Lankan society. It has rarely been the focus of research or discussions in scientific forums from professionals in the fields of health, education, and social sciences. For example, published data are lacking with regard to the prevalence of stuttering in Sri Lanka. We also do not have clear understanding about what people know about stuttering, how they view the problem, and how they react to people who stutter.

Accordingly, the present study aimed to explore the level of knowledge about stuttering among a group of primary school teachers and their attitudes toward children who stutter.

Method

Setting

The study was conducted in the Lyceum International School located in Colombo, Sri Lanka, after receiving approval by the ethical clearance committee of the Faculty of Medicine, University of Kelaniya. The island-wide group of eight Lyceum International Schools, with the parent or main school located in Colombo, are regarded as leading international schools in Sri Lanka.

The parent school had a student population of approximately 3,000 girls and boys. Its primary section had 125 teachers, the majority of whom were females. The "pre-grade" and "primary" grades contained two teachers in each class. The school followed an inclusive education system with the goal of providing equal opportunities to all children, including children who have disabilities and special needs. This involved being educated in their age-appropriate classes alongside their normal peers, but with the help of special services and access to needed facilities. The children with special needs received services as needed from occupational therapists and/or speech-language therapists during their school days. All instruction was provided in English.

Study Sample and Method of Sampling

The proposed sample size was 100 primary school teachers who were employed in the school. The principal investigator first explained the aim of the study and its method to all teachers in the primary section ("pre-grade," and "primary") and invited them to participate in the study. Teachers who expressed their willingness to be participants in the study received printed consent forms and the questionnaire.

Questionnaire

A self-administered, structured questionnaire, developed for a similar study of primary school teachers in India (Pachigar, Stansfield & Goldbart, 2011), was used for this investigation. The questionnaire consisted of two parts: Part 1 assessed knowledge and attitudes of the respondents about children who stutter, while Part 2 collected demographic information regarding the respondents. The questionnaire was pre-tested in a pilot study of three teachers in the primary section who did not participate in the main study. These three teachers were also asked to comment on the length of the statements, the meaning of the words, and to suggest alternate vocabulary that might more easily be understood by teachers to be sampled. Their comments informed the final questionnaire.

Data Collection

Data collection commenced on July 1, 2012, and continued for a period of one month, excluding school holidays. All teachers who consented to participate in the study were given a detailed explanation, either individually or in small groups, about the questionnaire and how to respond to the two parts. Then the questionnaire (inside an envelope) was distributed individually to the 100 teachers. Each participant was given approximately two days to complete the questionnaire and asked to return the completed questionnaire by putting it into a "postal box" kept in the staff room.

Data Analysis

All completed questionnaires were collected and data were entered electronically into an Excel worksheet. The descriptive statistics were done using Excel software while significance testing (using Chi-Square) was carried out on the "Mini tab 14" statistical software using an alpha level of $p < 0.05$ for statistically significant differences.

Results

Of the 100 teachers who participated in the study, 84 returned the completed questionnaire for a response rate of 84%. Demographic profiles (Part 2) of the respondents are shown in Table 12.1. All the teachers were female and 31% were pre-grade teachers, with lower representations from grades 1 through 5 (2% to 24%). Of the total sample, 41% had no previous experience in teaching a child who stutters, while 24% had experience in teaching only one such child. Fifteen percent had taught three or more students who stutter. Sixty-one percent of the sample had read some information about stuttering, while 2% had received some formal training covering the fluency disorder. Fourteen percent of the teachers stated that they had discussed—or received instructions about—stuttering from a speech and language specialist. Ten teachers (12%) reported having a family member or a close relative who stuttered. The highest level of education of the respondents was: high school (4%), one- or two-year university degree or special training in early childhood and primary education (81%), and four-year university degree, mostly in education (13%).

Table 12.1: Selected Background Characteristics of the Study Participants

Description	Responded						Omitted	Total
Level of Education	School		Degree	—	—	—	—	—
	3 3.6%	68 80.9%	11 13.1%	—	—	—	2 2.4%	84 100%
Grade Currently Teaching	Pre-grade	1	2	3	4	5	—	—
	26 31%	20 23.8%	20 23.8%	9 10.7%	7 8.3%	2 2.4%	0 0%	84 100%
Teaching Experience (Years)	0–3	4–6	7–11	12–20	≥ 21		—	—
	28 33.3%	22 26.2%	18 21.4%	8 9.5%	6 7.2%	—	2 2.4%	84 100%
Number of CWS Taught	None	1	2	3	4	≥ 5	—	—
	34 40.7%	20 23.8%	9 10.7%	8 9.5%	2 2.4%	3 3.6%	8 9.5%	84 100%

Key: CWS = children with stuttering

Knowledge and Attitudes about Stuttering and Children Who Stutter

Part 1 of the questionnaire explored knowledge and attitudes about stuttering using 14 statements (Table 12.2). One statement (no. 15) explored teachers' opinions about how they believe the general public would react to stuttering. Table 12.2 summarizes the levels of agreement expressed by teachers to each statement.

Sixty-nine (82%) teachers responded to all statements. All teachers responded to statements 6 and 8 while a minimum number of 77 (92%) teachers responded to statement 11. The participants responded to 12 statements on average.

A majority (57%) of teachers agreed or strongly agreed that stuttering does not affect a child's IQ level, while a sizable minority (29%) disagreed or strongly disagreed. Nearly half of the sample was of the opinion that many students who stutter are shy and quiet. A vast majority (90%) did not agree that punishment will help to improve a child with stuttering behavior. Many teachers thought that children with stuttering have potential to overcome the problem (86%), and the child's everyday environment is an important factor in reinforcing or reducing one's stuttering (90%).

Sixty-five percent believed that a teacher should not exempt a child who stutters from talking in front of the class. Further, nearly all (96%) also believed that they should avoid making children who stutter aware that they are different

Table 12.2: Frequency and Percentages of Teachers' Responses to Knowledge and Attitudes Statements

Statement	Desirable	Neutral			Undesirable	
	Strongly Agree	Agree	Neutral	Disagree	Strongly Disagree	No Response
1 Stuttering* does not affect a child's IQ level	11 13.1%	37 44.0%	9 10.7%	18 21.4%	6 7.1%	3 3.6%
2 Teachers should avoid calling attention to a stuttering child's speech	12 14.3%	20 23.8%	11 13.1%	27 32.1%	8 9.5%	6 7.1%
3 Children are more fluent when a teacher puts the child at ease before speaking	25 29.8%	45 53.6%	8 9.5%	1 1.2%	1 1.2%	4 4.8%
4 A child's everyday environment is an important factor in reinforcing or reducing his/her stutter	33 39.3%	43 51.2%	4 4.8%	3 3.6%	0 0%	1 1.2%
5 A teacher should exempt a child who stutters from talking in front of the class	3 3.6%	10 11.9%	13 15.5%	31 36.9%	24 28.6%	3 3.6%
6 Most students who stutter can be described as "shy" and "quiet"	2 2.4%	38 45.2%	14 16.7%	25 29.8%	5 5.9%	0 0%
7 Teachers should make children repeat words until they can speak them fluently	8 9.5%	36 42.8%	16 19.0%	20 23.8%	3 3.6%	1 1.2%
8 Children who stutter should be made aware that they are different from other children	0 0%	3 3.6%	0 0%	28 33.3%	53 63.0%	0 0%
9 A child who stutters should be taught to accept and expect "ridicule"	1 1.2%	9 10.7%	10 11.9%	22 26.2%	39 46.4%	3 3.6%
10 Teachers have relatively little influence on the development of the child's stutter	1 1.2%	23 27.4%	18 21.4%	25 29.7%	14 16.6%	3 3.6%
11 Punishing stuttering behavior will increase fluent speech	1 1.2%	4 4.8%	2 2.4%	22 26.2%	54 64.2%	1 1.2%
12 Teachers have relatively little influence on how the child perceives his/her own stutter	0 0%	26 30.9%	17 20.2%	30 35.7%	4 4.8%	7 8.3%

CONTINUED

Table 12.2 *continued*: Frequency and Percentages of Teachers' Responses to Knowledge and Attitudes Statements

Statement	Desirable		Neutral			Undesirable
	Strongly Agree	Agree	Neutral	Disagree	Strongly Disagree	No Response
13 Teachers should be more lenient in grading a stuttering child's written academic performance	6 7.1%	14 16.7%	15 17.8%	38 45.2%	7 8.3%	4% 4.8%
14 Stuttering is a condition that cannot be "cured"	2 2.4%	0 0%	7 8.3%	44 52.3%	28 33.3%	3 3.6%
15 Ridicule is a common human reaction to stuttering	7 8.3%	17 20.2%	20 23.8%	19 22.6%	19 22.6%	2 2.4%

*In the questionnaire, the term "stammer/stammering" was used instead of "stutter/ stuttering."

from other children. A large majority (83%) also felt that children are more fluent when a teacher puts the child at ease before speaking.

The study explored the variability of the responses about stuttering among different categories of teachers in the sample (tables 12.3 and 12.4). Higher levels of knowledge and more desirable attitudes were observed among teachers who reported having a family member or a close relative who stutters. However, the difference was not statistically significant on a Chi-Square analysis (X^2 = 3.15; p = 0. 07). Teachers who had experience in teaching three or more students with stuttering gave significantly more desirable answers than those who had less or no experience in teaching students who stutter (X^2 = 4.5; p = 0.03).

Our study also inquired whether ridicule is a common human reaction to stuttering. Forty-five percent of the sample did not believe that it was common; however, 20% remained neutral regarding the statement.

Discussion

Teacher Attitudes

The present study showed that Sri Lankan primary school teachers held desirable attitudes toward certain aspects of stuttering; however, inadequate knowledge and undesirable attitudes about the disorder were also present. Before considering the specific findings, we emphasize that the context of the study

Table 12.3: Comparison of Responses of Teachers Who Had or Did Not Have a Family Member (FM) or a Close Relative (CR) with Stuttering

	Number of Desirable Responses	Number of Neutral and Undesirable Responses	Total
Teachers who had a FM or a CR who stutters (n = 10)	99 71%	41 29%	140 100%
Teachers without a FM or a CR who stutters (n = 74)	653 63%	383 37%	1036 100%

Table 12.4: Comparison of Responses of Teachers Who Had Experience in Teaching Three or More Students with Stuttering and Those Who Had Less or No Experience with Stuttering Students

	Number of Desirable Responses	Number of Other Responses	Total
Teachers who taught ≥ 3 students with stuttering (n = 13)	129 71%	53 29%	182 100%
Teachers who taught ≤ 2 students with stuttering (n = 71)	623 63%	371 37%	994 100%

participants' background characteristics and working environment no doubt affected their knowledge and attitudes about stuttering. The study was conducted in an urban setting using an English-speaking study sample in a workplace with available resources on stuttering at the workplace, the Lyceum International School in Colombo. Thus, the sample by and large represents a relatively affluent group among the teacher population on the island.

A majority of teachers in the sample had access to some information about stuttering in the past. For example, 61% reported that they had read some information about stuttering. Further, a substantial number of teachers had received formal training covering the subject of stuttering or discussed stuttering with a subject specialist. It is unlikely that such resources are available to all teachers in general in Sri Lankan schools. Thus, the levels of agreements to statements may differ among those teachers.

This study also confirmed that many teachers had limited experience in teaching children who stutter. About 40% had never taught a single child with stuttering. One plausible reason for this observation is that nearly 60% of the sample had less than six years of total teaching experience. Another reason might be that some teachers were not sufficiently informed about stuttering to identify such students in their classrooms. Similarly, variability of responses was observed among different subgroups having different exposures to people who stutter. For example, previous experience in teaching children with stuttering was significantly associated with improved knowledge and desirable attitudes about stuttering, and a trend for improved knowledge and more desirable attitudes toward stuttering was associated with teachers who had family members or close relatives who stutter.

Since the same questionnaire was used in our study as by Pachigar et al. (2011), results of two studies were compared. A majority of both study populations had positive responses to many statements on the questionnaire. However, in contrast to our study, a majority of Indian teachers did not agree that the children with stuttering were quiet and shy. They also believed ridicule was a more common human reaction to stuttering. We also observed that the teachers' responses to children's stuttering in the Kuwaiti study (Abdalla & St. Louis, 2012) were quite compatible with those of the present study. It was interesting to observe many similarities in the responses given by teachers from the three different study populations.

Limitations and Conclusions

Generalization of the results from this study should be tempered by the following limitations. The sample size was respectable but not large. More importantly, the study sample was fully comprised of an urban population and the school was one of the best educational institutions in the country. Accordingly, the findings should not be generalized to the teacher population at large in Sri Lanka. It is believed that use of a mixed quantitative and qualitative research model would provide a broader and perhaps more accurate understanding of respondents' attitudes and stereotypes (Panico, Healey, Brouwer, & Susca, 2005).

In spite of these limitations, the information gathered from this study suggests that training programs designed to eliminate negative reactions and promote positive attitudes toward stuttering among teachers in Sri Lanka have the potential to help children who stutter. A logical next step would be to conduct in-depth interviews or focus group discussions to better understand what knowledge would contribute to more positive teacher attitudes. In this way, the training offered would involve collaborative efforts and be more likely to bring about the desired effect, namely, a change in attitudes and ultimately a change in classroom behavior toward the more helpful inclusion of stuttering children.

Acknowledgments

The authors thank all the study participants and the following resource people: Ms. T. Chilton (Speech and Language Therapist, UK), Dr. K. A. S. Jayawardena (Ministry of Health, Sri Lanka), and Mrs. K. Grero (Coordinating Principal, Lyceum International School, Sri Lanka), for their support and guidance.

Chapter 13

A Comparison of Stuttering Knowledge and Attitudes of Polish SLPs and SLP Students

Katarzyna Węsierska, Marta Węsierska
Kenneth O. St. Louis, Ann Beste-Guldborg

ABSTRACT

This study documented and compared attitudes and knowledge of Polish speech-language pathologists (SLPs) and SLP students toward stuttering and people who stutter, using a Polish version of the *Public Opinion Survey of Human Attributes–Stuttering* (*POSHA–S*). Overall, both groups showed similar profiles, but with a number of statistically significant differences. Common to other *POSHA–S* studies of SLPs, both groups in this study displayed more favorable attitudes and levels of knowledge about stuttering when compared to the *POSHA–S* database medians of numerous sample means. Still, a belief in the stuttering stereotype, a lack of knowledge about stuttering, and a general sense of discomfort remain.

Introduction

Stuttering is a communication disorder that affects between 1% and 5% of the population and can have a destructive impact on the quality of life of an individual (Bloodstein & Bernstein Ratner, 2008; Craig, 2010). Cross-cultural research shows an abundance of stigma and stereotypes toward both stuttering and people who stutter (Abdalla & St. Louis, 2012; Alghazo & Gaad, 2004; Boyle & Blood, Chapter 2; Heite, 2000; Ip, St. Louis, Myers, & An Xue, 2012; Özdemir, St. Louis, & Topbaş, 2011a; Pachigar, Stansfield, & Goldbart, 2011; St. Louis,

Filatova, Coşkun, Topbaş, Özdemir, Georgieva, McCaffrey, & George, 2011; St. Louis, Chapter 1; St. Louis & Roberts, 2010; Xing Ming, Jing, Yi Wen, & Van Borsel, 2001). Similar attitudes have been found in the general public of Poland, where a recent study found social exclusion and stigma are as likely toward Poles who stutter as among most other populations studied (Przepiórka, Błachnio, St. Louis, & Woźniak, 2013).

Speech-Language Pathologists' Views of Stuttering

Furthermore, researchers have found negative attitudes toward stuttering among speech-language pathologists (SLPs) (Cooper & Cooper, 1996; Crichton-Smith, Wright, & Stackhouse, 2003; Lass, Ruscello, Pannbacker, Schmitt, & Everly-Myers, 1989; Ragsdale & Ashby, 1982; Silverman, 1982; Woods & Williams, 1976) and speech-language pathology students (St. Louis & Lass, 1981; St. Louis, Przepiórka, Beste-Guldborg, Williams, Błachnio, Guendouzi, Reichel, & Ware, 2014). Early investigations indicated widespread negativity among SLPs toward stuttering, as well as a belief in the stuttering stereotype (Cooper & Rustin, 1985; Maviş, St. Louis, Özdemir, & Toğram, 2013; Turnbaugh, Guitar, & Hoffman, 1979; Yairi & Williams, 1970). In 1982, Ragsdale and Ashby concluded that the category of "stutterer" evoked negative feelings in clinicians. Negative attitudes are known to adversely influence the efficacy of stuttering treatment (Quesal, 2010; Yaruss, 2010), impact treatment outcomes (Andrews & Cutler, 1974; Guitar & Bass, 1978), and are predictive of treatment failure (De Nil & Brutten, 1991).

The treatment of stuttering is reportedly one of the least popular aspects of the SLP's job (St. Louis & Durrenberger, 1993), and many feel inept conducting therapy with people who stutter (Crichton-Smith et al., 2003). Among commonly cited explanations are that stuttering is difficult to treat and that experiences associated with it engender negative feelings (Brisk, Healey, & Hux, 1997; Cooper & Rustin, 1985; St. Louis & Durrenberger, 1993). Today, although improvements in SLP attitudes have been noted, a belief that stuttering is difficult to manage persists, as does the stuttering stereotype (Cooper & Cooper, 1996; Crichton-Smith et al., 2003). Two recent studies of Polish SLPs reported a lack of knowledge, experience, confidence, and perceived competency in working with people who stutter, as well as a reluctance to treat them (Tarkowski, 2005; Węsierska, 2012).

Purpose

Accordingly, to improve the therapeutic process and treatment outcomes for stuttering people in Poland, there is a need to better understand the knowledge and attitudes of both SLPs and SLP students toward stuttering. The primary aim of this study was to answer the question: Are there attitudinal and knowledge differences between the practicing SLPs and the professionals in training (students) in Poland with regard to stuttering and people who stutter? A secondary aim dealt with the question: Are stuttering attitudes of Polish SLPs and SLP students different from those of the general public?

Method

Survey Instrument

The *Public Opinion Survey of Human Attributes –Stuttering (POSHA–S)* was designed to provide a standard measure of public attitudes toward stuttering within the context of a variety of human attributes and conditions (St. Louis, 2012c). A Polish translated version of the *POSHA–S* was administered to measure Polish SLP and SLP student attitudes toward stuttering. Previous research has shown that the *POSHA–S* is translatable, reliable, valid, user-friendly, and efficient (St. Louis, 2005, 2012c; St. Louis, Lubker, Yaruss, & Aliveto, 2009; St. Louis, Reichel, Yaruss, & Lubker, 2009; St. Louis & Roberts, 2010; St. Louis, Williams, Ware, Guendouzi, & Reichel, 2014).

The *POSHA–S* is a questionnaire that asks respondents about beliefs and reactions related to stuttering. It begins with an extensive demographic section to categorize participants and then goes on to ask for information about stuttering. Respondents are asked about their knowledge of the disorder, and attitudes toward it, including behaviors they would exhibit during an interaction with a person who stutters. Additionally, it compares respondents' impressions and desire to stutter in relation to other "anchor" attributes, including intelligence, left-handedness, mental illness, and obesity. The instrument consists of closed questions and a rating scale that requires approximately 10 minutes to complete.

Participants

Potential participants were recruited through practicing SLPs and college lecturers from 10 Polish provinces at various workshops, conferences, and classes. Provinces included in the study were: Wielkopolskie, Małopolskie, Łódzkie, Mazowieckie, Opolskie, Podkarpackie, Pomorskie, Śląskie, Warmińsko-Mazurskie, Zachodniopomorskie. Figure 13.1 is a map of Poland with the included provinces highlighted. A cover letter explaining the study was given to all potential respondents. Those who chose to participate signed a consent form and were made aware of their right to refuse to answer any questions or withdraw from the study at any time without penalty. Participation was voluntary.

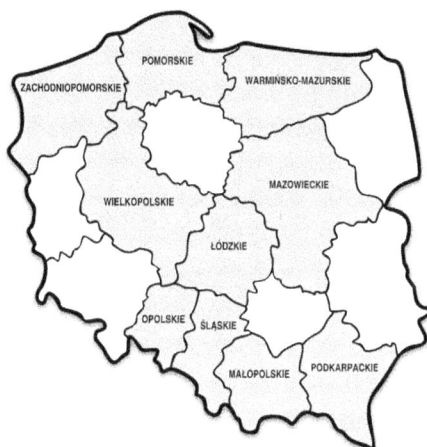

Figure 13.1: Polish provinces represented in the study.

Due to the long distances between sampling sites in Poland, other SLPs and lecturers assisted the researchers in data collection. These professionals were trained in research protection and process, as well as in survey-delivery methods. They were asked to follow strict written procedures to explain the research, ensure confidentiality, administer the survey, and to return completed questionnaires to the researchers.

A total of 543 participants thoroughly completed the survey: 188 SLPs and 355 SLP students. The participants were almost exclusively female (98% of the SLPs and 99% of the students) with a mean age of 39.5 years for the SLPs and 30.8 years for the SLP students. The mean number of years of education was 17.9 for the SLPs and 16.6 for the students. The student group contained mostly postgraduate diploma students who had already obtained a master's degree in linguistics, pedagogy, or psychology. This accounted for the relatively low age and educational discrepancy between the students and SLPs. Most respondents were married (74% of the SLPs and 54% of the SLP students) and currently employed (99% of the SLPs and 76% of the students). The SLPs worked in a variety of professional settings, including education, health service, and private practice. More SLPs described themselves as parents than did SLP students (71% versus 46%). Virtually none reported themselves as a person who stutters (0% of SLPs and <1% of SLP students), and less than one-third of the respondents knew someone who stuttered (15% of SLPs and 32% of SLP students). The participants represented both urban and rural areas of Poland. Figure 13.2 provides selected *POSHA–S* demographic information for the SLP and SLP student samples (St. Louis, 2012c).

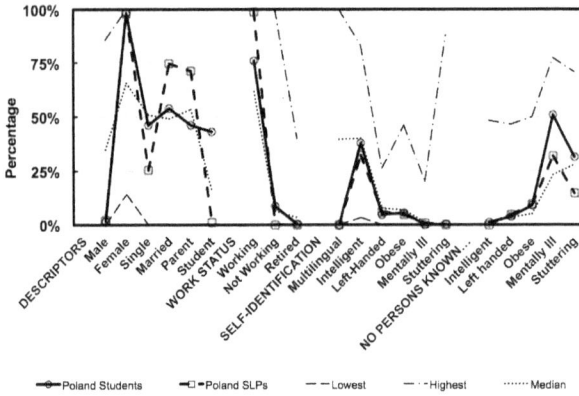

Figure 13. 2: Demographic results summarizing percentages of SLPs and SLP students according to sex, marital/parental/work status, and self identification of—or familiarity with—five human attributes.

Data Analysis

Data were compiled and converted to a -100 to +100 scale (0 = neutral), then analyzed according to *POSHA–S* guidelines (St. Louis, 2012c). Responses were clustered and averaged into components and subscores, two reflecting stuttering and one measuring obesity and mental illness. Both the Beliefs about People Who Stutter (BEL) and Self Reactions to Stuttering (SR) subscores were averaged to determine an Overall Stuttering Score (OSS) for the SLPs and the SLP students. Similarly, the *POSHA–S* subscore for Obesity/Mental Illness (O/MI) was calculated. Results were then analyzed for significance with the use of independent *t*-tests using Bonferroni correction p ≤.00417. Cohen's *d* effect sizes were calculated for significant differences (Cohen, 1988).

Results

Of the 60 standard *POSHA–S* rating comparisons (including items, components, subscores, and OSS), 17 of the *t*-tests (28%) were statistically significant between the SLPs and SLP students. Cohen's *d* effect sizes ranged from .26 "small" to .63 "moderate" with a mean of .41 "moderate." This, according to St. Louis (2012c), reflects a substantial difference between the two samples.

Figure 13.3 represents mean converted *POSHA–S* component scores, subscores, and Overall Stuttering Scores (OSS) for both the SLP group and the SLP student group in comparison with the highest, lowest, and median sample means

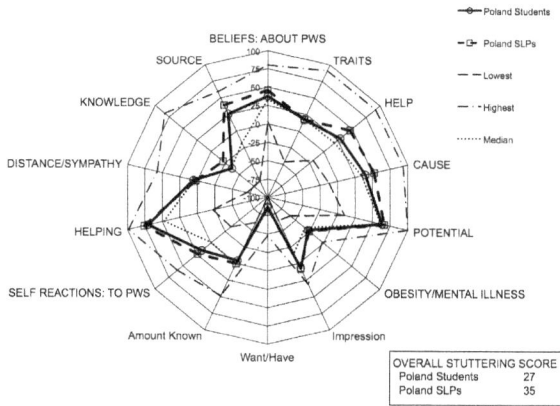

Figure 13.3: *POSHA–S* Summary graph for the SLPs and SLP students, showing component scores, subscores, and Overall Stuttering Scores.

in the *POSHA–S* database representing 188 samples from 8,144 respondents (circa July 2013). Points closer to the periphery indicate more positive and accurate perceptions while those closer to the center reflect more negative and inaccurate responses (St. Louis, 2011a). Visually, the profiles are similar with the SLP group showing slightly higher (more positive) scores than the SLP student group across most *POSHA–S* categories (SLPs: OSS [+35], BEL [+46], SR [+24], and O/MI [-26]; SLP students: OSS [+27], BEL [+37], SR [+16], and O/MI [-28]). Consistent with other *POSHA–S* studies of SLPs and SLP students (Gottwald, Warner, Hartley, Fraas, Hawver, & St. Louis, 2011; St. Louis et al., 2014), the Polish SLPs and students had mean ratings slightly to somewhat higher than average ratings compared to more than 180 *POSHA–S* database samples around the world. Overall Stuttering Scores (OSS) for both groups were moderately positive with Belief Scores (BEL) much higher than Self Reaction Scores (SR), a consistent phenomenon across all *POSHA–S* studies. The Obesity/Mental Illness subscore was quite low for both groups, another common finding among *POSHA–S* studies.

Figure 13.4 presents typical profiles (presented in mean ratings) for the five attributes in the general section of the *POSHA–S* (St. Louis, 2012c). As above, the profiles were very similar between the two groups. Visibly the SLPs and SLP students had better impressions of stuttering (SLPs = +36, SLP students = +27) than mental illness (SLPs = +8, SLP students = -2) or obesity (SLPs = +6, SLP students +16). When asked whether they would want to be someone who stutters, both the SLPs and SLP students responded quite negatively (-65, -70, respectively), but better than when asked if they would want to be mentally ill (-87, -90) or

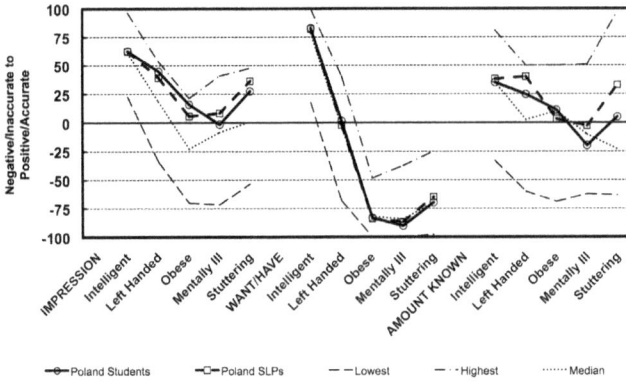

Figure 13.4: Mean *POSHA–S* general section results for SLPs and SLP students, including components contributing to the Obesity/Mental Illness subscore.

obese (-84, -83). Finally, when asked to rate the amount known about stuttering, not surprisingly, SLPs knew significantly more than SLP students (SLPs = +33, SLP students = 5).

Figure 13.5 displays mean scores for all the items and the four component scores that make up the *POSHA–S* Belief subscore (BEL). SLPs had more positive overall beliefs (+46) about stuttering than SLP students (+37). Examination of the trait component score indicated a general understanding among both groups that people who stutter are not to blame for their condition (SLPs = +97, SLP students = +96); however, a belief in the stuttering stereotype was evident by neutral to inaccurate responses to the questions: people who stutter are nervous or excitable (+2, +11) and shy or fearful (-46, -54).

Both SLPs and SLP students understood that speech-language pathologists (+99, +98, respectively) could help with stuttering. There was less agreement on whether a person who stutters could be of assistance, with SLPs (+69) having a more accurate understanding than SLP students (+29). When asked about the cause of stuttering, SLPs seemed to have more accurate knowledge than SLP students (+52, +40). Significant differences existed between the groups in response to genetic factors (+67, +41) and rejecting virus/disease (+67, +38) as causes of stuttering.

Finally, both groups were asked about the potential of people who stutter, and results were positive (SLPs = +67, SLP students = +63). There was a belief that people who stutter could make friends (+99, +98, respectively) and lead a normal life (+97 for both), but less certainty about people who stutter holding

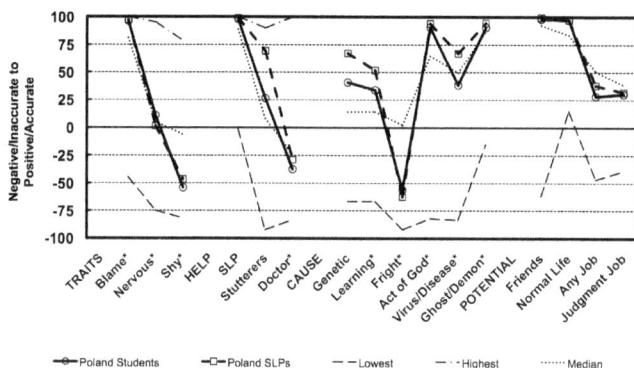

Figure 13.5: Mean item and component scores contributing to the *POSHA–S* Beliefs about People Who Stutter subscore (BEL) for SLPs and SLP students.

"any job" they want (+38, +28) or one that requires judgment or decision-making (+32, +30).

Figure 13.6 shows similar mean scores for all the items and the four component scores that make up the *POSHA–S* Self Reaction Subscore (SR). Comparable to all previous *POSHA–S* studies, Self Reaction subscores were less positive than Belief subscores for both SLPs (+24) and SLP students (+16). Both groups showed good understanding of how to help a person who stutters (SLPs = +76, SLP students = +70), but still felt they would tell a person who was stuttering to "slow down" or "relax" (+27, +10, respectively). Even though both groups had lower scores on this item, there was a trend for the SLP group to score higher.

When asked about their feelings regarding interactions with people who stutter, both groups exhibited neutral scores (SLPs = +2, SLP students = +5). There was a general feeling of discomfort and worry regarding the disorder as evidenced by responses to comfort level when interacting with a stuttering individual (-31, -41, respectively), as well as a sense of apprehension if they themselves (-80, -76) or a sibling began to stutter (-63, -45). In addition, the amount of knowledge reported by the SLPs and SLP students in this sample was low (-21, -37). Neither group reported much experience with (-86, -89) or knowledge about stuttering (-10, -27). Finally, the sources of information about stuttering that SLPs and SLP students reported were varied with printed material (+88, +52), the Internet (+68, +39), and school (+31, +50) being the biggest sources of information for both groups. Interestingly, specialists were not highly reported as a source of information about stuttering by either Polish SLPs or SLP students (+3, +24).

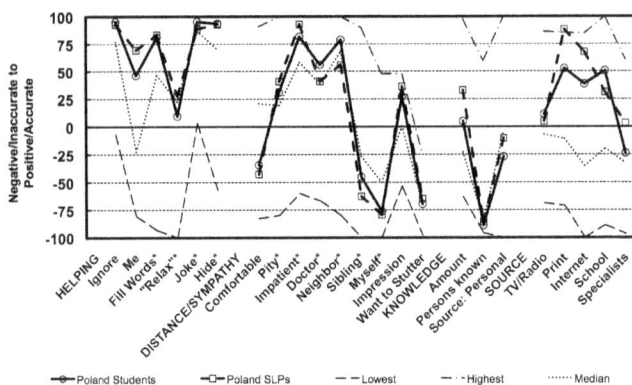

Figure 13.6: Mean item and component scores contributing to the *POSHA–S* Self Reactions to People Who Stutter subscore (SR) for SLPs and SLP students.

Discussion and Conclusion

Compared to the *POSHA–S* database median values of more than 180 sample means, speech-language pathologists and SLP students in this sample had higher-than-average ratings that reflect more favorable attitudes and higher levels of knowledge, a finding seen in all *POSHA–S* studies of comparable groups (Gottwald, et al., 2011; St. Louis et al., 2014). Similarly, both Polish SLPs and SLP students on average scored higher than the Polish general public (Przepiórka et al., 2013). Not surprisingly, the primary finding in this study was for SLPs to have greater and more accurate knowledge of stuttering than students preparing to become speech-language pathologists.

Even though respondents in this study have higher *POSHA–S* scores than the general public, some areas of concern remain. There is still at least a modest belief in the stuttering stereotype by SLPs and SLP students. Both groups reported with commonality that people who stutter are nervous, shy, and fearful. This finding corroborates recent research that, while attitudes about stuttering and people who stutter may be shifting positively over time, negative or stigmatizing attitudes still exist and more work must be done (Abdalla & St. Louis, 2012; Cooper & Cooper, 1996; Crichton-Smith et al., 2003). In addition, the reported lack of knowledge about stuttering and experience with people who stutter by SLPs and SLP students is disturbing. Not only does it stand to reason that professionals who treat stuttering people should have the most current and accurate knowledge available, studies indicate that familiarity with people who stutter can have a positive impact on attitudes toward stuttering (Gabel, Hughes, Forney, 2011; Gabel, Schlagheck, Eyestone, & Emch, 2006; Klassen, 2001).

Certain cautions are in order. First, the convenience sampling strategy used in this study did not reach all provinces of Poland. Therefore, despite the fact that the sampling represented widely distant areas of the country, an argument could be made that the results may not be generalizable to the entire population of SLPs and SLP students in Poland. Second, the danger in any questionnaire, and especially in one involving students, is that participants may give socially acceptable responses rather than admit to their actual beliefs. Speech-language pathologists and students of speech-language pathology may have felt that reporting negative attitudes toward people who stutter or stuttering would be unacceptable for their profession. Still, the results of this study are comparable to others carried out with the *POSHA–S* and thus can be seen as informative to the professional body. Continued educational opportunities to enhance the knowledge, skills, and attitudes of SLPs and SLP students are warranted. Future studies should focus on effective ways to improve attitudes especially with regard to the stuttering stereotype.

Acknowledgments

The Polish translation was made available by Aneta Przepiórka and Agata Błachnio. The authors would also like to thank colleagues who supported the researchers in the process of data collection.

Chapter 14

Effects of Fluency Disorders Coursework on Students' Stuttering Attitudes in Two Countries

Lejla Junuzović-Žunić, Mary E. Weidner, Isabella K. Reichel, Susanne Cook, Kenneth O. St. Louis, Mercedes B. Ware

ABSTRACT

Previous research has shown that attitudes toward stuttering are amenable to change, but not always in the desired direction. There have been several calls to address speech-language pathology students' stuttering attitudes during their academic training to mitigate any potentially stereotypic behavior or biases that would interfere in their future work with people who stutter.

The primary aims of this study were: (1) to investigate the impact of fluency disorders coursework on the attitudes toward stuttering of students in a variety of settings in the United States (U.S.) and Bosnia and Herzegovina (B & H) and (2) to compare student stuttering attitudes cross-culturally. Students' stuttering attitudes were investigated before and after participation in a fluency disorders course using the *Public Opinion Survey on Human Attributes-Stuttering (POSHA–S)*. The classes were half of an undergraduate fluency disorders course in the United States, several similar graduate fluency disorders classes in the United States, and an undergraduate fluency disorders class in B & H. The length and specific content of the coursework varied widely. Students' attitudes in all three classes improved similarly following participation in fluency disorders coursework as measured by the *POSHA–S* Overall Stuttering Scores. Pre versus Post results of each class reached statistically significant levels from 7% to 13% of the *POSHA–S* ratings. Depending on the coursework and setting, either students' Self Reactions, Beliefs, or both were notably amenable to change following the coursework.

Introduction

Several studies have reported that speech-language pathologists may hold negative attitudes toward stuttering and frequently identify stuttering as one of the most challenging disorders to treat (e.g., St. Louis & Durrenberger, 1993). Some reasons for this may be their discomfort with addressing the affective components of stuttering (Manning, 2001; Shapiro, 1999) and their limited exposure to people who stutter during their academic and clinical training (Murphy & Quesal, 2004). Lass, Ruscello, Pannbacker, Schmitt, and Everly-Myers (1989) found that speech-language pathologists (SLPs) generated a higher percentage of negative adjectives than positive or neutral to describe stutterers. Among the most frequent negative adjectives were: shy, nervous, and frustrated. From a decade-long series of studies, Cooper and Cooper (1996) found that although SLPs indicated some improvement in the overall beliefs about stuttering and stutterers, evidence of negative attitudes toward stuttering remained.

As with practicing clinicians, negative stuttering attitudes and misconceptions among SLP students have also been reported. St. Louis and Lass (1981) reported that a majority of students perceived stutterers to have underlying psychological problems such as difficulty with relationships and feelings of inferiority. University students who were not in speech-language pathology, surveyed by Betz, Blood, and Blood (2008), rated their perceptions of a hypothetical preschool child uniformly more negatively (i.e., more guarded, nervous, and tense) when the child was identified as stuttering versus when not so identified. On a self-report scale, SLP graduate students felt that watching a video of stuttered speech was more unpleasant and uncomfortable, with feelings of embarrassment and emotional arousal, compared to watching fluent speech (Guntupalli, Nanjundeswaran, Dayalu, & Kalinowski, 2012). Guntupalli et al. went further to measure physiological responses and showed that the students demonstrated measureable, visceral reactions during the stuttering viewing experience. Specifically, they showed increased skin conductance responses and acceleration in heart rate when viewing severe stuttered speech samples versus fluent speech samples.

It has been suggested that increased knowledge and exposure to stuttering may have a positive effect on students' understanding of the multifactorial nature of stuttering, as well as their stuttering attitudes (Hughes, Gabel, Roseman, & Daniels, Chapter 15; Klein & Amster, 2010; Lees & Stewart, 2001).

In a study of high school students, Flynn and St. Louis (2011) found that adolescents' attitudes toward stuttering changed positively on the *Public Opinion Survey on Human Attributes–Stuttering* (*POSHA–S*) after watching a professionally prepared video for teens (MTV *True Life®: I Stutter*) but improved even more following an oral presentation by one of the featured people from the episode who stuttered moderately to severely in the presentation. With a modified and Arabic version of the *POSHA–S*, Abdalla and St. Louis (2014) found that stuttering attitudes of students in teacher training programs improved following an educational video on stuttering, but practicing teachers maintained their negative pre-intervention attitudes. Their findings are consistent with those of Gottwald, Warner, Hartley, Fraas, Hawver, and St. Louis (2011) and Gottwald, Kent, St. Louis, and Hartley (2014), who found watching a video about the personal experiences of stutterers positively improved attitudes of respondents who had limited personal experience with—or knowledge about—stuttering. It must be noted that not all studies attempting to improve attitudes, especially with adolescents, have resulted in expected results (see Abdalla, Chapter 5). Recently, St. Louis, Przepiórka, Beste-Guldborg, Williams, Błachnio, Guendouzi, Reichel, and Ware (2014) demonstrated that undergraduate and graduate SLP students hold more positive *POSHA–S* measured attitudes toward stuttering than students in other majors. The authors attributed the better attitudes to a "halo effect" related to wishing, planning, or otherwise preparing for a career in speech-language pathology. Similarly, practicing SLPs have also been found to hold relatively high stuttering attitudes prior to a program aimed to improve their attitudes (Gottwald et al., 2011).

The findings from these studies are particularly important because they suggest that stuttering attitudes may be improved by increased knowledge and exposure to stuttering and may be mitigated during training programs. However, because different interventions and measurement tools were used to examine attitudinal change in different populations, judgments and comparisons related to the efficacy of each approach cannot be ascertained. As such, there is a need to closely examine the impact of various intervention approaches using one standardized measurement tool in different populations.

Informed by the results of the aforementioned studies, it was hypothesized that one potential way to improve stuttering attitudes in SLP students is participation in a fluency disorders course that clearly aims to increase stuttering knowledge, including understanding and appreciating the personal experience of stuttering. Instructors in the area of fluency disorders are challenged with the task of teaching students the theoretical underpinnings of the disorder, as well as adequately preparing them to work clinically with people who stutter.

Curriculum development in the United States is, by necessity, guided by American Speech-Language-Hearing Association (ASHA) standards that mandate providing students with a comprehensive understanding of—and exposure to—stuttering. Addressing negative stuttering attitudes in training programs might better equip students with the knowledge and skills to treat clients who stutter. Doing so in the long term could be expected eventually to dilute negative stuttering attitudes among practicing SLPs.

For this study, the impact of curriculum instruction as measured before and after either a graduate level or undergraduate level fluency disorders class using the *POSHA–S* was investigated. Three different fluency courses conducted by different instructors at different universities, two in the United States and one in Bosnia and Herzegovina (B & H), were targeted in order to provide a comprehensive and global understanding of the impact of fluency disorders–related coursework on students' stuttering attitudes. The study addressed the research question: Can SLP student attitudes be improved by participation in fluency disorders coursework at the undergraduate or graduate level in a wide variety of educational settings?

Method

Measurement Instrument

The Public Opinion Survey on Human Attributes (*POSHA–S*) (St. Louis, 2011a) was selected to measure attitudes toward stuttering before and after a stuttering coursework because it provides accurate comparisons among geographically and culturally diverse groups, as well as among people who speak different languages (e.g., Abdalla & St. Louis, 2012, 2014; Boltužić, Jelčić Jakšić, & St. Louis, 2013; Ip, St. Louis, Myers, & An Xue, 2012; Przepiórka, Błachnio, St. Louis, & Wozniak, 2013; St. Louis & Roberts, 2010). As such, the results of this study could be used to critically evaluate the effectiveness of fluency coursework in the process of stuttering attitude change. For the B & H class, the *POSHA–S* was translated into the Bosnian-Herzegovinian national languages, Bosnian, Croatian, or Serbian, which are similar but with different names and different standards. Respondents completed either paper-and-pencil or online versions of the instrument. Paired *t*-tests were conducted for all within-group *POSHA–S* items, including subscores and Overall Stuttering Score using a Bonferroni correction of $p \leq .05/12$ or $.00417$ to reduce the likelihood of both Type I and Type II errors. Cohen's *d* effect sizes were determined for differences that were statistically significant.

Participants and Procedure for Each Sample

BOSNIA AND HERZEGOVINA UNDERGRADUATE. Table 14.1 provides a summary of selected demographic information and compares the data to the *POSHA–S* database. Students in the B & H sample consisted of 27 fourth-year undergraduate speech-language pathology and audiology majors at the University of Tuzla. They were sampled before any fluency disorders coursework (Pre) and after a basic course (Post 1) and again after a more advanced course (Post 2), all on paper-and-pencil *POSHA–S*s that were handed out in class. Students were instructed to use anonymous codes recorded on cards they kept to assure anonymity. The students' mean age was 22.9 years, and they had a mean of 16.5 years of schooling at the time of the pre-test. All students (96% female and 4% male) self-identified as Caucasian and were predominantly Muslim (70%), but with 7% Christian (evenly split between Catholic and Orthodox). All of them listed single or combinations of Bosnian, Serbian, or Croatian as their native language, and two-thirds reported knowing at least one other language. Their incomes relative to their own families and friends, as well as to all the people in their country, were below average (i.e., -20 compared to a median sample value of 1 on a -100 to +100 scale in the *POSHA–S* database).

The students' stuttering attitudes were measured on three occasions: (1) prior to Fluency Disorders I, a course that covered stuttering theories, facts, and assessment; (2) following completion of Fluency Disorders I; and (3) following Fluency Disorders II, a course that focused exclusively on stuttering therapy. Both courses were taught by the first author. As noted, paired *t*-tests were run for Pre and Post analyses between the three comparisons: Pre versus Post 1, Pre versus Post 2, and Post 1 versus Post 2.

U.S. UNDERGRADUATE. Participants in the U.S. undergraduate sample consisted of fourth- or senior-year undergraduate speech-language pathology and audiology students from West Virginia University in their final semester. They responded to non-mandatory invitations to fill out the *POSHA–S* online on three occasions: (1) three months before the coursework (Pre 1), (2) immediately before the coursework (Pre 2), and (3) immediately after it (Post) eight weeks later. Anonymity was assured by the use of special questions at the end, e.g., "What was the name of your first elementary school?" Although 19 of 45 students filled out the Pre 1 survey, 29 filled out the Pre 2 survey, and 22 filled out the Post Survey, only 13 students filled out all three versions. The results from the latter group only are reported here. Their mean age was 21.5 years and they had 15.9 mean years of schooling at the time of the initial pre-survey.

Table 14.1: Demographic Characteristics of B & H, WV, and NYC Respondents, as well as Median Values from the *POSHA–S* Database Samples (205 Samples circa March 2014 Reflecting *POSHA–S* Administrations for 9,294 Respondents)

POSHA–S Variable	B & H Pre	B & H Post 1	B & H Post 2	WV Pre 1	WV Pre 2	WV Post	NYC Pre	NYC Post	POSHA–S Database Median
Number in sample	27	27	27	13	13	13	86	86	55
Age (year)	22.9	23.2	23.6	21.5	21.9	22.0	27.1	27.3	35.6
Education (year)	16.5	16.5	16.5	15.9	15.8	16.2	17.7	17.7	14.7
Student/Working (%)	100/0	100/0	100/0	100/31	100/46	100/46	98/57	91/62	17/61
Married/Parent (%)	11/0	11/0	11/0	0/0	0/0	0/0	44/5	44/5	49/48
Income Score (-100 to +100)	-20	-11	-16	19	10	23	-2	-17	1
Sex (Male/Female) (%)	4/96			0/100			6/94		34/66
Race (Caucasian/ Hispanic/African American/Asian) (%)	100/0/0/0			100/0/0/0			79/15/4/2		—
Religion (Christian/ Jewish/Muslim/ Other) (%)	26/0/70/4			100/0/0/0			30/66/0/4		—
English as native language (%)	—			100			73		—
Bosnian, Serbian, or Croatian language (%)	100			—			—		—
Self Identification (%)									
Multilingual	67	63	63	8	8	0	69	67	39
Stuttering	0	0	0	0	0	0	0	0	0
Mentally ill	0	0	0	0	0	0	1	1	1
Obese	0	0	0	0	0	0	7	9	7
No People Known (%)									
Stuttering	11	7	4	15	38	15	19	17	30
Mentally ill	15	26	22	31	8	8	40	35	23
Obese	0	4	0	0	0	0	2	1	5
Completion time (minutes)	9.7	9.6	7.0	11.7	11.2	14.2	15.1	16.1	11.0

All of them reported being unmarried, Caucasian, Christian, and native English speakers. Only two (8%) reported knowing another language, and, compared to the *POSHA–S* database median, their relative incomes were above average. The undergraduate fluency disorders coursework occurred during the first half of a required course taught by the fifth author. The eight-week stuttering component focused on stuttering theories, facts, personal experiences of stutterers, and an overview of stuttering assessment and treatment. The second half, which followed the post-coursework *POSHA–S*, was devoted to voice disorders.

U.S. GRADUATE. Graduate student participants in the United States consisted of 86 speech-language pathology students enrolled in six different required graduate-level fluency disorders courses—four courses were conducted at Long Island University and one each at Lehman College and Touro College—all in metropolitan New York City. All the courses were taught by the third author, and the sampling consisted of handing out paper-and-pencil versions of the *POSHA–S* on (1) the first day (Pre) and (2) the last day (Post) of each course, coded for anonymity. A longer experimental version of the *POSHA–S* was used at Long Island University and Lehman College, and the final *POSHA–S* was used at Touro College. A total of 161 students were enrolled in the classes, but 86 were available for pre- and post-survey comparisons, primarily due to loss of post-survey data for the Touro College class of 67 students, which required online follow-up surveys that were completed by only 17 of them. The sample of 86 students (94% female and 6% male) had a mean age of 27.1, and 17.7 years of schooling at the time of the pre-survey. Of these students, 44% were married, and 5% were parents. Most (79%) were Caucasian; the rest were Hispanic, African American, or Asian. Two-thirds (66%) were Jewish, and 30% were Christian. Seventy-three percent listed English as their native language, with nearly 70% indicating they spoke more than one language. The graduate courses focused on standard advanced stuttering knowledge related to assessment and treatment. Most, but not all, of these courses also integrated research in the form of specially designed curricula and laboratory experiences with people who stutter that focused on relevant aspects of allied fields, such as emotional intelligence, mindfulness, stigma, counseling, and cultural awareness, described in detail by Reichel and St. Louis (2004, 2007, 2011). None or virtually none of the U.S. graduate students in these three samples reported stuttering or being mentally ill, and only 7–9% of them reported being obese.

232

Results

Table 14.2 shows mean results of each *POSHA–S* item, component, subscore, and Overall Stuttering Score (OSS) for each of the three groups in each pre- or post-coursework condition. We ran paired *t*-tests between Pre and Post responses for each sample. Additionally, we compared the Post 1 versus Post 2 for the B & H sample and Pre 1 versus Pre 2 for the West Virginia (WV) sample; none of these comparisons was statistically significant. In fact, relatively few Pre versus Post comparisons were statistically significant using the conservative Bonferroni correction ($p \leq .00417$), due principally to the small sample sizes for B & H and WV. Shaded mean ratings in Table 14.2 show these significant differences, all between some combination of Pre versus Post. Of the 60 possible *POSHA–S* ratings, 7% were significant between Pre versus Post 1 for B & H, with Cohen's *d* effect sizes between .86 and 1.44 or "very large." Eleven percent were significant between the B & H Pre versus Post 2 ratings (d = .86 to 1.99; "very large"). The WV undergraduate sample comparisons were: Pre 1 versus Post—8% significant (d = 1.32 to 1.82; "very large") and Pre 2 versus Post—6% significant (d = 1.47 to 2.63; "very large"). Thirteen percent of the U.S. graduate (NYC) sample Pre versus Post comparisons were significant (d = .52 to 1.09; "moderate to very large").

The radial graphs in figures 14.1 to 14.3 represent the *POSHA–S* components, subscores, and Overall Stuttering Scores for each sample. The graph is arranged so that more positive ("better") attitudes are closer to the periphery and less positive ("worse") attitudes closer to the center.

Given the variability in the coursework (instructors, content, level, and auxiliary material), as well as differences in sampling procedures (invited with no expectation of responding versus handed out in class), we analyzed results only between conditions *within* each of the three sample groups. We did not compare one sample to another except in terms of subscores and OSSs.

BOSNIA AND HERZEGOVINA UNDERGRADUATE. Figure 14.1 illustrates that undergraduate B & H students demonstrated consistent improvement in stuttering attitudes over the duration of their fluency coursework for a majority of component scores and the OSS. Specifically, improvement was noted from Pre scores (i.e., prior to any fluency coursework) to Post 1 scores (i.e., following Fluency 1), and an additional improvement to Post 2 scores (i.e., following Fluency 2) for the following components: Helped by (whom), Accommodating/Helping (a stuttering person), Knowledge/Experience (about stuttering), and Knowledge Source. There was marginal improvement for the Beliefs subscore (3 units) but marked improvement for the Self Reactions subscore (12–20 units).

Table 14.2: *POSHA–S* Mean Ratings of B & H, WV, and NYC Respondents as well as Median Values from the *POSHA–S* Database Samples (205 Samples circa March 2014 Reflecting *POSHA–S* Administrations for 9,294 Respondents) (Significant Differences Between Pre versus Post Ratings Are Shaded)

POSHA–S Variable	B & H Pre	B & H Post 1	B & H Post 2	WV Pre 1	WV Pre 2	WV Post	NYC Pre	NYC Post	*POSHA–S* Database Median
OVERALL STUTTERING SCORE	25	33	37	31	32	46	9	20	17
Beliefs About People Who Stutter	29	32	32	60	60	77	33	37	34
Traits/Personality	-10	-26	-28	28	33	46	10	13	18
Have themselves to blame[a]	-7	-44	-42	100	100	92	100	75	83
Nervous or excitable[a]	37	22	26	-8	15	23	-23	-5	6
Shy or fearful[a]	-59	-56	-67	-8	-17	23	-46	-32	-7
Stuttering Should Be Helped by:	34	48	53	69	64	92	54	58	19
Speech and language therapist	100	100	100	100	100	100	95	98	89
Other people who stutter	-36	-7	8	31	23	85	23	35	11
Medical doctor[a]	38	52	52	75	69	92	44	43	-25
Stuttering Is Caused by:	29	53	43	50	51	73	40	37	34
Genetic inheritance	-8	56	44	-31	-38	69	43	48	15
Learning or habits[a]	36	59	48	23	31	75	8	2	15
A very frightening event[a]	-54	-27	-33	62	38	38	-21	-21	-1
An act of God[a]	33	37	8	46	77	54	27	21	65
A virus or disease[a]	77	96	88	100	100	100	83	79	50
Ghosts, demons, spirits[a]	92	96	100	100	100	100	99	92	87
Potential	62	54	58	92	92	98	28	38	62
Can make friends	93	93	93	100	100	100	-30	-23	93
Can lead normal lives	85	85	89	100	100	100	69	75	85
Can do any job they want	19	0	7	92	100	100	39	58	50
Should have jobs requiring good judgment	50	37	44	77	69	92	35	44	37

CONTINUED

Table 14.2 *continued*: *POSHA–S* Mean Ratings of B & H, WV, and NYC Respondents as well as Median Values from the *POSHA–S* Database Samples (205 Samples circa March 2014 Reflecting *POSHA–S* Administrations for 9,294 Respondents) (Significant Differences Between Pre versus Post Ratings Are Shaded)

POSHA–S Variable	B & H Pre	B & H Post 1	B & H Post 2	WV Pre 1	WV Pre 2	WV Post	NYC Pre	NYC Post	POSHA–S Database Median
Self Reactions to People Who Stutter	22	34	42	1	4	16	-15	3	0
Accommodating/Helping	56	80	88	70	69	83	50	69	47
Try to act like the person was talking normally	78	93	89	100	92	100	43	42	77
Person like me	52	85	92	8	23	31	29	82	-22
Fill in the person's words[a]	70	85	100	92	75	92	42	73	46
Tell the person to "slow down" or "relax"[a]	-52	26	56	46	62	92	33	56	22
Make joke about stuttering[a]	89	96	100	100	100	100	94	87	88
Should try to hide their stuttering[a]	96	96	93	77	62	85	61	77	70
Social Distance/Sympathy	16	8	19	14	3	16	-23	-10	5
Feel comfortable or relaxed	81	81	93	31	8	54	-13	8	19
Feel pity[a]	100	100	100	-25	-33	0	-9	14	19
Feel impatient (not want to wait while the person stutters)[a]	100	100	100	46	38	58	50	61	58
Concern about my doctor[a]	44	19	15	62	100	92	5	21	39
Concern about my neighbor[a]	15	-15	0	85	100	100	31	32	69
Concern about my brother or sister[a]	-70	-70	-48	31	-8	-8	-84	-76	-24
Concern about me[a]	-70	-93	-63	-31	-92	-77	-90	-84	-51
Impression of person who stutters	28	33	41	15	8	8	-1	15	2
Want to have stuttering	-88	-81	-69	-85	-92	-85	-92	-84	-70
Knowledge/Experience	-27	-14	-8	-44	-48	-29	-60	-45	-36

Table 14.2 *continued*: *POSHA–S* Mean Ratings of B & H, WV, and NYC Respondents as well as Median Values from the *POSHA–S* Database Samples (205 Samples circa March 2014 Reflecting *POSHA–S* Administrations for 9,294 Respondents) (Significant Differences Between Pre versus Post Ratings Are Shaded)

POSHA–S Variable	B & H Pre	B & H Post 1	B & H Post 2	WV Pre 1	WV Pre 2	WV Post	NYC Pre	NYC Post	POSHA–S Database Median
Amount known about stuttering	2	52	70	-19	-35	50	-21	29	-23
People who stutter known	-86	-85	-87	-81	-86	-84	-86	-84	-86
Personal experience (me, my family, friends)	4	-8	-8	-31	-23	-54	-73	-81	-1
Knowledge Source	42	59	68	-35	-6	-8	-30	0	-15
Television, radio, films	26	30	50	-54	8	-54	-52	-42	-5
Magazines, newspapers, books	56	85	92	-69	-38	-8	-17	10	-12
Internet	58	85	93	-100	-31	-69	-44	8	-35
School	46	100	100	69	85	100	20	56	-15
Doctors, nurses, other specialists	23	-4	4	-23	-54	-8	-56	-32	-33
Obesity/Mental Illness Subscore	-21	-20	-8	-40	-47	-44	-37	-29	-34
Overall Impression	14	7	23	-10	-29	-33	-18	-7	-15
Obese	-88	-78	-76	-96	-100	-100	-96	-92	-83
Mentally ill	26	15	31	15	-15	-31	-17	-6	-9
Want to be	-87	-81	-75	-96	-100	-100	-97	-95	-84
Obese	-88	-78	-76	-96	-100	-100	-96	-92	-83
Mentally ill	-85	-83	-74	-96	-100	-100	-97	-98	-85
Amount Known about	11	15	29	-13	-12	2	3	14	0
Obese	11	7	13	-4	-12	8	16	20	10
Mentally ill	11	22	44	-23	-12	-4	-11	8	-10

[a]The signs of the mean ratings for this item are reversed so that higher scores reflect "better" attitudes and lower scores "worse" attitudes.

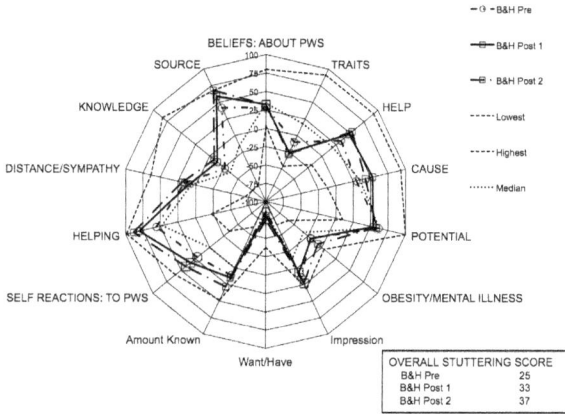

Figure 14.1: *POSHA–S* components, subscores, and Overall Stuttering Scores for B & H comparisons (before coursework, after the first undergraduate fluency disorders course, and after the second undergraduate fluency disorders course).

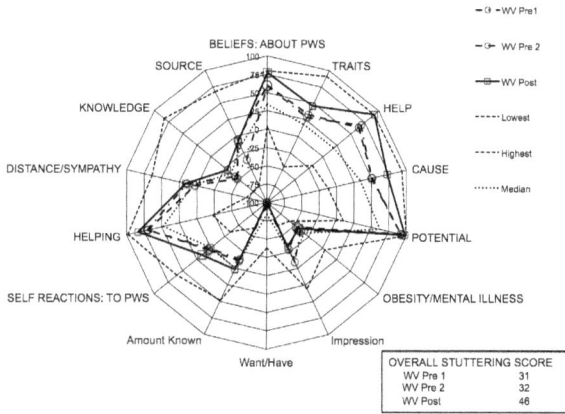

Figure 14.2: *POSHA–S* components, subscores, and Overall Stuttering Scores for WV comparisons (three months before coursework, immediately before undergraduate coursework, and after the eight weeks of fluency disorders coursework).

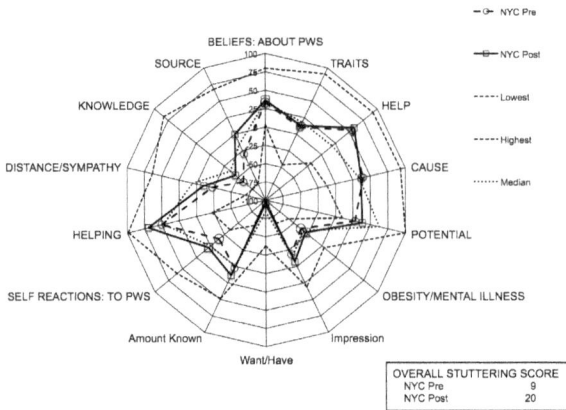

Figure 14.3: *POSHA–S* components, subscores, and Overall Stuttering Scores for NYC comparisons (before graduate fluency disorders courses and after the one-semester courses).

Overall Stuttering Scores increased by 8 units from 25 to 33 (Pre to Post 1), and another 5 units from 33 to 37 (Post 1 to Post 2). Overall results indicate modest attitudinal changes after completion of Fluency 1, which were further improved after clinical exposure and experience in the Fluency 2 course. As noted, none of these latter improvements was significantly different.

U.S. UNDERGRADUATE. As expected, there was virtually no change between Pre 1 and Pre 2 *POSHA–S* scores following a three-month period during which time no stuttering training was provided. By contrast, Figure 14.2 illustrates a substantial improvement in Post scores following eight weeks of undergraduate fluency coursework. Improvement between Pre 2 and Post scores was noted for the following components: Traits/Personality, Helped by, Causes, Potential, Accommodating/Helping, Social Distance/Sympathy, and Knowledge/Experience. Both stuttering subscores improved, Beliefs by 14–15 units and Self Reactions by 12–15 units.

Overall Stuttering Scores increased by only 1 unit from 31 to 32 (Pre 1 to Pre 2), but improved by 14 units from 32 to 46 (Pre 2 to Post). As was hoped, there was a substantial improvement in students' stuttering attitudes following the fluency coursework for virtually all components, subscores, and OSS of the *POSHA–S*.

U.S. GRADUATE. Following completion of a graduate-level fluency disorders course, improved *POSHA–S* ratings occurred for virtually all components, including: Traits/Personality, Helped by, Potential, Accommodating/Helping, Social Distance/Sympathy, Knowledge/Experience, and Knowledge Source (Figure 14.3). The Beliefs subscore increased by 4 units, and the Self Reactions subscore increased by 18 units. Overall Stuttering Score increased by 11 units, from 9 to 20. It should be noted that the Pre to Post results for each of the three NYC schools investigated (not shown in the table) were similar, ranging from 10 to 12 units. Overall, results indicate a positive change in stuttering attitudes following completion of a graduate-level fluency course as measured by the *POSHA–S*.

Discussion

Summary

These three independent investigations provide robust evidence that attitudes of speech-language pathology students toward stuttering can be improved on a standard measure following coursework in fluency disorders at both the undergraduate and graduate level, as well as interculturally, similar to the cross-sectional findings of St. Louis et al. (2014), who investigated attitudes of SLP and non-SLP students at undergraduate and graduate levels. Even though the *POSHA–S* scores from the samples in this study differed before the courses, all groups manifested attitude change in the desired direction and to a similar measured degree. Overall Stuttering Scores for B & H, WV, and NYC improved by 12, 15, and 11 units, respectively. A large-scale multinational study that seeks to isolate variables related to international and intercultural differences may help explain the variability of the Pre scores in the different samples. Nevertheless, the similar change in stuttering attitudes is particularly notable, given the vastly different coursework experiences of the three groups.

Importantly, the *lack* of change between the Pre 1 and Pre 2 means for the U.S. undergraduate students provides evidence that the *POSHA–S* measures what it is intended to measure. The fact that attitudes did *not* change during the three months between these administrations, but did change after eight weeks of fluency disorders coursework, confirms other research showing minimal positive effects on stuttering attitudes of simply filling out the instrument more than once (St. Louis, Lubker, Yaruss, & Aliveto, 2009; St. Louis, 2012c).

Attitude Change

Results of this study provide encouraging support for prior investigations aimed to mitigate stuttering attitudes (e.g., Abdalla & St. Louis, 2014; Flynn & St. Louis, 2011). It is important to remember, however, that the degree to which SLP student attitudes improved may have been tempered by their prior exposure to—and interest and experiences in—the field of speech-language pathology. Respondents in all groups had more positive scores at baseline for most *POSHA–S* items, components, and subscores when compared to the median values of the *POSHA–S* database of 9,294 respondents. For example, the Accommodating/Helping subscore prior to any fluency instruction in B & H, WV, and NYC were respectively 56, 70, and 50, which are all higher than the *POSHA–S* median value of 47. St. Louis et al. (2014) explained this finding by ascribing a "halo effect" to SLP students. They suggested that SLP students may, by virtue of their choice of profession, have more positive stuttering attitudes prior to direct fluency instruction. This means that any improvements in attitudes might not appear as substantial as the attitudes of students with lower baseline scores and no exposure to or interest in the field of speech-language pathology. Improvements in stuttering attitudes in this study were much less dramatic than those of the high school students studied in Flynn and St. Louis (2011). Flynn and St. Louis found that, although students' attitudes improved by 25 units after watching a live presentation given by a stutterer (compared to an average 13-unit improvement in the present study), the high school students' pre-intervention OSS was much lower than the OSS of students in any of the three groups of this study. An analysis to control for pre-intervention scores may be considered in future investigations. In the same vein, fluency coursework may be more susceptible to widely varying, multiple, and even contradictory influences on attitudes that would dilute positive changes observed after a carefully prepared presentation and video (e.g., Abdalla & St. Louis, 2014; Flynn & St. Louis, 2011). In any case, the present study provides evidence that participation in coursework at the undergraduate or graduate level has the potential to improve students' stuttering attitudes. Interestingly, method of instruction and specific curriculum appear to have had less influence on such changes in attitude than might have been expected.

Coursework

It is reasonable to conclude from this study that coursework in fluency disorders has the potential to improve students' stuttering attitudes. However, the impact of any positive change will be in the permanence of that change and if attitudinal improvement will enhance the treatment experience of people who stutter. While this study primarily investigated changes in Pre versus Post attitudes following coursework, it did not account for the possible variability of attitudes that may have taken place throughout the course. In this regard, we are unable to determine the linearity of their attitude change. For example, in the case of the NYC group (Reichel & St. Louis, 2004, 2007, 2011), it would be interesting to examine how the specific curricula integrated into regular fluency disorders courses and lab experiences impacted students' attitudes. Also, it is of particular interest that the scores from the B & H group were most improved following coursework related to stuttering treatment, as well as personal contact with stutterers. This finding supports previous investigations in which select attitudes were improved following exposure to and clinical experience with stuttering (e.g., Delaney, 2001; Leahy, 1994). While facts and discussion alone related to stuttering may be enough to result in some attitudinal improvement as with the WV sample, providing opportunities to interact with people who stutter either through personal or therapeutic exchanges may further augment the positive effect. Finally, specific coursework may have accounted for the differences in specific *POSHA–S* items that were not captured in the OSS. For example, in the item relating to "stuttering causes," the WV group had a Post rating of 73, while the Post rating of the NYC sample was 37. This clearly could have been a function of the fact that the WV instructor is the author of the *POSHA–S*, even though no attempt was made to modify a course that had been taught similarly for many years. Additional research will need to explicitly examine whether or not differences in coursework accounts for the variability in responses for specific *POSHA–S* items.

Conclusion and Future Research

This study provides encouraging support that coursework related to the nature and causes of stuttering may be a potential medium to improve SLP students' attitudes toward stuttering. Given the vast differences in curricula, instruction, and samplings, however, intergroup comparisons were inappropriate. As such, it is difficult to determine the underlying curricular nuances or identify specific modules or course content that may have been responsible for attitudinal change. Larger and more representative sample sizes, along with highly controlled instruction across different classes, should be considered for future investigations in this area. Specifically, studies should attempt to determine what information or experiences are particularly influential on students' stuttering attitudes and for how long those improved attitudes are maintained. One such example is Chapter 15 in this volume by Hughes, Gabel, Roseman, and Daniels. The ultimate goal of such studies would be to develop the most impactful and meaningful fluency curricula so that the future quality of stuttering treatment is enhanced optimally.

Chapter 15

———————

An Interdisciplinary Training Program in Stuttering: Raising Awareness and Changing Attitudes

Stephanie Hughes, Rodney M. Gabel,
Christopher P. Roseman, Derek E. Daniels

ABSTRACT

This pilot research program explored ways to foster collaborative relationships between school counseling and speech-language pathology (SLP) graduate students. Students in SLP and school counseling programs at the University of Toledo were recruited to participate in an intensive eight-day stuttering clinic for children who stutter. Participants received preliminary training about stuttering and the roles of school counselors and speech-language pathologists. They engaged in collaborative experiences at the stuttering clinic to raise awareness of stuttering, improve attitudes toward stuttering, and identify ways speech-language pathologists and school counselors can collaborate to serve children who stutter. Post-clinic qualitative and quantitative data indicated that student participants learned factual information about stuttering, recognized the socio-emotional needs of children who stutter, and began to consider how school counselors and SLPs can work together to provide services to this population.

Introduction

Effects of Stuttering on Children Who Stutter

Though stuttering is not generally believed to be caused by psychological or emotional disturbance, people who stutter experience high levels of anxiety and stress related to speaking and social experiences (Craig, Hancock, Tran, Craig, & Peters, 2003; Ezrati-Vinacour & Levin, 2004). The difficulties that people who stutter have in producing fluent speech are compounded by societal reactions to stuttering. Researchers have consistently found that stuttering individuals of all ages are viewed in a negative and stereotypical manner by a variety of professionals, including speech-language pathologists (SLPs), teachers, and rehabilitation counselors (e.g., Craig et al., 2003; Evans, Healey, Kawai, & Rowland, 2008; Hughes, Gabel, Irani, & Schlagheck, 2010a). These negative views of stuttering are unfortunate, especially for children who stutter who face many challenges during their school years. Students who stutter seem to be at particularly high risk for poor social relationships with fellow students. Peers perceive CWS to be less popular than classmates who do not stutter (Davis, Howell, & Cooke, 2002). Furthermore, a growing body of research indicates that the lives of CWS are adversely affected by school bullying (Blood & Blood, 2004, 2007; Davis et al., 2002; Hugh-Jones & Smith, 1999; Langevin, Chapter 3; Langevin, Bortnick, Hammer, & Wiebe, 1998; Langevin & Prasad, 2012). Children who are bullied tend to experience depression, physical illness, anxiety, and sleep disorders (Forero, McLellan, Rissel, & Bauman, 1999; Salmon, James, & Smith, 1998); they also have high absenteeism rates from school (Swearer, 2011) and are at increased risk for poor academic performance (Glew, Fan, Katon, Rivara, & Kernic, 2005).

School seems to be a challenging environment for stuttering children to navigate, even if they are not bullied. In a retrospective study of kindergarten to Grade 12 school experiences, Daniels, Gabel, and Hughes (2012) found that adult participants reported that stuttering affected their academic performance, classroom participation, relationships with teachers and peers, and social relationships. Moreover, 16 of the 21 participants reported that their school speech therapy would have been more beneficial if it had addressed the socio-emotional consequences of stuttering. These findings emphasize the need for schools to provide more support to children who stutter.

School Counselors, Speech-Language Pathologists, and Stuttering

Given concerns with bullying and peer relationships, school counselors would seem to be a natural source of support for children who stutter in school settings. Over the last decade, the American School Counselor Association (ASCA) has adopted and actively promoted national standards that more clearly define the role of professional school counselors. School counselors are trained specifically to work with mental health and substance abuse issues that develop from a comprehensive biopsychosocial perspective. In terms of working directly with SLPs, professional school counselors are prepared to develop and implement curricula across several developmental areas such as self-concept, self-esteem, and social skills. School counselors also assist with the establishment and implementation of behavior plans, counsel families, and operate as a primary referral source (Murphy & Kaffenberger, 2007). Few, if any, studies, however, have been conducted on the attitudes of school counselors toward stuttering and people who stutter.

Also lacking are studies that investigate SLPs' attitudes toward interdisciplinary collaboration when providing services to children who stutter in schools. In one notable exception, St. Louis and Lass (1981) found that most university students in SLP training programs did not believe that school counselors were aware of the psychological ramifications of stuttering. They believed that counseling stuttering children should be the exclusive domain of SLPs. Such findings are troubling given the emotional support that school counselors are qualified to provide to such students. Even more troubling is that many SLPs report being uncomfortable or ill-prepared to work with people who stutter (Brisk, Healey, & Hux, 1997; St. Louis & Durrenberger, 1993). This lack of comfort and preparation may be due to a continuing reduction in education and clinical preparation of SLPs in the area of stuttering (Yaruss & Quesal, 2002). Tellis, Bressler, and Emerick (2008) called for more systematic training in fluency disorders, citing SLPs' lack of knowledge and skills when assessing and treating fluency clients.

Purpose

To address the need for interdisciplinary services for children who stutter in schools, the project discussed in this chapter investigated how collaborative relationships between SLPs and school counselors could be facilitated in the context of an intensive clinic for stuttering children. The overarching goals of the project were to educate graduate students in SLP and school counseling programs about stuttering in general, help them to recognize the potential for collaboration between SLPs and school counselors, and provide them with the opportunity to see first-hand the social and emotional effects of stuttering for children and their parents.

Methods

Setting: The University of Toledo's *Intensive Stuttering Clinic for Children and their Families*

In the summer of 2013, the first and second authors offered an eight-day clinic at the University of Toledo for children who stutter. This clinic, the *Intensive Stuttering Clinic for Children and their Families* (ISCCF), was designed to provide services for older children ages eight to 12 and their parents. As is consistent with the evidence base for providing treatment for children who stutter, the program focused on teaching children about stuttering, addressing negative attitudes and feelings about speaking, learning better means of coping with stuttering, and using techniques for speaking more fluently (Langevin, Kully, & Ross-Harold, 2007; Runyan & Runyan, 2007). The ISCCF also fostered social skills development, promoted emotional resiliency, and ameliorated the negative effects of bullying for children who stutter (Langevin et al., 2007; Murphy, Yaruss, & Quesal, 2007a, 2007b). Parent counseling, an important component of fluency therapy for school-age children (DiLollo & Manning, 2007), was also provided during the clinic. Enjoyable activities such as crafts, scientific experiments, outdoor activities, and games were integrated into group and individual therapy.

Participants

Participants were eight graduate students in an SLP program and eight graduate students in a school counseling program. The SLP students (all female) were assigned to the ISCCF as a clinic placement in which they provided about 50 hours of therapy to children at the clinic. The school counseling students (two male, six female) were recruited on a voluntary basis from counseling classes taught by the third author. Note that while the SLP students were assigned to the ISCCF as part of their clinical education, participation in the study was voluntary as it necessitated additional training and time above and beyond their regular clinical duties. All eight of the SLP students decided to participate in the study. Every student participant received a $150 gift card to the campus bookstore for his or her participation in the project.

Clinical Training and Activities

The eight SLP students, all of whom had taken a graduate fluency course, began preparing for the ISCCF about five weeks prior to the start of the clinic. The first and second authors reviewed therapy techniques with students, discussed possible therapeutic activities, and reviewed the agenda for each day of the clinic during this time. About two weeks before the start of the clinic, students attended an hour-long seminar on the roles and responsibilities of school counselors presented by the third author, a state-licensed and nationally certified counselor. The SLP students were informed that school counseling students were only obligated to observe therapy and did not have to actively participate, but that school counselors could serve as "friendly listeners" for children at the clinic and could answer questions SLP students may have had about the emotional, mental, or social health of their clients. During the ISCCF, the eight SLP students conducted six hours of supervised fluency therapy daily to fulfill their assigned clinical duties.

To prepare for their role in the ISCCF, school counseling students watched the film *Transcending Stuttering* and viewed a narrated PowerPoint presentation on stuttering created by the first and second authors, who are SLPs. School counseling students who participated in the study were required to observe 10 hours of fluency therapy in total. While observing was the only requirement, students were told that they were also welcome to engage in games and conversation with the children, and that they could ask questions of the SLP students regarding therapy or stuttering in general. As many of the school counseling students worked during the day or were taking graduate classes, they did not have set hours for attending the ISCCF. The school counseling students arranged their hours ahead of time with the first author, who then introduced the counseling students to SLP students and their clients as appropriate. While observing, many counseling students actively engaged with clients in a variety of ways, such as playing a game of "*Jeopardy!*" related to stuttering facts, eating lunch with the children, and in one particularly memorable occasion, diffusing a tense situation in which tears were shed over the correct way to play kickball. One client revealed that he saw a counselor at his school and, with parent permission, the school counseling student to whom he had confided was able to provide some focused, supervised counseling services related to bullying. Toward the end of the ISCCF, the SLP students and a school counseling student developed and played a game with the children about differences that was designed to improve self-esteem. The extent to which individual school counseling students chose to participate in therapeutic activities and engage with the children seemed to vary depending on their extroversion and the expectations of the SLP student(s) with whom they were observing.

Data Collection and Analysis

Prior to the study, all participants completed a qualitative pre-clinic survey that asked for their perceptions of stuttering and the roles of SLPs and school counselors when treating children who stutter. At the end of the clinic, both school counseling and SLP students took a post-clinic survey that included both qualitative and quantitative questionnaire items and wrote a reflection paper about their experiences. For brevity's sake, and due to overlapping content in survey data and the reflection paper, this chapter discusses findings from only the quantitative portion of the post-clinic survey and from qualitative analyses of students' reflection papers, written at the conclusion of the ISCCF. The surveys were administered electronically via Survey Monkey and consisted of a Likert-type questionnaire, some open-ended questions, and demographic items. For the reflection papers, SLP students were asked to simply write about their experiences with the ISCCF, including the collaboration with school counseling students. School counseling students wrote their reflection papers to fulfill a counseling class assignment. As such, they were told to address topics in their papers such as their prior understanding of children who stutter, stereotypes about stuttering, roles of SLPs, professional and personal changes in perspectives before and after the clinic experience, and how they as future school counselors could collaborate with SLPs to help youngsters who stutter.

Students' reflection papers were analyzed using qualitative data procedures consistent with phenomenological analysis. Each of the four authors reviewed the reflection papers, noting similarities among responses and grouping individual students' statements into themes that represented the data set. Consensus on themes was obtained among the authors for validity and credibility purposes; the fourth author was not directly involved in the ISCCF and did not know any of the SLP or school counseling students who were involved in the project. As such, this author contributed an unbiased perspective during the data-analysis process.

Results

Quantitative Results

Analysis of post-clinic Likert-type survey items indicated unanimous agreement from participants that stuttering children can benefit from the services of both school counselors and SLPs. With the exception of one SLP student, all participants felt that they knew more about stuttering after participating in the clinic. A small majority of SLP and school counseling students (five out of eight for each group) felt that they could lead an in-service workshop about stuttering for coworkers in the future. The remaining three students in each group mostly selected the "neither agree nor disagree" option. Only one school counseling student disagreed that he or she could lead an in-service workshop in the future. Figure 15.1 shows the extent to which participants agreed or strongly agreed with four out of five of the questionnaire items. The fifth item, "I feel *un*prepared to work professionally with children who stutter," indicated 100% disagreement (disagree or strongly disagree) from all SLP students and six school counseling participants. The two remaining school counseling participants selected the "neither agree nor disagree" option for this question.

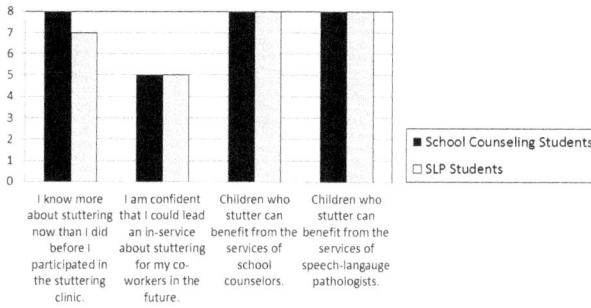

Figure 15.1: Number of students agreeing/strongly agreeing with questionnaire items.

Qualitative Results

Two major themes from students' reflection papers emerged and are presented in the following sections.

THEME 1: SLP STUDENTS RECEIVED SUPPORT FROM STUDENT COUNSELORS. Some of the SLP students noted that the stuttering children who participated in the ISCCF demonstrated challenging behaviors or had difficult family lives. As such, they appreciated the support that the student counselors could provide, not just to the clients, but also to the SLP students. "When I had concerns about my client's home life, [the school counseling students] were there to answer my questions . . . it was very nice to have an additional support system for those topics that [SLP] students are not as familiar with," wrote one SLP student. Similarly, another SLP student reported that the school counseling students were "very helpful on the day that bullying was addressed. They assisted in setting up role-playing activities which were very beneficial for the children." In general, the SLP students believed that the school counseling students contributed to the overall success of clients in the ISCCF: "Overall, I had a good experience with the counselors and felt they had great ideas for getting the children to express more about their feelings and emotions." Finally, SLP students appeared to recognize the mutual benefits of having school counseling students in the clinic. One student summarized her perceptions as follows:

It was great to learn about the role of school counselors can play with a child who stutters in the school setting. I think many of the school counseling observers learned something new about stuttering and ways of helping future children in schools with communication disorders.

The ultimate goal of this program was to help SLP and counseling students recognize the potential to form collaborative professional relationships between the two disciplines. One SLP student and counseling student established a particularly positive working relationship. This student summed up her experience as follows:

> Having the opportunity to have the graduate school-counseling students around was great. I quickly teamed up with a school-counseling student and was able to coordinate daily sessions with my client and her. With her help and suggestions, these daily sessions ended up benefiting my client and made him feel more comfortable talking about negative situations with regards to his fluency. I looked at this as a total breakthrough and new beginning for my client. . . .

THEME 2: STUDENT COUNSELORS LEARNED MORE ABOUT STUTTERING AND THEIR ROLE IN PROVIDING SERVICES TO CHILDREN WHO STUTTER. The school counseling students reflected upon what they did not know about stuttering prior to participating in the ISCCF. As one student wrote:

> Before I began my observations, I was under the impression that individuals who stutter had this disorder due to social anxiety. I admit I was a bit naïve to the mechanics of the disorder and had little experience with it. Within the first 15 minutes at the clinic when the clients were playing group "*Jeopardy!*" I discovered that I was dead wrong.

In addition, school counseling students also seemed to believe that their participation in the ISCCF would be useful in their future professional work: "I learned a lot about stuttering from them, both technically and emotionally. I am hoping to take this experience with me and remember what I need to implement in my school as a future counselor."

Several of the counseling students expressed that they felt they did indeed see a need for their intervention with children who stutter. One student summarized the need by suggesting: "Many of these children had mentioned that they are bullied at school because of their stutter. Bullying can lead to low self-esteem, and also a lowered urge to want to join in at school no matter what the activity may be." Another student noted that: "after a few days of observing, it turns out that most students had other issues in conjunction with their stuttering. I was able to answer questions that [SLP students] had about social behaviors, ADHD, and other counseling related questions." From these comments, it was evident that the counseling students were able to identify a role they can play in helping children who stutter.

Discussion

This project engaged SLP and school counseling students in an eight-day clinic for children who stutter. Students from these disciplines observed each other demonstrating clinical skills that could be used in future professional work involving children with stuttering and other communication disorders in schools. Data were collected to determine the extent to which participation in the clinic had a meaningful effect on students in terms of increased knowledge of stuttering in general and greater appreciation for the collaborative potential between school counselors and SLPs.

Quantitative results from a post-clinic survey indicated that the majority of participants increased their knowledge of stuttering and agreed that both school counselors and SLPs can play an important role in providing services for the stuttering child. The Likert-type items on the questionnaire were administered only once, after the clinic was complete. These questions will be administered both pre- and post-clinic during future iterations of this project.

Qualitative analysis of participants' reflection papers at the end of the clinic revealed two major themes that centered around: (1) support that SLP students and children who stutter received from school counseling students, and (2) school counseling students' increased understanding of stuttering and how school coun-selors can support children who stutter in schools. The SLP students indicated that at times their clients' secondary problems involving social skills and disrup-tive home environments were challenging. They appreciated the school counseling students' willingness to tackle some of these broader issues that were not neces-sarily related to stuttering but had an effect on progress during the stuttering clinic. For their part, the school counseling students expressed that many of their initial impressions of stuttering were incorrect. They identified areas in which school counselors could help stuttering youth navigate the school experience, particularly in the areas of social skills, self-esteem, and preventing or coping with bullying.

In summary, school counseling and SLP graduate students seemed to develop a new appreciation for each other's disciplines during an intensive clinic for children who stutter. Both groups of students expressed an interest in working together in the future and agreed that school counselors and SLPs can collaborate in the provision of services for these children in schools. These sentiments suggest that the unease that SLP students feel about allowing school counselors to counsel youngsters who stutter (as noted in the work of St. Louis and Lass, 1981) can be ameliorated by providing information about school counseling and access to school counselors.

One caveat for future researchers is that this was a pilot study, in which the projected role of school counseling students was to serve primarily as friendly adult observers who could converse with stuttering children while learning more about stuttering and the services that SLPs provide. While the majority of school counseling students did just that, two students were very quiet observers who did not become involved in games or converse much with the SLP students or the clients. Conversely, two other students took on a more direct counseling and planning role. Qualitative responses indicated some confusion over the role that student counselors should take when interacting with SLP students and young clients at a stuttering clinic. Future iterations of this study should clarify the roles and expectations of student counselors for everyone, including SLP students.

Part Four

RESEARCH: ATTITUDES OF PEOPLE WHO STUTTER
AND/OR THEIR FAMILY OR FRIENDS

Chapter 16

The *Appraisal of the Stuttering Environment (ASE)*: A New Clinical Tool to Measure Stuttering Attitudes in the Client's Environment

Kenneth O. St. Louis, Chelsea D. Kuhn, Lindsey Lytwak

ABSTRACT

Adults who stutter and parents of children who stutter have been shown to hold more positive attitudes toward stuttering than the non-stuttering majority. Moreover, differences have been found within stuttering groups or parents of children who stutter. This study sought to develop a clinical instrument to measure the stuttering attitude environment. Specifically, it was designed to determine the extent to which stuttering attitudes of stuttering adults are different from those of their family members and close friends, and how these attitudes are different from those of the general public. A prototype of a new clinical instrument, the *Appraisal of the Stuttering Environment (ASE)*, was developed by adapting an experimental prototype of the *Public Opinion Survey of Human Attributes–Stuttering (POSHA–S)*. The *ASE* was completed by convenience samples of stuttering adults, their family members, their close friends, and unrelated adults. Additional information describing the stutterers was also obtained. The *ASE* results were compared with adapted *POSHA–S* results. Overall, statistically significant differences indicated that the stuttering adults manifested the most positive attitudes toward stuttering on the *ASE*, followed next by their families and friends (which were quite similar), and followed finally by the public. Even so, some *ASE* items revealed different profiles, e.g., some attitudes of the families and friends were more positive than those of the stuttering adults. *ASE* and *POSHA–S* profiles were quite similar. The *ASE*, when finalized, shows considerable promise as a clinical instrument for use by speech-language pathologists to assess the attitudes among friends and family of their stuttering clients.

Introduction

Rationale

BACKGROUND. A large and burgeoning evidence base confirms that public attitudes toward stuttering are negative, as is reported Boyle and Blood (Chapter 2), Gabel (Chapter 4), and Langevin (Chapter 3). Recent evidence also indicates that such attitudes can be effectively quantified (e.g., St. Louis, Chapter 1). St. Louis and colleagues have reported extensively on the development of the *Public Opinion Survey of Human Attributes–Stuttering* (*POSHA–S*) (e.g., St. Louis, 2005, 2011a, 2012c; St. Louis, Lubker, Yaruss, Adkins, & Pill, 2008; St. Louis, Williams, Ware, Guendouzi, & Reichel, 2014). Two different rating scales were used in experimental versions, and the second one (referred to in St. Louis [2012c] as the *POSHA–E2*) utilized a 1–9 Likert scale for all ratings. The 1–9 scale was found to be effective and also comparable to the final *POSHA–S*, which used a 1–5 rating scale for the general section comparing stuttering to four other attributes (intelligence, left-handedness, obesity, and mental illness) and a 1–3 rating scale converted from "no," "not sure," and "yes" responses (St. Louis, 2012c). The 1–9 scale, even though it was no doubt more sensitive to attitudes of individual respondents, was not used in the final *POSHA–S* because it required more respondent time to complete and generated data that was not necessary for epidemiological studies of *population attitudes* rather than *individual attitudes*. The so-called *POSHA–E2* also had many more items than the final *POSHA–S* that were winnowed down through a systematic and multi-faceted item analysis process (c.f. St. Louis, 2012c).

Throughout the developmental work on the *POSHA–S*, it became increasingly apparent that the quantified measurement of attitudes toward stuttering could have clinical implications beyond documenting changes in attitudes of non-stuttering populations. Group studies have shown that attitudes can be improved (Abdalla & St. Louis, 2014; Flynn & St. Louis, 2011; Junuzović-Žunić, Weidner, Reichel, Cook, St. Louis, & Ware, Chapter 14). It is reasonable to assume, therefore, that attitudes of individual stuttering clients or their families are changeable as well. For example, if the family attitudes of a stuttering client were found to be especially negative, clinical care of that client should logically include providing information and discussions with family members to attempt to reduce any stigma at home.

There are currently no measures of stuttering attitudes designed specifically for clients and their families and close friends. A number of instruments are used by speech-language pathologists (SLPs) to assess stuttering clients' self-reports of their thoughts, perceptions, and emotions (e.g., the *Overall Assessment of the Speaker's Experience with Stuttering* [*OASES*] [Yaruss & Quesal, 2008], the *Perceptions of Stuttering Inventory* (*PSI*) [Woolf, 1967], and the *St. Louis Inventory of Life Perspectives and Stuttering* [*SL♦ILP-S*] [St. Louis, 2001]). Also, a few instruments measure similar constructs of the immediate families or peers of those who stutter but are quite limited in focus, such as to address teasing and bullying in children (e.g., the *Peer Attitudes Toward Children Who Stutter Scale* [*PATCS*] [Langevin & Hagler, 2004]).

ATTITUDES OF PEOPLE WHO STUTTER. Differences in attitudes of those who stutter regarding stuttering would suggest that past or current environments may play a role in those differences. One especially revealing finding from previous research using the *POSHA–S* has been that people who stutter have attitudes that are more accurate (i.e., based on the current stuttering literature on the nature of stuttering) and sensitive (i.e., more positive) than the non-stuttering majority (St. Louis & George, 2008). The best attitudes reported so far for the final *POSHA–S* items were from leaders of the stuttering self-help movement in North America and Western Europe. Somewhat less positive attitudes were observed from individuals who stuttered—or used to stutter—who were recruited through clinical and nonclinical populations. And even less positive were attitudes of non-recruited adults in general public samples, all taken from the *POSHA–S* database, who had indicated that they themselves stuttered (St. Louis & George, 2008). Table 16.1 displays the *POSHA–S* Overall Stuttering Scores (OSS), Belief and Self Reactions subscores, and components of these groups. The stuttering members of the public reported by St. Louis and George were updated by recent additions to the *POSHA–S* database (circa July 2013) containing 188 samples from 8,144 people representing 29 countries and 20 languages. Table 16.1 also features results of a sample of parents of stuttering children, recruited primarily from individuals attending the National Stuttering Association's annual convention (Daniels & Hughes, 2011).

It is apparent that the OSS and the Self Reaction subscore, along with its components, were highest or most positive for the self-help leaders, followed by

Table 16.1: *POSHA–S* Attitudes of Three Groups of Stuttering Adults (Leaders in the Self-Help Movement, Adults Recruited by Students from Clinical and Nonclinical Populations, and Adults in Public Samples Identifying Themselves as Stutterers) and One Group of Parents of Children Who Stutter

POSHA–S Variable	Self-Help Leaders[a]	Recruited: Clinical and Nonclinical[a]	Not Recruited: POSHA–S Database	Parents of Stuttering Children[b]	POSHA–S Database Median
Number	25	25	122	47	188 Samples
Overall Stuttering Score	65	39	23	58	16
Beliefs About People Who Stutter	71	47	34	73	33
Traits	68	6	16	49	18
Help (from)	73	58	23	76	19
Cause	73	54	35	82	34
Potential	70	72	61	86	62
Self Reactions to People Who Stutter	60	31	13	43	-1
Accommodating/Helping	93	78	33	80	47
Social Distance/Sympathy	57	30	12	54	4
Knowledge/Experience	83	37	30	33	-36
Knowledge Source	6	-21	-21	4	-18
Obesity/Mental Illness	-27	-40	-33	-32	-34
Impression	-14	-12	-21	-15	-15
Want/Have	-70	-93	-74	-82	-84
Amount Known	3	-16	-5	2	1

[a]Data originally reported by St. Louis and George (2008)
[b]Data from Daniels and Hughes (2011) and later supplemented by additional respondents

parents, then by the clinically and nonclinically recruited stutterers, and finally by self-identified stutterers from population samples. Belief subscores and three-fourths of its components were highest for parents, followed by the self-help leaders. With few exceptions, the median sample means from the *POSHA–S* database were lower than the four groups for the stuttering ratings. By contrast, most of the Obesity/Mental Illness ratings of the stutterers and parents were similar to the database medians from the general public. Very likely the information received from speech-language pathologists (SLPs), the extant literature, or interactions with others who stutter could be partly responsible for the differences in attitudes observed for the adult stutterers; however, it is possible that differences in attitudes in their environments play a role as well. The parental data suggest that experience with children who stutter may sensitize parents, resulting in better than average attitudes. Whether this would foster better attitudes in their stuttering children is not known, but is certainly a reasonable hypothesis.

Purpose

Clinically, SLPs would find it useful to document and potentially change the attitudes in their clients' environments. Accordingly, this study reports the first step in the development of a measure of the stuttering environment, the *Appraisal of the Stuttering Environment* (*ASE*). Its primary purpose was to compare attitudes of stutterers with those of their family members and close friends, as well as with the public to determine if attitude environments that involved a stuttering person would be different from those without such an influence. Secondary purposes of the study were to identify preliminary patterns of attitude differences among the four groups (i.e., stutterers, family members, friends, and the public) and to compare results of the *ASE* with results from the *POSHA–S*.

Method

ASE Instrument

A first prototype of the *ASE* was generated by adapting the *POSHA–E2* (second experimental version of the instrument) containing its 1–9 scale, but using the same demographic and general items that are in the final *POSHA–S*. The rationale for using the 9-point scale was that it would be more sensitive to changes in *individual* attitudes in clinical uses than the 1–3 or 1–5 scales in the *POSHA–S*. The rationale for including most of the items of the *POSHA–E2* relates to individual client/family differences. Based on factor analysis and other criteria (St. Louis, 2012c), many of these items were deemed redundant and therefore deleted in the final *POSHA–S*. Nonetheless, they were retained in this *ASE* prototype because they might show selective differences in individual clients' attitude environments, especially if efforts to change attitudes were to be undertaken. Thus, the *ASE* prototype adds 50 individual items to the 45 in the *POSHA–S* for a total of 95. Those clustered into the same 11 components, 3 subscores, and the OSS as the *POSHA–S* yields 110 total ratings.

Participants

The authors recruited a convenience sample of 32 adults who stutter from clients, acquaintances, and referrals. After giving informed consent, each stutterer was asked to supply names and contact information of four close family members and four close friends within five years of his or her age who could be contacted. Of all those contacted by e-mail, mail, and/or telephone, 47 of 128 (32 × 4) family members and 41 of 128 friends responded and filled out questionnaires, either on paper copies or online versions through an Internet link, *with the stuttering referrer in mind*. Additionally, but carried out one year earlier, an anonymous control group of 45 adults were recruited with the only exclusion criterion being that no SLPs or SLP students could be included.

Other Stuttering Measures

The following measures were obtained from the study groups: (1) stuttering adults: the *ASE* (mostly paper-and-pencil version), the *OASES* (paper-and-pencil version), the *SL♦ILP–S* (paper-and-pencil version), the request for names/contact information of family and friends, and the percent syllables stuttered (%SS) of a 150- to 500-word spontaneous speech sample; (2) family and friends: the *ASE* (paper-and-pencil or online version), an adapted *SL♦ILP–S* pertaining to the stuttering adult who referred them (paper-and-pencil or online version), and a short questionnaire about the stuttering adult's frequency of stuttering symptoms (e.g., repetitions, prolongation, avoidance, accessory behaviors) (paper-and-pencil or online version); and (3) control adults: the *ASE* (paper-and-pencil version). St. Louis (2012b) documented that *POSHA–S* online administrations were basically equivalent to paper-and-pencil administrations.

Data Analysis

For this brief report, only partial summary results for the *SL♦ILP–Ss*, *OASESs*, stuttering questionnaires, and %SS are presented. The report focuses instead on the results of the first prototype of the *ASE*. As with the *POSHA–S*, all ratings for the *ASE* were converted to a mean rating scale ranging from -100 to +100 (0 = neutral). Ratings for some items are inverted so that, uniformly, higher scores reflect more positive attitudes, and lower scores less positive attitudes. Since the *ASE* ratings were derived from previous *POSHA–E2* items, the results for the stutterers, family members, friends, and unrelated controls were compared to mean values from 22 samples representing 1,103 respondents from eight countries and six languages who filled out that experimental version. It should be noted that we added the 165 respondents from this study to the previous total of 18 samples from 938 respondents. Our rationale was that for numerous items, the samples here represented the highest values observed to date, and those were necessary to calculate percentile comparisons (see below).

All pair-wise independent *t*-test comparisons were run for the 110 ratings between the four sample groups. These included individual items; components (clusters of items); subscores (clusters of components); subscores (Beliefs about people who stutter, Self Reactions to people who stutter, and Obesity/Mental Illness); and the OSS (mean of the two stuttering subscores) as has been done in numerous *POSHA–S* studies (St. Louis, 2012c). The Bonferroni correction was also applied (p ≤ .00417 [.05/12]), and Cohen's (1988) *d* effect sizes for statistically significant differences run, as has also been documented previously (Fagerland, 2012; St. Louis, 2012c).

As noted, the *ASE* contains all the items of the *POSHA–S*, plus 50 additional items. Excluding the added items, we generated *POSHA–S* tabular profiles for the four sample groups and compared them to parallel *ASE* profiles containing the same—but expanded—components, subscores, and OSS.

Results

Demographic Characteristics

Table 16.2 summarizes selected demographic results from the four groups. Average ages were from low thirties to high forties, with the stuttering adults being the youngest, i.e., 31 years, and the family members being the oldest, i.e., 49 years. Not surprisingly, with higher mean ages, fewer student and more working respondents, as well as more married individuals who were parents, characterized the samples. Education levels, race, and religion were comparable and unremarkable. More female than male respondents comprised the family, friend, and control groups as is typical of most *POSHA–S* convenience samples, but the reverse was true, as expected, for the stuttering group. By definition, the stuttering group stuttered, yet 22% of them did not self-identify as such, presumably because they may have perceived themselves not to be stuttering at the time of the survey. Only 4% of the family members reported stuttering, as did 1% of the friends, and none of the controls. A higher percentage of stutterers identified themselves as mentally ill (13%) compared to the other three groups (0–2%). Twelve percent to 28% of the four groups knew no one who was mentally ill, and 36% of the controls did not know someone who stuttered compared, by design, to 0% for the stutterers, family members, and friends.

Table 16.2: Demographic Means for Four Samples

Demographic Variable	Stuttering Adults	Family	Friends	Controls
Number	32	47	41	45
Age (year)	31.6	49.1	35.6	41.2
Education (year)	14.8	14.6	15.2	14.1
Male/Female (%)	71 / 29	22 / 78	43 / 57	42 / 58
Student/Working (%)	41 / 63	15 / 49	41 / 34	33 / 67
Married/Parent (%)	38 / 28	79 / 70	37 / 39	56 / 56
Income Score (-100 to +100)	5	12	12	6
Race (Caucasian/African American / Other) (%)	87 / 10 / 3	95 / 5 / 0	87 / 5 / 8	98 / 0 / 2
Religion (Christian/Other/n/a) (%)	69 / 27 / 4	77 / 5 / 18	58 / 17 / 25	100 / 0 / 0
Self-Identification (%)				
Obese	19	4	15	16
Mentally Ill	13	2	2	0
Person Who Stutters	78	4	2	0
No People Known (%)				
Obese	0	0	0	4
Mentally Ill	16	28	12	18
Person Who Stutters	0	0	0	36

Stuttering Characteristics

Table 16.3 provides a summary of experimenter, self, and family/friend ratings for the 32 stuttering adults relative to their stuttering severity, symptoms, and self-perceptions. Unfortunately, speech samples were not available for nearly half of the stuttering adults. Percent stuttered syllables (%SS) for 16 of them ranged from 0.9% to 15.6% with a mean of 6.4%. According to the *OASES* Total Impact Scores for the 32 stutterers, 7% were mild, 36% were mild-moderate, 36% were moderate, 18% were moderate-severe, and 4% were severe. The mean severity on a 5-point scale, from "mild" to "severe," was 2.8 or between "mild-moderate" and "moderate" on the *OASES* scale. Impact scores for the four-item categories of the *OASES*, i.e., "general information," "reactions to stuttering," "communication in daily situations," and "quality of life," were similar to the Total Impact Score. On the *SL♦ILP–S*, the total score, or sum of all 13 items (with five items inverted so that higher scores consistently reflect more severe scores) was 47.3, ranging from 8–77. The Total Effect Score mean for the stuttering adults was

Table 16.3: Stuttering-Related Measures for the Stuttering Adults: %SS (Experimenter-Rated), *OASES* (Self-Rated), Adapted *SL♦ILP–S* (Self-Rated), and Questionnaire Means (Family- and Friends-Rated)

	Stuttering Adults	Family	Friends
Percent Stuttered Syllables (%SS)	6.4%	—	—
OASES Total Impact (Higher = more severe)	48.3	—	—
OASES General Information Impact (Higher = more severe)	49.8	—	—
OASES Reaction to Stuttering Impact (Higher = more severe)	51.0	—	—
OASES Communication in Daily Situations Impact (Higher = more severe)	51.2	—	—
OASES Quality of Life Impact (Higher = more severe)	41.1	—	—
SL♦ILP-S Total (Higher = more severe)	47.3	53.4	47.8
SL♦ILP-S Total Effect Score (Higher = more severe)	31.7	38.7	31.1
SL♦ILP-S Help Others Score (Lower = more help)	7.0	7.7	9.1
SL♦ILP-S Health/Life Satisfaction Score (Lower = more)	9.3	8.2	8.2
Questionnaire Total (1–5; Higher = more symptoms) (n = 18)	—	2.8	2.6
Repetitions	—	3.2	3.2
Prolongations	—	2.9	2.7
Blocks	—	3.3	2.9
Struggle/Tension	—	3.3	2.7
Avoiding	—	2.3	2.0
Accessory Behaviors	—	2.4	2.5
Substitutions	—	2.5	2.4

31.7 (range = 7–64), the Help Others Score was 7.0 (range = 2–18), and the Health and Life Satisfaction Score was 9.3 (range = 3–21). On the *SL♦ILP–S* self-judged severity item, ratings were as follows: 16% for 1 ("none"), 16% for 2 ("very mild"), 25% for 3, 15% for 4, 16% for 5 ("moderate"), 9% for 6, 6% for 7, 3% for 8, and 3% for 9 ("very severe"). The *SL♦ILP–S* ratings from the close friends were similar to those of the stutterers, but the Total Effect Scores of the family members were significantly higher than the stutterers' or friends' ratings using independent *t*-tests (p < .05).

These data are consistent with scores on the seven-item stuttering-related symptom questionnaires filled out by family and friends on 5-point scales ranging from "never" to "always" observed. Family members sent in question-naires for 22 stutterers, and friends did so for 21 stutterers. Eighteen of these stutterers had at least one family member and one friend fill out a question-naire. In all 18 cases, at least one person rated the person as having at least one symptom beyond "1" or "never" observed. In most cases, at least half of the symptoms were identified. Table 16.3 shows that the means for each symptom clustered around "3" or "sometimes" observed, and for 5/7 of the ratings, parents identified slightly more symptoms than friends did.

Clearly, the *OASES*, *SL♦ILP–S*, symptom questionnaire, and %SS results sum-marized in Table 16.3 demonstrate that the stuttering participants did in fact stutter overtly and also believed they did. The data also showed that their stut-tering severity spanned the range of severity from "mild" to "severe," but that the large majority of them were within the "mild" to "moderate" range, which is typical (Soderberg, 1962).

Group Comparisons

The Appendix displays all mean *ASE* ratings for the four groups. It also provides a comparison of those ratings with the median sample means from 22 samples in the 1–9 scale database of 1,103 respondents that contained virtually all of the *ASE* items. The long table shows in brackets after each identifier which of the pair-wise comparisons, if any, were significantly different (p ≤ .00417). Specific comparison codes are shown at the bottom of the table.

Figure 16.1 shows the components and subscores for the four groups graphi-cally, in comparison to the highest, lowest, and median sample means observed to date for *ASE* and *ASE*-related (i.e., *POSHA–E2*) samples (circa July 2013).

The number (and percentages) of the 110 pair-wise comparisons significantly different (detailed in the Appendix) were as follows: adults who stutter versus family members—22 (20%), adults who stutter versus friends—27 (25%), adults who stutter versus controls—29 (27%), family versus friends—3 (3%), family versus controls—33 (30%), and friends versus controls—43 (39%). Cohen's *d* effect sizes for individual ratings ranged from 0.62 to 4.14 ("moderate" to "very large"). Considering the mean Cohen's *d* for each of these groups, comparisons ranged from 1.03 to 1.38 or all "very large."

Percentile ranks of the four means were generated relative to the 22 data-base samples. Thirteen percent of the control means were in the lowest quartile

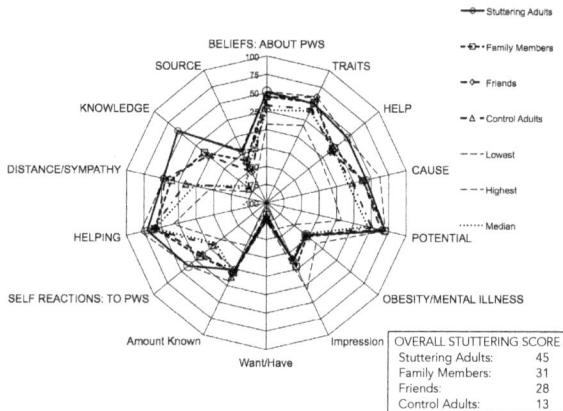

Figure 16.1: ASE profiles for the stuttering adults, their family members and friends, and the controls.

(0–25th percentile) associated with the most negative attitudes, 64% were in the second and third quartiles (25th–75th percentile or interquartile range), and 24% were in the highest quartile (75th–100th percentile). Since one would expect the large majority of percentiles to be in the interquartile range, these results confirm that our controls were generally about average in their attitudes. Percentages of the adults who stutter in the lowest quartile, interquartile range, and highest quartile were, respectively, 6%, 29%, and 65%, or much more positive than average. Families' and friends' values were quite similar and also somewhat less positive than the stutterers. The 1st, 2nd–3rd, and 4th quartile percentages for families were 12%, 26%, and 62%, and for friends were 15%, 24%, and 62%.

Patterns for Various *ASE* Ratings

Overall, as seen in the OSS values, the stuttering adults had the most positive attitudes (which were well above average), followed by their families and friends (which were more positive than average and quite similar to each other), and finally by the controls (which were about average). Figure 16.1 generally reflects this pattern. It is not clear why the stutterers' families and friends had more significant differences from the controls than did the stutterers themselves, i.e., 30% and 39% versus 27%, even though the OSSs were greater for the stutterers.

The same pattern of means characterized exactly half of the *ASE* ratings (55/110), most of which were significantly different (Appendix). These ratings were highest for stutterers, next highest and similar for family or friends, and lowest for controls. Examples included: the Beliefs and Self Reactions subscores, help from component, help from other stutterers or not from a medical doctor (items), help by "me" (i.e., the respondent) item, knowledge/experience component, amount known (item), people known (item), personal experience with stuttering (item), and Internet as the source of knowledge (item).

Other patterns emerged as well, however. For 15 of the 110 ratings, stutterers and their family members and friends all had relatively similar positive attitudes but much more positive attitudes than the controls. Such profiles occurred with: rejecting physical or emotional abuse or physical injury or accident as cause (items); ability to speak without stuttering, communicate effectively, interact socially, make friends, get a job, or do well at work (items); concern or worry if one's doctor, child's teacher, religious leader, son/daughter, or sibling stuttered (items); and overall impression of a person who stutters (item).

One item, virus/disease causation for stuttering, was much more soundly rejected by the adults who stuttered than by the other three groups, which all had quite similar ratings. By contrast, one item, i.e., making a joke about stuttering, was of least concern to the stutterers, but of much higher and equal concern to the other groups.

Another interesting pattern in 10 ratings featured attitudes of friends and family members being more positive than those of the stuttering adults and controls on items such as: stutterers not being nervous/excitable or shy/fearful; stutterers should get help; rejecting pressure/tension at home, psychological, and parental overreaction to children's speech mistakes as causes; should have jobs requiring much talking; not feeling impatient or pity when talking to a stuttering person; and identifying family or friends as the source of stuttering knowledge.

The opposite pattern also occurred in 11 ratings, i.e., wherein family and friends were more negative than the stutterers and controls. Examples of items were: stuttering being associated with lower-than-average intelligence, should be helped by others who stutter, SLPs, or (not) religious leaders; causes from problems in brain function, physical makeup/body function, or not becoming bilingual in childhood; should have influential jobs; waiting patiently or not telling the person to "slow down" or "relax" during one's stuttering; and feeling curious when talking with a stuttering person.

Family and friends of the adults who stutter were significantly different on only three items, all favoring attitudes of the family members, i.e., should have jobs with lots of talking, amount known, and source of knowledge from others who stutter (items). Four others, although non-significant, also showed this pattern: rejecting help from a psychologist/psychiatrist (item), genetic causation (item), concern if I stuttered (item), and overall impression of person who stutters (item). Trends for the opposite pattern also occurred in four items, i.e., attitudes of close friends being better than those of family members occurred for: stutterers being nervous or excitable, should not be helped by a physical or occupational therapist, and not being concerned if a son/daughter or sibling stuttered.

Comparison of *ASE* with *POSHA–S*

Finally, we compared components, subscores, and the OSS for *ASE* with *POSHA–S* ratings in the four sample groups in Table 16.4. The Obesity/Mental Illness subscore, components, and items, as well as the Knowledge/Experience component in the Self Reactions subscore are unchanged in the *ASE*, so those ratings obviously are identical. Otherwise, it can be seen that the two measures are quite comparable, although there would be no *a priori* reason to assume this should be the case, given the addition of 50 items in the *ASE*. The *ASE* OSSs for family, friend, and control groups were only 2–3 points higher than the *POSHA–S* OSSs. For the stuttering adults, the *ASE* OSS was 6 points higher. Belief subscores differed by only 2–5 points, and the Self Reactions subscores differed by 9–11 points. Trait, Cause, and Social Distance/Sympathy components varied the most between the two measures.

Discussion

This study clearly demonstrated differences in the stuttering environments of individuals who have had considerable closeness to—or interaction with—adults who stutter versus those who have not. The specific results in this study suggest that a person's stuttering can improve attitudes of those associated with him or her, as was shown for friends versus controls. The same may be true for family members of a person who stutters, although the effect could be in the other direction, i.e., positive attitudes of family members could improve attitudes of stutterers. It is likely that the effect goes both ways.

In spite of evidence from earlier *POSHA–S* results (Table 16.1) and this study that attitudes of stutterers and their close associates are more positive than average, it cannot be assumed that attitudes of stutterers and their family or friends would necessarily be more positive than the non-stuttering majority. Anecdotal reports from around the world, and some solid evidence, suggest that stuttering generates negative attitudes and stigma in affected individuals and their close associates (Ip, St. Louis, Myers, & An Xuc, 2012; Özdemir, St. Louis, & Topbaş, 2011b; Reese, Hoffmann, & Li, 1999; St. Louis & Roberts, 2010). If documented, it would be in cases such as these that the *ASE* would have considerable potential to understand the reasons for—and dynamics of—such negative attitudes.

Table 16.4: Comparison of *ASE* Versus *POSHA–S* Attitudes of Four Groups: Stuttering Adults, Their Family Members, Their Close Friends, and Adults in a Control Group

POSHA–S Variable	Stuttering Adults		Family		Friends		Controls	
	ASE	*POSHA–S*	*ASE*	*POSHA–S*	*ASE*	*POSHA–S*	*ASE*	*POSHA–S*
OVERALL STUTTERING SCORE	45	39	31	28	28	26	13	10
Beliefs About People Who Stutter	52	50	45	50	44	49	33	38
Traits	50	18	52	42	60	59	42	26
Help (from)	43	53	21	23	13	12	16	27
Cause	43	56	38	57	38	53	23	40
Potential	70	72	70	78	64	74	51	58
Self Reactions to People Who Stutter	38	29	17	7	13	3	-7	-18
Accommodating/ Helping	70	58	60	48	56	42	63	42
Social Distance/ Sympathy	47	34	36	27	44	37	15	1
Knowledge/ Experience	57	57	10	10	3	3	-69	-69
Knowledge Source	-23	-33	-36	-58	-53	-69	-37	-43
Obesity/Mental Illness	-29	-29	-28	-28	-30	-30	-28	-28
Impression	-13	-13	-4	-4	-16	-16	-14	-14
Want/Have	-77	-77	-84	-84	-80	-80	-82	-82
Amount Known	1	1	5	5	5	5	12	12

The results indicate that the *ASE* shows promise as a clinical instrument. When finalized, it could be used by SLPs, who could give it to the family members and friends of their stuttering clients in order to obtain a measure of the stuttering environment. Several specific uses suggest themselves. First, the *ASE* could be given before and at regular intervals during speech therapy to determine if changes, hoped for or not hoped for in the client, were related to changes in the stuttering environment. Second, the *ASE* could be used to compare stuttering environments for different clients, especially those who responded well to speech therapy versus those who did not, to gain potentially valuable insight into the reasons for success or lack thereof. Third, if the *ASE* becomes widely used and the results documented, the instrument might well become part of a battery of measures used routinely in diagnostic evaluations to assist in prognostic appraisals.

The next step is to finalize the *ASE*. As part of that process, investigations should be undertaken to replicate these preliminary findings with other samples, especially with people who stutter who have never had any speech therapy or self-help. Once a final version is completed, it should be made available to SLPs, who could then begin the process of determining the extent to which improving the stuttering environment will affect stuttering severity, quality of life of those who stutter, and response to treatment. International comparisons using translated versions of the *ASE* should be carried out as well. Finally, since subscores and OSS on the *ASE* corresponds quite closely to parallel values on the *POSHA–S*, it would be possible to compare clients' stuttering environments using the *ASE* with those of the surrounding community using the *POSHA–S*.

Appendix

Mean ratings for *ASE* Overall Stuttering Scores, subscores, components, and items, as well as the median sample mean for 22 different samples representing 1,103 respondents. Statistically significant pair-wise comparisons are shown in bracket (see notes below).

ASE Variable	Stuttering Adults	Family	Friends	Controls	1–9 POSHA–E2 Database Median
OVERALL STUTTERING SCORE [1,2,3,5,6]	45	31	28	13	7
Beliefs About People Who Stutter [3]	52	45	44	33	27
Traits [6]	50	52	60	42	39
Are to blame[a]	63	83	90	93	86
Nervous or excitable[a] [6]	2	15	40	-10	8
Shy or fearful[a] [2,6]	-11	28	47	-6	7
Lower intelligence[a] [1,2,5,6]	79	12	13	76	76

CONTINUED

ASE Variable	Stuttering Adults	Family	Friends	Controls	1–9 POSHA-E2 Database Median
Can speak without stuttering [5,6]	71	81	77	43	52
Can communicate effectively [5,6]	70	69	81	37	36
Are pleasant	80	78	72	58	51
No different from anyone else	48	47	64	47	48
Help (from) [1,2,6]	43	21	13	16	20
Should get help[a] [1,5,6]	48	82	74	42	59
Others who stutter [1,2]	46	-29	-28	9	14
Person's family [5,6]	30	48	33	24	33
Other stutterers	46	31	28	12	2
SLP [1,2,5,6]	66	16	-1	81	81
Medical doctor[a] [3]	48	21	7	-12	-17
Psychologist/psychiatrist[a] [3,5]	20	29	-3	-30	-42
Physical/occupational therapist[a] [3]	35	2	30	-16	2
Religious leader[a] [1,2,5,6]	51	-15	-22	34	54
Cause [3,6]	43	38	38	23	16
Genetic	19	1	-29	-7	-11
Brain function [1,2,5,6]	45	-28	-23	32	31
Physical makeup/body function [1,2]	-11	-59	-57	-21	-28
Learning[a]	31	38	40	7	15
Imitation[a]	84	76	70	61	48
Talk fast[a]	27	-1	17	-7	-7
Bilingual in childhood[a] [1,2,5,6]	77	3	16	63	31
Psychological[a]	-8	14	18	-20	-18
Pressure/tension at home[a] [1,2,5,6]	21	75	74	-6	-2
Parents overreacting to mistakes in child's speech[a]	39	52	57	37	24
Emotionally traumatic event[a] [5]	56	72	64	25	-3
Physical or emotional abuse[a] [3,5,6]	42	59	47	-4	42
Act of God[a]	55	73	75	56	48
Virus/disease[a]	84	61	68	65	57

CONTINUED

ASE Variable	Stuttering Adults	Family	Friends	Controls	1–9 POSHA-E2 Database Median
Injury or accident[a] [3,5,6]	36	73	68	-7	6
Ghost/demons/spirits[a]	89	96	100	93	89
Potential [3,5]	70	70	64	51	45
Can interact socially [3,5,6]	84	83	93	57	68
Can make friends [6]	92	92	96	74	84
Can do well in school	94	90	95	79	79
Can get a job [6]	90	92	96	75	74
Can do well at work [6]	94	89	97	79	84
Can raise a family [3]	99	93	97	86	87
Can lead a normal life	82	93	94	77	78
Can do any job they want	59	73	71	51	54
Should have jobs requiring lots of talking [1,4,5,6]	-9	57	10	-36	-36
Should have jobs requiring good judgment	54	53	36	30	20
Should have jobs requiring earning trust of others	52	47	28	31	18
Should have influential jobs [1,2,3,6]	52	-20	-43	4	-8
Self Reactions to People Who Stutter [1,2,3,5,6]	*38*	*17*	*13*	*-7*	*-11*
Accommodating/Helping [2]	70	60	56	63	59
Ignore	58	79	58	74	39
Wait patiently [1,2,5,6]	74	-18	-33	66	61
Helped by me [2,3]	33	-9	-17	-37	-19
Say "It's OK to stutter"[a]	4	34	26	25	10
Say "stop stuttering"[a]	92	97	97	97	92
Joke[a]	66	95	95	94	89
Walk away[a]	98	99	99	96	91
Find another speaker[a]	100	84	94	93	87
Hit[a]	100	96	99	100	97
Fill words[a]	66	69	70	39	42

CONTINUED

ASE Variable	Stuttering Adults	Family	Friends	Controls	1–9 POSHA–E2 Database Median
Say "slow down" or "relax"[a] [1,2,5,6]	78	-31	-28	40	23
Imitate[a]	94	98	99	94	94
Hide[a] [1,5,6]	48	82	74	42	59
Social Distance/Sympathy [3,5,6]	47	36	44	15	3
Comfortable [6]	28	37	51	9	9
Relieved [2]	-1	-23	-47	-38	-43
Curious [1,2,3]	41	-36	-41	-16	-6
Surprised[a]	53	76	82	53	62
Embarrassed[a]	61	62	74	61	61
Frustrated[a] [6]	69	72	83	52	69
Impatient[a] [5,6]	66	85	91	47	56
Annoyed[a]	88	68	82	81	80
Pity[a] [5]	29	45	32	-3	20
Doctor[a] [3,5,6]	75	64	75	19	15
Child's teacher[a] [3,5,6]	63	57	67	-12	-35
Child's friend[a]	79	70	82	60	-7
Spouse[a] [3]	77	64	70	31	-39
Neighbor[a]	86	77	90	69	46
Religious leader[a] [3,6]	93	71	86	52	32
Son/daughter[a] [6]	13	-13	17	-35	-51
Sibling[a] [3,6]	35	4	41	-15	-49
Myself[a] [3,6]	8	-35	11	-47	-52
Impression [3,5]	29	30	6	-8	3
Want to stutter	-52	-62	-62	-65	-73
Knowledge/Experience [1,2,3,5,6]	57	10	3	-69	-63
Amount [2,3,4,5,6]	69	53	2	-32	-23
People known [1,2,3,5,6]	26	-63	-54	-86	-86
Personal experience [3,5,6]	77	40	62	-90	-80

CONTINUED

272

ASE Variable	Stuttering Adults	Family	Friends	Controls	1–9 POSHA–E2 Database Median
Knowledge source [2]	-23	-36	-53	-37	-44
Other people who stutter [2,3,4]	45	11	-56	-29	-15
Family/friends [1,2,5,6]	-23	62	48	-11	-42
Famous people who stutter	-36	-68	-71	-38	-65
TV/radio [5,6]	-46	-60	-56	-5	-38
Print [2]	-30	-44	-71	-51	-42
Internet [1,2,3]	-3	-56	-79	-63	-67
School	-39	-72	-56	-36	-47
Specialists	-47	-59	-81	-62	-54
Obesity/Mental Illness	*-29*	*-28*	*-30*	*-28*	*-33*
Impression	-13	-4	-16	-14	-15
Obese	-23	-17	-24	-24	-22
Mentally ill	-2	9	-7	-3	-10
Want/have	-77	-84	-80	-82	-83
Obese	-76	-80	-83	-81	-82
Mentally ill	-77	-87	-78	-84	-86
Amount known	1	5	5	12	5
Obese	5	13	19	21	20
Mentally ill	-2	-3	-8	3	-9

[a]The signs of the mean ratings for this item are reversed so that higher scores reflect "better" attitudes and lower scores "worse" attitudes.

Note: [x . . .] refers to significantly different pair-wise comparison (p ≤ .00417) for:

[1] = Stutterers versus Family
[2] = Stutterers versus Friends
[3] = Stutterers versus Controls
[4] = Family versus Friends
[5] = Family versus Controls
[6] = Friends versus Controls
No brackets = None

Children's and Parents' Perspectives about the Psychosocial Impact of Stuttering and Stuttering-Related Bullying

Susanne Cook and Peter Howell

ABSTRACT

Psychosocial impact and bullying were assessed in 15 children who stutter and their parents using two newly developed German questionnaires. The *Speech Questionnaire* measured the psychosocial impact of stuttering on the child's life; the *Bullying Assessment* measured stuttering-related bullying. Factors measured in the *Speech Questionnaire* were perspectives on stuttering in general, feelings about stuttering, different speaking situations, and impact of stuttering. Factors measured in the *Bullying Assessment* were bullying, frequency, and types of bullying. There were significantly different perspectives between children and their parents in the areas "Impact of Stuttering" and "Bullying." The clinical implications of the results are discussed.

Introduction

Stuttering can be characterized as a speech fluency disorder, but its effects extend beyond speech. Studies have shown that children who stutter are at risk of being bullied and that stuttering has an impact on the psychosocial outlook of the person who stutters (e.g., Benecken & Spindler, 2004; Blood & Blood, 2004; Hugh-Jones & Smith, 1999; Langevin, Chapter 3; Yaruss & Quesal, 2006).

Psychosocial impact refers to how well a person adjusts to the diagnosis and the extent of psychological impairment caused by the condition. "Psychosocial" is also sometimes used interchangeably with the term "quality of life" (Keeffe, 2005). Questionnaires and interview techniques have been used to assess psychosocial impact and bullying in children who stutter (e.g., Blood & Blood, 2004; Cook, Donlan, & Howell, 2013; Langevin, Bortnick, Hammer, & Wiebe, 1998, Yaruss, 2010). Such questionnaires provide information only from the child's perspective (for example, as the target of bullying). The attitude of parents toward the stuttering of their child and the impact that bullying has on both the child and the parent are also important factors in planning therapy and, potentially, its success. Clinicians not only deal with children but also with their parents, and these two groups may have different expectations and attitudes about the care the child is given. For example, a parent might be more concerned about the professional future of his or her child than the child is at some point in time. Differences in expectations were revealed through in-depth interviews in a recent qualitative study (Landau, 2011) wherein the opinions of 10 children who stutter were compared to those of their parents on a range of factors, including bullying, stuttering awareness, worries about future prospects, and acceptance. Landau reported significant differences in the opinions of the children and the parents for 75% of the topics that were addressed, e.g., parents rated the stuttering of their children as more severe and more serious than did the children, and they also expressed more concern with regard to the future than did their children.

The difference in impact that stuttering has on a child and a parent has rarely been examined in research and, when it has, concordance of impact is usually reported. Against this background and in the light of Landau's report of widespread differences between parents and children, the current study was carried out to measure the perspectives of parents and children who stutter on the psychosocial impact of stuttering on the child's life and on bullying. In order to measure psychosocial impact of stuttering and the experience of bullying, two new questionnaires were used: (1) the *Speech Questionnaire (Fragebogen zum Sprechen)*, which assesses the psychosocial impact of stuttering on the child's life (Cook & Howell 2014); and (2) the *Bullying Assessment (Fragebogen zum Mobbing)*, which obtains information about stuttering-related bullying. Both questionnaires (described in more detail below) were developed for German participants and permitted quick data collection during therapy. In their original forms, the *Speech Questionnaire* and *Bullying Assessment* were written from the child's perspective. For this study, both instruments were also rewritten from the viewpoint of the parents so that data for children and their parents could be collected.

Speech Questionnaire

Instruction. This questionnaire contains seven sets of statements. For each statement tick the answer that applies to you.

A General	Strongly agree	Agree	Somewhat agree	Somewhat disagree	Disagree	Strongly disagree
1. My speech sounds perfectly natural to me.	☐	☐	☐	☐	☐	☐

B When I think about my stuttering, I feel	Strongly agree	Agree	Somewhat agree	Somewhat disagree	Disagree	Strongly disagree
1. helpless.	☐	☐	☐	☐	☐	☐

C Different speaking situations	Strongly agree	Agree	Somewhat agree	Somewhat disagree	Disagree	Strongly disagree
1. I don't avoid activities, speaking situations or certain people, even when I think I might stutter more.	☐	☐	☐	☐	☐	☐

D Impact of Stuttering	Strongly agree	Agree	Somewhat agree	Somewhat disagree	Disagree	Strongly disagree
1. My life is much affected by how other people react to my stuttering.	☐	☐	☐	☐	☐	☐

Figure 17.1: Speech Questionnaire (sample statements for children).

Bullying Assessment

E Bullying	Always	Very often	Often	Sometimes	Rarely	Never
1. I get bullied at school.	☐	☐	☐	☐	☐	☐

F Frequency of bullying	Never	Not more than other kids	A bit more than other kids	Often	Very often	All the time
1. How much do you get bullied now?	☐	☐	☐	☐	☐	☐

G Forms of bullying	Always	Very often	Often	Sometimes	Rarely	Never
1. I was/am called names.	☐	☐	☐	☐	☐	☐

Figure 17.2: Bullying Assessment (sample statements for children).

Based on Landau's (2011) study, it was hypothesized that, using these questionnaires, the perspectives of children and their parents would differ. Sample extracts from English versions of the child forms are provided in figures 17.1 and 17.2, and from the parent forms in figures 17.3 and 17.4.

Method

Participants

Fifteen German-speaking children and adolescents who stutter (10 boys and 5 girls) between 9.0 and 17.7 years of age ($M = 14.1$, $SD = 2.9$) and one parent of each child participated in the study. No restriction was placed on which parent completed the questionnaires. All children and adolescents participated in an intensive summer therapy program.

Speech Questionnaire

Instruction. This questionnaire contains seven sets of statements. For each statement tick the answer that applies to you.

A General	Strongly agree	Agree	Somewhat agree	Somewhat disagree	Disagree	Strongly disagree
1. The speech of my child sounds perfectly natural to me.	□	□	□	□	□	□

B When I think about my child's stuttering, I feel	Strongly agree	Agree	Somewhat agree	Somewhat disagree	Disagree	Strongly disagree
1. helpless.	□	□	□	□	□	□

C Different speaking situations	Strongly agree	Agree	Somewhat agree	Somewhat disagree	Disagree	Strongly disagree
1. My child doesn't avoid activities, speaking situations or certain people, even when s/he thinks s/he might stutter more.	□	□	□	□	□	□

D Impact of Stuttering	Strongly agree	Agree	Somewhat agree	Somewhat disagree	Disagree	Strongly disagree
1. My child's life is much affected by how other people react to his/her stuttering.	□	□	□	□	□	□

Figure 17.3: Speech Questionnaire (sample statements for parents).

Bullying Assessment

E Bullying	Always	Very often	Often	Sometimes	Rarely	Never
1. My child gets bullied at school.	□	□	□	□	□	□

F Frequency of bullying	Never	Not more than other kids	A bit more than other kids	Often	Very often	All the time
1. How much does your child get bullied now?	□	□	□	□	□	□

G Forms of bullying	Always	Very often	Often	Sometimes	Rarely	Never
1. My child was/is called names.	□	□	□	□	□	□

Figure 17.4: Bullying Assessment (sample statements for parents).

Instruments

Cook's (2013) *Speech Questionnaire*, which measures the impact of stuttering on the child's life, consists of 27 statements in four categories that relate to the four areas specified in the International Classification of Functioning, Disability, and Health (ICF) (World Health Organization, 2001). The *Speech Questionnaire* dimensions are: "A: General" with five statements (e.g., "My speech sounds perfectly normal to me"); "B: Feelings towards stuttering" with seven statements (e.g., "When I think about my stuttering I feel helpless"); "C: Different speaking situations" with eight statements (e.g., "I don't avoid activities, speaking situations or certain people, even when I think I might stutter more"); and "D: Impact of stuttering" with seven statements (e.g., "My life is much affected by how other people react to my stuttering"). Responses to each statement are rated on 6-point Likert scales ranging from "strongly agree" to "strongly disagree," with higher scores indicating greater impact of stuttering on the child's life. The child form of the *Speech Questionnaire* is a reliable and valid instrument. Cook (2013) and Cook, Donlan, and Howell (2013) reported Cronbach's alpha = .855; test-retest reliability correlation for 22 participants, which was highly significant with $r = .925$ and p < .001. The Kaiser-Meyer-Olkin Measure of Sampling Adequacy (KMO) was .833, which, according to Field (2009), is a good result. The overall score, summed over the 27 statements, ranged from 27 to 162 and provided a measure that reflects severity of the experienced impact of stuttering on the child's life.

The *Bullying Assessment* (Cook & Howell, 2014) measured the child's experiences of bullying. The assessment consists of 13 statements in three categories. The categories are: "A: Bullying" with five statements (e.g., "I get bullied at school"); "B: Frequency of bullying," with two statements (e.g., "I never get bullied now"); and "C: Type of bullying" with six statements (e.g., "I was/am called names"). The statements in category C involve responses to two different points in time, i.e., "when the child was younger" and "today." This permits one to document bullying that occurred in the past, even when the child is no longer bullied. Responses from 196 German children who stutter were used to assess reliability and validity of the *Bullying Assessment*. Split-half reliability, calculated on all 196 children who stutter, gave a Cronbach's alpha of .883, which is a good result (Field & Hole, 2003). Test-retest reliability was assessed on 22 participants, and this was highly significant with $r = .923$, p < .001. The overall score of the *Bullying Assessment* for three categories (Bullying, Frequency of bullying, Types of bullying) ranged from 13 to 78. These values reflect the severity of experiences of bullying with higher numbers indicating a more severe bullying experienced by the child.

The two measures were compared for criterion validity by calculating and correlating the raw scores of the *Bullying Assessment* with the raw scores of the *Speech Questionnaire*. The correlation was significant ($r = .347$, p < .001).

Children and parents separately completed the *Speech Questionnaire* and the *Bullying Assessment* before the children received therapy intervention. Although separate instruments, the two questionnaires were distributed together to respondents.

Results

The overall results (mean scores and standard deviation) of the scores of the *Speech Questionnaire* and the *Bullying Assessment* are given in Table 17.1. The scores are reported first as overall scores (summed across all items for all the categories) and then for the separate categories (summed across all items within each), and finally the responses to the individual statements within the categories are examined.

Table 17.1: Mean Overall Scores and Category Scores, Followed by Standard Deviations and Standard Errors of the Means for the *Speech Questionnaire* (*SQ*) and the *Bullying Assessment* (*BA*) Completed by 15 Children Who Stutter and 15 of Their Parents

	Group	Mean	Standard Deviation	Standard Error Mean
SQ Overall score	child	82.33	22.79	5.884
	parent	91.27	21.11	5.451
BA Overall score	child	25.07	7.45	1.923
	parent	28.53	10.02	2.587
SQ "General"	child	15.33	4.78	1.233
	parent	17.73	3.88	1.002
SQ "Feelings Toward Stuttering"	child	21.93	7.75	2.001
	parent	22.13	8.64	2.232
SQ "Different Speaking Situations"	child	25.67	7.12	1.838
	parent	26.40	7.06	1.823
SQ "Impact of Stuttering"	child	19.40	7.55	1.949
	parent	25.00	4.74	1.223
BA "Bullying"	child	10.47	4.17	1.077
	parent	14.33	5.25	1.355
BA "Frequency of Bullying"	child	4.80	1.57	.405
	parent	4.67	1.40	.361
BA "Type of Bullying"	child	9.80	3.45	.890
	parent	9.53	4.75	1.226

Overall Scores

Speech Questionnaire: Generally, the overall scores (summed across all items and categories) of the parents indicated that the psychosocial impact stuttering has on their children was higher than was reported by the children (91 versus 82). Nevertheless, there were no significant differences between the questionnaires completed by the children and by their parents using an independent sample *t*-test: $t(28) = -1.114$, p $= .275$, *ns*.

Bullying assessment: As a group, parents thought that their children experienced more bullying than was reported by the children (29 versus 25). Again, these scores did not differ significantly: $t(28) = -1.075$, p $= .291$, *ns*.

Scores for Categories

Speech Questionnaire: To gain more detailed insight into the perspectives of the children and their parents, results of the categories (summed across each set of individual items) of the *Speech Questionnaire* were compared. There was a significant correlation between the perspectives of the children who stutter and

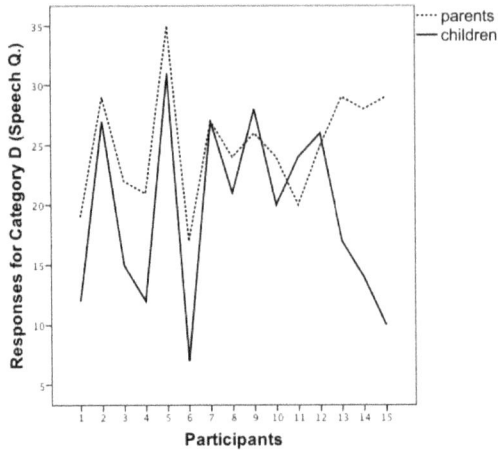

Figure 17.5: Comparison of children's and parents' responses for category D: "Impact of Stuttering" of the Speech Questionnaire.

their parents for category D: "Impact of Stuttering" (r = .536, p =.040), which indicated that scores tended to correspond (e.g., if a parent had a high score, his or her child was also likely to score high), but for this category there were also significant differences of the perspectives of the children who stutter and their parents: $t(28)$ = -2.434, p = .022. Figure 17.5 shows this relationship graphically and indicates that results of parents and children generally went in a similar direction, but parents tended to rate the impact stuttering had on the lives of their children higher than the children.

Bullying Assessment: No significant correlations between individual parent and child scores within any of the categories of the *Bullying Assessment* were found. Category A (Bullying) of the *Bullying Assessment* showed significant mean differences between the perspectives of the children who stutter and their parents: $t(28)$ = -2.234, p = .034. The experiences of bullying reported by the children were less what parents thought their children were experiencing.

Responses to Individual Statements

Speech Questionnaire: Finally, responses to individual statements were examined by conducting an independent samples *t*-test to compare the responses of the children who stutter with the responses of the parents (not shown in Table 17.1). There was a significant difference in the perspective of children ($\overline{X}$ = 2.67, SD = 1.839) and parents ($\overline{X}$ = 5.07, SD = 1.387) with respect to statement D2 of the *Speech Questionnaire:* "My ability to succeed at school is not really influenced by my stuttering" ($t(28)$ = -4.036, p < .001). These results suggested that parents rated this statement significantly more negatively than the children.

Bullying Assessment: With respect to individual item comparisons on the *Bullying Assessment*, a significant difference between the responses of children ($\overline{X}$ = 2.13, SD = 1.685) and parents ($\overline{X}$ = 3.80, SD = 2.007) occurred for the statement A4: "The bullying affects my stuttering" ($t(28)$ = -2.463, p = .020). This indicated that parents rated the impact of bullying on stuttering higher than their children. The other significant difference between children ($\overline{X}$ = 1.40, SD = 1.121) and parents ($\overline{X}$ = 2.73, SD = 1.907) was found for statement A5: "I find it hard to make friends at school" ($t(28)$ = -2.334, p = .027). Parents again rated this statement more negatively than their children.

Discussion

Overall scores of the *Speech Questionnaire* completed by children and parents did not show significant differences, and neither did three of the category scores, which means the hypothesis that the perspectives of children and their parents would differ was not supported. Only for category D of the *Speech Questionnaire*, "Impact of Stuttering," did a discrepancy between the perspectives of children and their parents occur, which suggests that parents rated the psychosocial impact stuttering has on their children higher than did the children. Statements relating to this category dealt with, for example, whether stuttering impacts the success at school (p = .003), or relationships with other people (p = .116). This is in line with the results of Landau's (2011) qualitative, retrospective study of experiences and expectations about therapy outcome of 10 dyads of children who stutter and their parents. Landau found a significant divergence of opinions between children who stutter and their parents with respect to experiences and expectations. The significant difference observed for statement D2 in this study showed that parents worried a lot about the impact stuttering had on their child's success at school and subsequent potential for their working life. Landau (2011) also found that parents mentioned concerns about the future significantly more often than did their children.

Regarding the *Bullying Assessment*, there was no significant difference between responses of the children who stutter and their parents with respect to the overall scores. Again, the hypothesis that perspectives of parents and children would differ was not supported. Looking at the categories, opinions of parents and their children in the current results differed significantly only for category A: "Bullying," which addressed issues such as whether the child was bullied at school, whether the bullying was directly related to the stuttering, or whether the bullying affected the stuttering. Child versus parent ratings for statement A4 ("The bullying affects my stuttering" / "The bullying affects the stuttering of my child") indicated that parents thought the effect of bullying on the child was greater than the child perceived it to be. This was also true for statement A5 of the *Bullying Assessment* ("I find it hard to make friends at school" / "It is hard for my child to make friends at school"). Results indicated that with respect to friendships, parents as a group thought it was harder for their child to make friends than did the children.

Limitations of the Present Study

One reason for the fact that the hypothesis was not supported could be that in this study, questionnaires only were used to collect data, which is less sensitive than the structured interviews Landau (2011) used. The versions for parents of the *Speech Questionnaire* and the *Bullying Assessment* were not validated for this study and should be addressed in a future study. For the current study, however, because the children's versions were reliable and valid, there was little reason to expect that this would not apply to the parent's version. However, until the parent version is validated, caution should be used in interpreting whether they give different responses to their children. Also, no information was collected concerning whether the mother or the father completed the parent versions. It did not seem appropriate to ask for only parents of one gender to complete the questionnaire as, in some cases, only one parent spoke German. Also, some single-parent families participated in the study. It is probable that in most cases, mothers completed the questionnaires, but parent gender should be considered in future work. Also, a major limitation in most studies about bullying and stuttering is that children who stutter have only been investigated as targets of bullying (e.g., Benecken & Spindler, 2004; Blood & Blood, 2004; Blood, Boyle, Blood, & Nalesnik, 2010; Hugh-Jones & Smith, 1999; Langevin, Chapter 3; Langevin et al., 1998). There is little doubt that children who stutter have a greater chance of being bullied, but it is also known that a child targeted for bullying is at risk to become a bully (Nansel, Overpeck, Pilla, Ruan, Simons-Morton, & Scheidt. 2001). At present, it is not clear the extent to which this situation applies to children who stutter. Parents might well know about their child bullying (from reports from schools), so questions related to this issue could be added to revisions of the *Bullying Assessment*.

Clinical Implications

It is important to be aware of the impact stuttering can have on a person's life and of stuttering-related bullying. Since parents perceived the psychosocial impact and experience of bullying as more severe than their children for some statements, discussing the impact of stuttering, school-related bullying, and related concerns could be important for both parents and children who stutter. One possibility would be to arrange for group counseling with parents of stuttering children of different ages. In this way, parents of older children could share how they dealt with education-related concerns and share strategies that have worked for them and their child. Another possibility would be to conduct therapy sessions with the parent and their child to highlight and align each individual's perspectives.

Chapter 18

_____

Stuttering in Women: Changes and Adaptations Throughout the Lifespan

Kathleen Scaler Scott and Dinamichele Boyer

ABSTRACT

Gender differences in attitudes and experiences of adults who stutter have been studied to a small degree. Qualitative analyses of adults who stutter have included women as part of their sample; however, no such analysis to date has specifically explored the experience of women who stutter at different points in their lifetime. This pilot study was designed as a preliminary look at the experiences of three women who stutter who were, respectively, in adolescence, young adulthood, and middle adulthood. Ethnographic interviews were conducted, and transcripts were culled for emergent themes. Specific identified themes included those related to outcomes of communication avoidance, preferences for listener reactions to stuttering, and shifting cognitive perceptions of stuttering with age. Clinical and research implications of findings are discussed.

Background

The experiences and perspectives of people who stutter have contributed significantly to the literature and have informed clinical practice. Qualitative research has helped us to gain in-depth knowledge (Tetnowski & Damico, 2001) of the experiences of people who stutter regarding treatment (Cream, Packman, & Llewellyn, 2004; Irani, Gabel, Daniels, & Hughes, 2012), life experiences (Daniels, Gabel, & Hughes, 2012; Daniels, Hagstrom, & Gabel, 2006; Klompas & Ross, 2004), recovery

(Finn & Felsenfeld, 2004), management (Plexico, Manning, & DiLollo, 2005; Plexico, Manning, & Levitt, 2009a, 2009b), and therapeutic relationships (Plexico, Manning, & DiLollo, 2010). One method of qualitative research deals with phenomenology. Unlike quantitative research wherein data are gathered regarding a specific question such as "What percentage of women who stutter choose to disclose their stuttering?", a phenomenological approach considers a phenomenon, such as the life experience of someone with stuttering, from the perspective of the participant (Cresswell, 1998). The data are gathered via recorded responses to open-ended questions, and findings emerge from the data analysis in the form of common themes. A "rich" picture of the important issues from the perspective of a participant (in this case, a person who stutters) is derived in this way.

Gender differences in attitudes and experiences of adults who stutter have been studied to a limited extent. Silverman and Zimmer (1979) found significant differences between stuttering women and men in scores on the short form of Erickson's S-scale, which measures communication attitudes. Silverman and Zimmer (1982) also reported gender differences in stuttering symptomatology and treatment experiences. Silverman (1982) found that clinicians considered stuttering to have a stronger negative impact upon females and children, whereas university students considered stuttering to have a stronger negative impact upon males, regardless of age. Qualitative analyses of adults who stutter have included women as part of their sample (Blood, Blood, Tellis, & Gabel, 2003; Corcoran & Stewart, 1998; Cream et al., 2004; Daniels et al., 2012; Irani et al., 2012; Klompas & Ross, 2004; Plexico et al., 2005; Plexico et al., 2010; Plexico et al., 2009a, 2009b); however, no such analysis to date has specifically explored the experience of women who stutter at different points in their lifetime.

This pilot study explored the experiences of women who stutter in late adolescence, early adulthood (i.e., twenties), and middle adulthood (i.e., forties). It was designed as a first step in using qualitative methodology to compare the experiences of women who stutter across different ages. The study sought to answer the following questions from the perspective of the participants: (1) What experiences are most salient to women who stutter at different points in their lives? and (2) What issues, if any, are unique to the experience of being a woman who stutters?

Method

Participants

Three females, one teen and two adults, who stuttered were interviewed for this study. All three participants were diagnosed with stuttering in early childhood by speech-language pathologists, and all three had previous fluency therapy, but were not currently enrolled in any therapy program. Average to above-average cognitive abilities was assumed based on completion of a bachelor's degree and doctoral degree for the two adults, respectively, and enrollment in honors coursework at a competitive high school for the teen. All participants were confirmed to exhibit patterns of stuttering by the first author, a speech-language pathologist with 20 years of experience and a Board-Certified Specialist in Fluency. All participants were administered the *Overall Assessment of the Speaker's Experience of Stuttering* (*OASES*) for adults (Yaruss & Quesal, 2008) or the *OASES-T* for teens (Yaruss, Quesal, & Coleman, 2010) to determine the overall impact of stuttering upon their life experience.

The teenager (TA) was a 17-year-old female completing her junior year in a competitive high school and taking Advanced Placement courses at the time of the study. TA was born in Guatemala, and was bilingual in Spanish and English. She began stuttering in early childhood and received therapy with her public school speech-language pathologist. Upon moving into a competitive private school in Grade 5, an increase in stuttering was noticed, so she sought private speech-language therapy to address this. TA reported that she felt her stuttering had limited impact upon her willingness to communicate in the early elementary years until she experienced a significant block while reading in front of her church and witnessed peers laughing. TA has not participated in any stuttering support groups. She scored a "moderate" overall impact (overall score 2.52) of stuttering upon her life on the *OASES-T*.

The young adult participant (YA), a 23-year-old female with a bachelor's degree in education, was employed as an English as a second language teacher. YA also began stuttering in early childhood. She had therapy throughout her elementary school years both from school-based and private practice speech-language pathologists. She was introduced to stuttering support in her late teens, and continued to play an active role in local and national stuttering support groups. She scored a "mild to moderate" overall impact (overall score 1.66) of stuttering upon her life on the *OASES*.

Participant MA (middle adulthood) was a 46-year-old female with a doctoral degree in criminal justice who was employed with a government agency as a grants manager. She reported that her stuttering began in early childhood and described herself as a covert stutterer working toward acceptance of more overt stuttering. She reported trying many techniques throughout her life to manage her stuttering, including combinations of speech therapy, counseling, and medication. She recently was introduced to stuttering support through the National Stuttering Association (NSA), and consistently attended annual conventions.

She scored a "moderate" overall impact (overall score 2.90) of stuttering upon her life on the *OASES*.

Data Collection

Data were collected via ethnographic interviews (Spradley, 1979). Each participant was interviewed in a quiet room by the authors. For the ethnographic interviews, "grand tour," "mini tour," and "example" questions were constructed. Grand tour questions are broad in scope and serve as a catalyst for participants to share their stories about their experience of stuttering from their own perspective. Primary grand tour questions for this study were: "What is your experience being a person who stutters?" and "What is your experience being a woman who stutters?" Mini tour questions are more focused, yet still broad enough for participants to speak on the given topic from their perspective. Mini tour questions consisted of the following: "How has your life been affected by stuttering?" and "What experiences regarding stuttering have stood out in your life?" Mini tour questions were followed up by questions seeking further examples as topics emerged from the interview (e.g., "You stated that how you react to stuttering has changed. Can you give some examples of ways your reactions have changed?").

Data Coding

Analysis of the interviews followed the recommendations of Smith and Osborn (2003) for Interpretive Phenomenological Analysis. Procedures included orthographic transcription of all interviews, reading of transcriptions by multiple coders, culling interviews for relevant themes, identifying and clustering emerging themes, triangulation among coders to establish reliability, and member checking to ensure validity.

Results

Emergent Themes

Three themes emerged from the analyses. After each, illustrative examples of commentary supporting it are presented and explained.

PRIVATE ATTITUDES TOWARD THE PUBLIC'S REACTIONS TO STUTTERING CHANGES WITH AGE. Included in this theme is the idea of a shift in the perception about the role of a person who stutters in educating the listener about stuttering. The teen's perception was that she preferred others to quietly accept her stuttering, allowing her flexibility in how much she wished to respond and communicate with others, and to refrain from seeking more information about stuttering. In short, the teen seemed to view it positively when others would accept her stuttering and "just let me be." She did not indicate that she viewed herself as playing a role in educating others about stuttering:

> *TA:* Teachers have definitely been very understanding and they don't pressure me to do anything or they don't ask me a billion questions about it to the point where it's it's kind of like as if they don't get it at all. They just kind of seemed to accept it and just let me be in class. . . .

This view of it being the listener's responsibility to understand and accept stuttering seemed to shift over time for the participant in her twenties. YA described her change in perception of others' reactions over time, indicating that whereas she once used negative listener reactions as a means to identify unkind listeners, she later developed a broader view of possible reasons for negative reactions. She also indicated that even though she did not always desire to do so, she felt responsible for educating misinformed listeners about stuttering:

> *YA:* . . . So one time I heard someone say that stuttering is like a jerk detector where it's like if you meet someone for the first time and you stutter and they do something stupid, like say you stutter on your name and they say "Oh, did you forget your name?" Because obviously, I just forgot my name. So it's like this person is probably a jerk so you can avoid them and not have to waste time becoming this person's friend . . . So, I feel like if anything it taught me to like weed out potential people.

> *YA:* One time, I was on a date with someone and my stuttering was kind of like my medium amount, like not too much, you know, the right amount of stuttering. I remember, he wasn't giving me eye contact, he might have finished my sentences a couple of times and I was starting to get really pissed off about it. Like, what are you doing? . . . But then what I realized later was he was just super nervous. . . . I think sometimes it's easy to judge people really harshly. Like, I think that this person finished my sentence once so this person is a jerk. Which I know what is something I'm sometimes guilty of doing. Sometimes, you just have to tell people how to respond because they don't know.

While TA saw the listener as responsible for knowing how to react to stuttering, and YA expressed a mixed view, Participant MA (i.e., forties) expressed a strong feeling of the importance of educating others.

> *MA:* So I kind of see it as, for something like this, the more people I tell I think the better. . . . The more people . . . Now they know someone who stutters where maybe they didn't know anyone.

> *MA:* Well, I kind of did this a little bit when I started disclosing at work to try and help them because people want to know how they should react, right? The same way with if you're in a wheelchair, do you want me to open the door for you, or is that patronizing? So, people generally want to know what's the appropriate thing to do.

REGRET OF AVOIDANCE CAN MOVE A PERSON WHO STUTTERS IN A POSITIVE OR NEGATIVE DIRECTION. The second theme relates to the fact that all three participants expressed regret about avoiding at least one communication opportunity. For TA and MA, this regret occurred at different points of their schooling, but was still brought up as a significant moment for the participants, shaping their feelings and/or events in later years.

> *TA:* Sometimes I have felt like I couldn't do things. For example, a big thing has been participating in classes and doing a big group presentation. In eighth grade every eighth grader has to have a speech and has to say it in front of the whole middle school and I didn't do it and I think that it has definitely held me back from doing some things. . . . I'm just like every eighth grader does it and I didn't so I feel like as if I didn't really complete eighth grade because of that.

> *MA:* It affected college in that . . . I think there was one presentation that I had to do for this one class where I don't remember how I did it, I think I told the professor that I stuttered but I did something where he let me go without doing the presentation and I had to do something else. . . . When I did that, I sent myself a message that there are certain things I can't do. And that was . . . I hated being limited, which, by the way, I think drove me to higher education because I felt at least if I had a PhD, no one could doubt my intelligence. I think that was one of the drivers of me going for my degree.

MA's regret of her decision to avoid shaped her educational and career path. She explains that currently she uses the idea of avoidance as a motivator to push her forward in communication situations:

MA: As I got older, I would have the little challenges for myself. I would say, "If I didn't stutter, would I do this?" If the answer was yes, I would do it. A lot of times I would be like, oh I can't do that because I stutter. I said, no, no. If I didn't stutter, would I still do this? Yes. So, then I would do it. It was just a little personal victory for me.

For YA, the regret is more in the "little moments" when she misses an opportunity to educate others. Like MA, the memory of avoidance drives her toward positive action:

YA: A couple of years ago I had gone to vote in some election I forgot what it was and . . . how after you vote you have to go to a volunteer and you give them like your street and your name and after that they look you up and give you a ballot and when you deposit it you do the same thing? Well, a police officer was manning the table and he was asking for street and name. I said my street okay and then, when I got to say my last name, I was stuttering. Not really, it was a block, it just wasn't coming out. So, the police officer, not a random person, was just like "Oh, did you forget your name?" I forget what he said exactly but it was just like some variation of that. The thing I was really proud of myself for in this moment is I think a lot of times it's really easy to shrug these things off and just be like, ha ha, because it's hard to react in the moment, but that time I said "No actually I stutter. I was stuttering." And he immediately was like, "Oh." And then immediately the volunteer sitting next to him was like "Oh he didn't mean anything by it." But I was like "Well, it's still hurtful so you should be more careful." It's a lot of situations like that really. . . . I feel like it's good to be able to feel proud of myself when I react the way I did when I was voting when I am able to actually respond.

TURNING POINTS SHIFTED PERSPECTIVES ABOUT STUTTERING. All participants spoke of specific turning points in their lives that shifted their perspectives regarding their stuttering (third theme). For TA, it was the acceptance of her stuttering by teachers and friends that seemed to help her worry less about her stuttering.

Interviewer: You said earlier that now you've learned to not make stuttering a big deal and to not worry about it so much. What things do you think made your view about that change over time?

TA: Probably all the support I had at school.

TA: I guess when I switched from public school to private and I met my new friends, I told them that I went to therapy for that and they seemed to accept it so I guess that was positive.

For YA and MA, turning points came when they were introduced to stuttering support in the form of NSA annual conventions. YA's turning point occurred when she was able to meet a positive role model through the convention, whereas MA's turning point occurred when she met others who stuttered, and realized that instead of stuttering being something she should hide, it was a positive aspect of people.

YA: One thing also, for me, at my first conference I met this girl named Kerry who was a teacher. I forget what grade she taught in elementary school and she stuttered. I guess this was a turning point actually. Basically, meeting her and talking to her made me realize that I could be a teacher and stutter. . . . In the back of my head I always had these ideas that maybe I can't do this. But then, when I talked to her and met her it made me realize that yeah, I can do this. It's not that crazy. . . . I think it's important for kids and other people to see themselves reflected in other people and to realize that they can be successful. That was probably a huge turning point for me.

MA: Going to my first full NSA conference, it struck me that when you're around stuttering all the time, that's the norm. That was normal to me. And everyone had their own style and their own personality through their stutter and it really became like a style. No two styles were the same. I remember so clearly being at the airport, waiting to go home, ordering some food, everyone talking fluently, and being like, wow, there's nothing. It's just so boring. No pizzazz. Nothing.

Discussion and Implications

From the perspectives of these three participants, it is evident that what may be viewed in the teen years and early adult years as negative listener reactions may later be perceived as an opportunity for educating others about stuttering. This difference raises potential implications about educating listeners on how to react when someone stutters. Blood et al., (2003) studied the disclosure practices of 48 adolescents who stutter. Sixty percent of them indicated that it was a rare occasion when they disclosed their stuttering to others. This avoidance of disclosure reflects the quiet acceptance wish expressed by TA in the current study. Although some of the existing material for listeners gives advice for nonverbal reactions that might apply across age ranges, we might consider different strategies for listeners of teens, such as quiet acceptance rather than frequent questioning, even if questioning is coming from a place of genuine interest. Clinically, a speech-language pathologist would want to determine whether a teen is ready to discuss and/or disclose stuttering and, if not, to continue to leave the door open for discussion when the time is right. This message may be an important one for parents of teens who stutter as well.

The finding that one's regret of avoidance can move those who stutter in a positive or negative direction carries important clinical implications. DiLollo and Manning (2007) have discussed using narrative therapy to have people who stutter tell their story and then reconstruct that story to change their view of stuttering's impact upon their life. In the current study, regret seemed to have moved both adults toward less avoidance of challenging communication situations. The adults seemed able to reconstruct their avoidance stories of past into future positive action. This type of story reconstruction could be used to help TA shape her future reality of attempts to approach communication challenges.

The adults in the current study expressed that support from the NSA marked a "turning point" in their thinking about stuttering. Yaruss, Quesal, and Murphy (2002) found similar perceptions among adults when they surveyed 200 adult members of the NSA. The investigators found that two of the resources rated highest for people who stutter were national stuttering support groups and/or educational groups regarding stuttering. These findings validate the need to consider stuttering support as a strong component in the therapeutic process for a person who stutters.

Future Areas of Research and Conclusion

This pilot study was designed to examine emerging themes among women who stutter at various ages. Although no gender-specific issues emerged from the perspective of this group, examination of these issues in a larger group of women of various ages would be appropriate. Such a study would help to determine whether the themes emerging in this study are representative of women who stutter in general, or were unique to the study participants. Also, themes that would emerge from larger samples of women should be compared to those that emerge from a parallel sample of men. As in-depth qualitative information continues to be amassed from the perspective of people who stutter, interventions and stuttering support can continue to be improved accordingly.

Chapter 19

_____

Qualitative Analysis of Covert Stuttering: Workplace Implications and Saving Face

Jill Douglass and John Tetnowski

ABSTRACT

The study investigated former covertly stuttering people within a qualitative research paradigm. Open-ended, ethnographic interviews were carried out with six adults who identified themselves as people who stutter and also who, for some time in their lives, covertly stuttered. The six participants shared their experiences of covert stuttering and their process of coming to terms with overt stuttering with three whose experiences related strongly with workplace issues. Emerging themes dealt with why some people maintain their covertness in the workplace, i.e., saving face and maintaining one's professional reputation. In contrast, the interviews elucidated why and how individuals with covert stuttering, through workplace penalties, can come to realize that hiding one's stuttering is unproductive. Considering parallels with other marginalized populations, recommendations for future directions in covert stuttering research are presented.

Introduction

"Covert stuttering" is discussed in the stuttering literature and appears in current textbooks related to fluency disorders (e.g., Manning, 2010); however, the topic has not attracted significant and systematic research. Bloodstein and Bernstein Ratner's (2008) careful review of the literature documented a paucity of systematic research for covert stuttering, and commented that "even with the passage of many years, this topic has not yet attracted a significant body of published research. 'Covert' stuttering appears to be a well-recognized clinical phenomenon with sparse research documentation" (p. 2).

From sparse published research regarding covert stuttering, we can derive a basic understanding of some of its core elements. Similar to Goffman's (1963) concept of *passing* as a normal person, Petrunik and Shearing (1983) mentioned that covert individuals may keep their stuttering a secret in an attempt to preserve their social identity as a typical fluent speaker. Many studies have documented the negative view of stuttering (e.g., Lass, Ruscello, Pannbacker, Schmitt, Kiser, Mussa, & Lockhart, 1994) held by people in positions of power. Knowledge of this perception may influence people who stutter to remain covert. Anecdotal reports exist that attempt to explain why some people who stutter become covert (e.g., Murphy, Quesal, & Gulker, 2007). These suggest that covertness is an attempt to preserve social identity, which may emerge after a listener's reprimand or disdain toward stuttered speech, e.g., a father telling his young daughter not to speak unless she speaks without a stutter.

Once an individual's stuttering has become covert, the person's attempts at remaining covert can go to extraordinary lengths. For some, being covert involves concealing their stuttering only in specific social situations (e.g., workplace) while others keep their stuttering a secret in any and all social interactions, even from those who are closest to them (e.g., a spouse, parent, or sibling). The cost of concealing stuttering can range from behavioral patterns as minimal as forgoing contributing to a conversation to those as complex as developing a pseudo-identity as a person who is considered "quiet" (since he or she minimally contributes) or "flaky" (since the person always seems to be at a loss for words and circumnavigates a topic) (Petrunik & Shearing, 1983).

Researchers who have acknowledged the existence of covert stuttering have highlighted the complex issue of definition and measurement. It is challenging to reliably measure a disorder that occurs intrinsically and should, therefore, be measured intrinsically (e.g., Douglass & Quarrington, 1952; Murphy et al., 2007; Perkins, 1990; St. Louis, 2006). Therefore, investigating unobservable behaviors (e.g., switching words before they are uttered) can play a key role in understanding this phenomenon.

Research findings suggest that the heightened anxiety associated with overt stuttering is comparable to that of individuals who seek treatment for anxiety disorders. Such anxiety in those who stutter is not regarded as the cause of stuttering; instead, it is viewed primarily as a result of stuttering (Iverach, O'Brian, Jones, Block, Lincoln, Harrison, Hewat, Menzies, Packman, & Onslow, 2009). The *Diagnostic and Statistical Manual of Mental Disorders* (American Psychiatric

Association, 2013) provides descriptive symptomology of covert symptoms of stuttering: "the disturbance [stuttering] causes anxiety about speaking or limitation in effective communication, social participation, or academic or occupational performance, individually or in any combination" (p. 46). With the known anxiety that people who stutter experience, it is reasonable to hypothesize that people who stutter covertly experience even greater anxiety from the pressure to pass as non-stutterers in their daily lives. In fact, Perkins (1990) wrote that individuals who report the greatest impact of stuttering on their life are those who rarely, if ever, allow others to see them stutter.

One aspect of life affected by overt stuttering is the workplace. In a number of studies (e.g., Gabel, Chapter 4; Klein & Hood, 2004; Palasik, Gabel, Hughes, Rusnak, 2012; Schlagheck, Gabel, Hughes, 2009), people who stutter have reported that their stuttering had negatively impacted their workplace experience, hindered their job prospects and workplace potential, and limited their responsibilities in the workplace. Most of these published findings regarding workplace experiences were conducted through survey methods, presumably concerning individuals whose stuttering was overt. The need exists to explore further the individual experience of workplace-related issues related to stuttering from a qualitative perspective and also to explore those perspectives for covertly stuttering people.

Purpose

Therefore, the purpose of the research described in this chapter was to systematically investigate the personal lives and experiences of individuals who self-reportedly stuttered covertly prior to being interviewed. As part of a research investigation on the transition from covert stuttering to overt stuttering, this chapter focuses on the question: What impact does covert stuttering have on a person's professional identity? Secondarily, it seeks to identify parallels between the covert to overt transition process of people who stutter and other marginalized populations, most notably lesbian, gay, bisexual, and transgender people (LGBT).

Method

Participants

Six participants (i.e., three males and three females) either identified themselves as people who formerly stuttered covertly and at the time of the interview identified themselves as people who stuttered overtly, *or* identified themselves as people who at the time of the interview were acknowledging their covert stuttering and in transition to stuttering overtly. They all met the following inclusion criteria: (1) reported having a history of stuttering as a child; (2 reported that he or she was, for some time, primarily a person who stuttered covertly and was in the process of openly identifying himself or herself as a person who stuttered overtly; and (3) were in early to middle adulthood (between the ages of 18 and 55).

Although not a criterion for inclusion, all of the participants were involved in the stuttering self-help community at a local or national level. They were recruited through personal contacts with the National Stuttering Association, Friends: The National Association for Young People Who Stutter, and by word of mouth. To protect their identities, the participants were de-identified in the data analysis (see below).

This study focused on the data and findings that highlighted the workplace implications of stuttering covertly. The three participants who provided the richest description of workplace implications included Annette (early forties), Chris (late thirties), and Elise (late thirties).

Qualitative Research Procedures

Semi-structured ethnographic interviews were conducted with the six individuals via the Internet-based program Skype. Electronic, live video interviews were completed in lieu of live face-to-face interviews due to geographical constraints of the participants' and the investigator's locations, and are widely accepted in this type of research (e.g., Johns, Chen, & Hall, 2003; O'Connor, Madge, Shaw, & Wellens, 2008).

Length of interviews ranged from 64 minutes to 87 minutes, with an average of 68 minutes. The semi-structured interviews began with a broad question, such as "Tell me about your speech." Following an interview technique termed "funneling" (Westby, 1990), participants were given extensive leeway and encouraged to continue with whatever content they provided. The investigator often took the role of listener and requested that participants provide examples or further descriptions when deemed appropriate.

Following the interviews, all data were transcribed orthographically for Interpretative Phenomenological Analysis (Smith & Osborn, 2003). This method is based on a double interpretation process, beginning with the participant interpreting his or her own thoughts, followed by the researcher creating interpretations based on the participant's personal interpretations. Interpretive Phenomenological Analysis broadly framed the study in order to flexibly explore details of the individual's personal and social experience as a person who stutters covertly. The interpretation element of the analysis identified common themes that emerged from their lived experiences, which provided evidence of similarities among the experiences of the six individuals transitioning from living a life of stuttering covertly to attempting the new role as an individual who stutters overtly. The researcher selected the themes that not only were reoccurring but, more importantly, themes that were represented by the richest passages that highlight them (Smith & Osborne, 2003). Accordingly, six themes were identified, of which two related to employment issues (see below). Subthemes were identified and provided explanatory details for each theme.

To recheck the accuracy of the interpretations and to ensure validity of the results, the investigator integrated the ethnographic procedure of member checking (Lincoln & Guba, 1985). Member checking was conducted with three of the participants, which involved reviewing key elements of each individual's interview transcript and discussing the investigator's interpretation along with the participant's interpretation. The back-and-forth negotiations of the interpretations led to validation of the final themes.

Results

Two themes regarding the impact of covert stuttering in the workplace emerged from the analysis of six covertly stuttering adults. They were: (1) *Justifying Covert Status* and (2) *Realizing That Hiding Is Professionally Unproductive*. Each is presented and followed by examples bearing on its relevant subthemes.

Theme: Justifying Covert Status

In their interviews, participants justified the lives they created for themselves. They often used the term "lifestyle" to capture the great extent to which covert stuttering affected their way of living and to make sense of a tumultuous time they were experiencing. The justification provided for being covert with stuttering in relation to their professional lives is reflected in the two subthemes, *Saving Face* and *Professional Reputation*.

SUBTHEME: SAVING FACE. The *Justifying Covert Status* theme contained the subtheme of *Saving Face* for Elise. Elise continued to battle with dissonance by having a covert mindset and perceived her own stuttering as a stigma, yet was knowledgeable about stuttering being classified as a disorder that is beyond an individual's control. Elise viewed others who stutter with compassion, though her perception of her own stuttering was intertwined with fears and self-judgment. Elise feared that if she were to stutter, she would be perceived as "a fool." She made an interesting parallel about her thoughts on stuttering:

For someone like me, and other coverts that I know, um, you don't know [they stutter] until [they] stumble, and then it takes people by surprise. You know, and I I kinda liken it to, you know, a woman wearing high heels, feeling confident, "I look good, I'm strutting down the road," and you're walking along and all of a sudden "boom!" and you fall because you're wearing high heels. And it's like, it's that jarring, you know. It's like you look normal, you look normal, you look normal, and all of a sudden "boom!" you're a fool.

Elise placed much pressure on herself not to look like "a fool" to outsiders. For Elise, the saving-face mentality was constantly on her mind. The fear of outside judgment with the dramatic possibility of others considering her a failure drove her to remain fairly covert. Elise compared her stuttering to something that is unattractive and unfeminine. She justified continuing to be covert for social appearance, i.e., *saving face*. She projected her reasons for stuttering covertly onto others who stutter covertly: "There's many reasons to become covert but some of the people who do are the ones who are concerned with their appearance and how they appear to others."

In the findings of Elise, we saw her actively attempting to save face by trying very hard to participate in society as a fluent member in order to maintain what she considered prestige in a "normal" social profile.

SUBTHEME: PROFESSIONAL REPUTATION. Elise's interview also reflected the subtheme *Professional Reputation* as a way to *Justify Covert Status*. Elise believed that if one is to maintain a respected reputation among colleagues, then there is no room for stuttering. She stated, "And, you know, to this day, you know, I see verbal communication as, or oral communication as crucial to be taken seriously as a professional, and, and stuttering is not part of that." Elise believed good communication and fluency are synonymous concepts.

Another participant, Annette, allowed herself to openly stutter at the workplace, although she continued to experience some covert stuttering insecurities, depending on the professional situation. As such, she, too, was affected by the *Professional Reputation* subtheme. She explained the following specific situation at work: "Well, I work at a [company] and there are some situations where I have to talk to a superintendent or a top-dog and I think I have to try to not stutter. I have to think because I worry about the image I am going to project." Both Elise and Annette clung to the mindset that their stuttering was a reflection of their characters, affecting their professional reputations (Schneider & Conrad, 1980).

Theme: Realizing That Hiding Was Professionally Unproductive

The realization that hiding was unproductive resonated in a number of ways. One of the covert strategies that the participants used was keeping their stuttering a secret from employers, friends, and relatives. The focus of this study is on workplace issues; hence, only one subtheme was relevant.

SUBTHEME: PROFESSIONAL PENALTIES. Participants Annette and Chris commented on professional penalties of their stuttering in the workplace. Descriptions ranged from noticing that avoidance strategies can negatively impact one's professional performance to losing one's job after overtly stuttering. The richest instances are further described.

For Annette, the realization of professional penalties emerged with many emotions and harsh realities. As she discussed her stuttering in relation to employment experiences, she reported the common fear of outsider judgment, a fear that was validated throughout her professional years. Her place of long-term employment was under new administration. This included a new male boss, who, prior to observing Annette working, had not appreciated her dedication to the advancement of the company. Annette was eventually fired after the boss witnessed her stuttering overtly during work. The following is the summary of this experience:

> To make a long story short, um, he heard me stuttering publicly sometimes on the job but I think that that would have been okay except that he heard it when I was covering [for a co-worker] (. . .) And that was an intimidating situation for me cause I had never [taken on this role of speaking in front of a group of children]. He felt that because he did not understand what stuttering was and because I had not told anybody because I was covert he thought that I was too nervous too anxious and not an effective role model [for children].

Annette's boss's immediate response to observing her stutter was to place her on a 90-day correctional plan. The plan appeared to be a delay tactic to her firing, e.g., setting goals that were unattainable. Annette reports the goals as "really ridiculous statistical goals that were set probably for me to fail. Because they were so ridiculously unattainable, that there was no way I could do it." After the 90-day correctional plan was over, she was then fired. Her boss's main reason for the firing was "ineffective communication skills and inability to be an effective role model [for children]." The harsh reality of being fired for lacking communication skills had no apparent grounds, causing Annette great confusion and distress. The termination of her long-term employment, together with a history of promotions for being proactive with the company, shocked her.

During that time in her life, Annette's stuttering was occasionally overt. She admitted to believing that by ignoring the overt stuttering, others would ignore it as well. At the time of the firing, she lived a covert lifestyle, hiding her stuttering during every communication interaction with every person she encountered, including friends, family, and coworkers.

In another example, Chris began realizing that hiding his stuttering was unproductive while he was in college and beginning to develop his professional reputation. He, like Annette, found that moments of stuttering were "sneaking out." Nevertheless, he frequently sacrificed his integrity to continue to keep his stuttering a secret. He shared one moment that occurred during a college internship:

> I had an internship at a court in [the city] and I got stuck in some really sticky situation where, uh, I had permission to be there but the judge asked me why I was in the room and I said I was volunteering with such and such a group. But I didn't say it just right and because—I didn't say it right because I was changing words. The judge figured something out and he said, "Well, you told me x, y, and z," and he got really upset with me. And I remember thinking, "This not stuttering is getting me into some really weird places."

In this case, Chris revealed his awareness that his covert stuttering no longer benefitted him. He witnessed the direct repercussions his covert strategies were having with his academic reputation and professional future. He saw the immediate impact of his covert stuttering with the reaction of a powerful figure, a judge. He clearly noticed that his covert strategies led him into professionally awkward situations; there was direct impact on his preprofessional experience and his relationship with respected figures.

Discussion

The present investigation's findings on workplace implications related to covert stuttering emerged from the data of a larger qualitative research project focused on the bigger-picture, transition process from stuttering covertly to stuttering overtly (Douglass, 2011), or "coming out of the stuttering closet." The above-described and other findings provided evidence of the direct impact of the stuttering-related stigma, as well as participants subscribing to that stigma, related to covert stuttering in the workplace. Goffman (1963) noted that as individuals go through a process of realizing they are disqualified according to the "normal point of view," they personally perpetuate the social stigma (i.e., self-stigma according to Boyle & Blood, Chapter 2). This is supported in the first theme, *Justifying Covert Status* wherein participants described why they chose to be or remain covert with their stuttering. Individuals observe ways in which society treats people with their difference and believe that they must live with their own secret differentness in a way that cannot be exposed without fear of rejection (Goffman, 1963). The experiences of Annette and Elise highlight the significance of workplace reputation as it might be affected by stuttering. They both felt that being a respected professional goes hand in hand with having fluent speech. Elise illustrated this in her question: "How can I appear confident [and] competent in the job if I'm stuttering?" Clearly, she viewed an uncontrolled element of herself as a legitimate character flaw (Schneider & Conrad, 1980). Remaining covert was justified consciously for occupational and social reasons.

The second theme, *Realizing That Hiding Was Professionally Unproductive*, reflected a mental journey that evolved over time, an awareness that emerged from the professional penalties that Annette and Chris experienced in the workplace. Annette's professional identity and experience were directly impacted by a coworker's blatant misunderstanding of an undisclosed difference. Ultimately, Annette's forced disclosure and firing was a significant professional penalty and personally traumatic time.

The psychological impact of each participant's transition process from covert stuttering to overt stuttering was often noted during the interview. In several interviews, participants cried, sighed deeply, or expressed anger during the recollection process. These felt emotions validated that the disclosure process from covert to overt stuttering can be a traumatic experience (Bohan, 1996; Goffman, 1963).

Linking Marginalized Populations' Experiences

Substantial parallels can be observed between workplace-related experiences of the participants related to their covert stuttering and individuals who must come to grip with other stigmatized problems. For example, the trauma related to disclosing that one stutters by someone who has hidden his or her stuttering for a long time might be further understood in relation to the "coming out" process of other marginalized populations such as lesbian, gay, bisexual, or transgendered individuals (or LGBT). Of course, the research conducted on the experiences of LGBT cannot be directly compared to the experiences of people who stutter because the experiences are vastly different and have vastly different etiologies. However, we can learn from a number of parallels between the two populations regarding social stigma and workplace implications. The legalities of discrimination at the workplace might be better understood by using a well-defined and researched marginalized population such as LGBT as a parallel. For example, disclosure of differences in the workplace requires an established inclusive work environment (Griffith & Hebl, 2002). This may not exist for either the LGBT populations or for people who stutter.

Annette's professional crisis occurred during a time when she had not come to terms with her stuttering identity. Similarly, individuals in the LGBT populations consider keeping their stigmatized differences hidden for fear of workplace retaliation. Griffith and Hebl (2002) found that people in the LGBT population who were open about their sexuality to close family members or friends were more likely to eventually disclose their sexuality to their coworkers than those who did not. This may also hold true for people who stutter. Further study is needed, but the current study sheds some light on why workplace disclosure may be so difficult for those who stutter.

Griffith and Hebl (2002) also report that the heightened anxiety of working with an unsupportive boss reduced the possibility of disclosure at the workplace. Research on LGBT individuals who disclose their sexual orientation at work suggests that a workplace that has thorough diversity training and a written nondiscrimination policy is likely to decrease the anxiety for disclosure in the workplace. With decreased anxiety, individuals are at ease that their coworkers and bosses are accepting of differences (Griffith & Hebl, 2002); policies such as this are nonexistent for stuttering. Once again, this is a fruitful area for future research.

Certainly, the findings of this study cannot be generalized to all people who stutter covertly; this is not the goal of qualitative research. However, these findings document the authentic impact of covert stuttering on workplace issues. In addition to the suggestions for future research that are noted earlier, questions raised by this study that future studies could address include (1) reasons why some individuals become covert with their stuttering while most do not, and (2) the impact of covert stuttering on individual experiences within other domains, such as school, family, and community.

Chapter 20

Changing Attitudes Toward Stuttering: What Children Liked about a Stuttering Education Resource

Marilyn Langevin

ABSTRACT

Stuttering-specific comments about what children liked and would change about a bullying-prevention and stuttering education program were drawn from a larger sample of comments made by children who participated in a large-scale intervention study. Although stuttering-specific comments were few in number, they suggest that school-age children are interested in learning about stuttering. As well, findings support earlier research that suggests stuttering children who are in an environment in which peers have learned about stuttering may be less vulnerable to bullying and be more accepted by the peer group.

Introduction

Empirical and anecdotal evidence indicates that the majority of school-age youth who stutter are mimicked and mocked, called names, and sometimes physically bullied (Hugh-Jones & Smith, 1999; Langevin, Chapter 3; Langevin, Bortnick, Hammer, & Wiebe, 1998). In addition, they are perceived negatively by their peers (Langevin, 2009; Langevin, Kleitman, Packman, & Onslow, 2009), have difficulty fitting in at school (Evans, Healey, Kawai, & Rowland, 2008), and appear to be at higher risk of being bullied than their typically fluent peers

(Blood & Blood, 2004, 2007; Blood, Blood, Tramontana, Sylvia, Boyle, & Motzko, 2011). Indeed, for some children who stutter, teasing and negative peer reactions to stuttering start in the preschool years (Langevin, Packman, & Onslow, 2009, 2010). Like typically fluent peers who are bullied, many victimized children who stutter experience short- and long-term consequences of bullying. Short-tem consequences include loss of confidence and self-esteem, embarrassment, difficulty making friends, negative effects on academic work, heightened anxiety, and diminished optimism and life satisfaction (Blood & Blood, 2004, 2007; Blood et al., 2011; Hugh-Jones & Smith, 1999).

In response to the persistent calls for programs to educate students about stuttering (e.g., Ruscello, Lass, & Brown, 1988), Langevin (2000) developed the *Teasing and Bullying: Unacceptable Behaviour* (*TAB*) program. *TAB* is a bullying-prevention program that also aims to improve attitudes toward children who stutter. With regard to bullying prevention, *TAB* contains units that help children (1) understand what bullying behaviors are, (2) develop or amplify existing empathy for victims, (3) change beliefs about differences (e.g., respecting and celebrating differences), (4) understand the importance of talking to an adult about the bullying (e.g., telling someone to get help), and (5) understand the difference between tattling and responsible telling. According to Debra Pepler (personal communication, 1999) and a Grade 4 teacher who shared his views with the author, "tattling is done to get someone into trouble, telling [in private and not in front of other students] is done to get someone [including oneself] out of trouble." Pepler and the teacher suggested that the reporting should be done in private rather than in front of classmates as often happens at the end of a recess period.

With regard to education about stuttering, *TAB* addresses the cause of a moment of stuttering (focusing on the physiological roots of stuttering), understanding stuttering (e.g., myths and facts), and how a listener can help a person who stutters (e.g., "Let them finish their sentences" or "Keep looking at them while they are they are talking even if they are having trouble"). In addition, *TAB* includes a video that depicts a girl who stutters who confidently talks about her stuttering, the physiology involved in speech production (including a segment showing the vocal folds in action), and her experiences with being teased about her stuttering. The video also includes a classroom scene in which a boy who stutters is teased about his stuttering. In a later scene the boy who stutters tell the classmate who is bullying him to "stop."

A feasibility study found that *TAB* has the potential to improve student attitudes toward children who stutter, particularly in the subgroup of children who did not know someone who stutters. Results also indicated that *TAB* has the potential to improve support for victims and reduce approval of bullying (Langevin & Prasad,

2012). Quantitative findings using a rating scale also revealed that the majority of children (66%) liked the program. As also would be expected, the majority of the children who did not like the program were those who were categorized as perpetrators of bullying based on self-report of involvement in bullying.

In order to gain a deeper understanding of aspects of *TAB* that were more or less meaningful to the children, the author also asked the children in the Langevin and Prasad (2012) study two open-ended questions: "What did you like about the teasing and bullying program?" and "What would you change in the teasing and bullying program?" The purpose of this report is to examine the frequency and nature of comments made that were specific to stuttering. Findings are presented within the context of frequency of comments made by all children in the Langevin and Prasad (2012) study in response to the two open-ended questions and the frequency of responses from children with differing bullying participant roles. Based on self-reports of involvement in bullying, participants in the Langevin and Prasad study were categorized as children who bullied, children who were victims of bullying, children who were dually involved in that they bullied and also were victims of bullying, and children who were not involved in bullying.

Method

Potential participants were drawn from 608 students (330 boys and 278 girls) from grades 3 to 6 (mean age = 9.7 years, SD = .85 years) from seven schools in a western Canadian province who participated in the Langevin and Prasad (2012) study.

Responses to the open-ended questions were reviewed multiple times by the author, and coding systems for each of the open-ended questions were developed. Responses to the question "What did you like about the teasing and bullying program?" first were coded as positive, negative (e.g., "Nothing"), or indeterminable (e.g., "Not sure"). Positive responses then were further coded into six subcategories, one of which pertained to the stuttering education unit. Negative items were not further coded because there were no subcategories of responses. Responses to the question "What would you change in the teasing and bullying program?" first were coded into five categories, one of which had recommendations for changes that related to the unit devoted to stuttering education. In total there were 1,012 open-ended comments from the 608 children to code. After independent coding by the author and a research assistant who also was independent of the study, inter-rater reliability (total agreements/total agreements plus disagreements × 100) for each of the coding systems was determined. Thereafter, disagreements were discussed until consensus on a code was reached. Inter-rater reliabilities ranged from 92.8% to 100%.

The children who responded with stuttering-specific comments to the two open-ended research questions consisted of 23 participants of which 18 provided one comment to the question about what children liked about the program and five about what could be changed about the program. They ranged in age from 9 to 11 (mean = 9.57), were in grades 4 to 6, and included 11 boys and 12 girls.

Results

What Children Liked about the Program

From the total sample of 608 participants, 83% of responses to the question that asked what children liked about the program were positive. Forty-seven percent of the positive comments were provided by the uninvolved participants whereas 6% of the positive comments were provided by children who were perpetrators of bullying. Thus, children who bullied provided the least number of positive comments.

Eighteen children made stuttering-specific comments. Two comments were coded as "indeterminable" (e.g., the response was simply "stuttering") and 16 were coded as positive. Positive comments came from children who were not involved in bullying (8), were victimized (6), and were dually involved (4). No children who bullied made stuttering-specific comments.

Participants providing stuttering-specific comments indicated that they like learning:

1. about stuttering, why children stutter, and about the physiology involved in speaking: for example, [I liked learning] "about bullying and stuttering", "why kids stutter," what "caused stuttering," "what happens when people stutter," and "how our bodies work when we're talking";
2. that children who stutter are like other "kids": for example, "Kids that stutters [sic] are not different from kids who don't stutter"; children also wrote about sorting out their feelings about children who stutter and befriending a child who stutters: "I like how it helps people on how they feel about people who stutter," and "I would love to have a friend who stutters";
3. that "stuttering isn't bad"; and
4. that "kids who stutter should not be teased."

With regard to a potential association between bullying participant role status and positive comments, only one association was notable. That is, a participant who was victimized commented that he liked the role model provided by the child who stuttered in the video and who responded assertively to the classmate who was bullying him; the participant wrote: "[I liked that the] boy that stuttered told [the] bully he didn't like being teased."

What Would You Change in the Teasing and Bullying Program?

From the total sample of 608 children, when asked what participants would change in the program, the majority of participants (62%) indicated that they would not change anything. Uninvolved participants provided the largest proportion of comments (50%), followed by victims (29%), and then by dually involved (16%) participants. Perpetrators of bullying provided the fewest comments (5%).

Regarding stuttering-specific comments, only five of the recommendations for change were specific to the stuttering unit. Comments that gave specific direction for change included children who wanted to learn "more things that tell you what causes stuttering," and two children who wanted the vocal folds segment to be removed from the video. These recommendations came from children who were not involved in bullying and children who were victimized. There were no notable associations between recommendations for change made and bully participant role status.

Discussion

Although the comments that were specific to stuttering were very few, they support the quantitative results of Langevin and Prasad (2012) and provide suggestions for change in future development of stuttering education programs. Consistent with reported improvements in attitudes toward children who stutter in Langevin and Prasad's (2012) report, comments suggest that participants came to understand that children who stutter are not different from other children and became more willing to affiliate with children who stutter. In Langevin and Prasad's (2012) report, the item on the *Peer Attitudes Toward Children Who Stutter Scale* (Langevin & Hagler, 2004; Langevin, 2009; Langevin et al., 2009) that showed the highest mean change score was "Kids who stutter are like normal kids." Items that reflect a willingness to affiliate with children in public (which is highly influenced by peer pressure) were also among those with the next highest mean change scores. Taken together, these quantitative and qualitative findings suggest that children who stutter may be more likely to be accepted by their peer group after the *TAB* program. The fact that at least one child who was a victim of bullying commented that he liked seeing the child who stutters in the classroom scene in the video stand up to the classmate who was bullying him is very positive. Children perceive assertiveness to be the most effective strategy for ending bullying (Camodeca & Goossens, 2005). This suggests that the children who stutter in the video, particularly the child in the classroom scene, could be remembered as positive role models. Finally, findings from this and Langevin and Prasad's report indicate that children who stutter may be less vulnerable to bullying after peers have participated in a stuttering education program that promotes an understanding of the commonalities among children who do and do not stutter and the potential befriending of children who stutter. From a young age, children are sensitive to differences in general (Katz, 2003), differences in fluency (Ezrati-Vinacour, Platzky, & Yairi, 2001), and prefer friends who are similar. A substantial body of research indicates that acceptance by peers and having friends and quality friendships protects against victimization (Bollmer, Milich, Harris, Maras, 2005; Boulton, Trueman, Chau, Whithand, & Amatya, 1999; Hodges, Boivin, Vitaro, & Bukowski, 1999).

Regarding suggested changes to the program, even fewer comments were specific to stuttering. It is encouraging to note that there was indication that children are interested in learning more about stuttering. It also is interesting to note that two children responded negatively to the inclusion of a segment of the video that showed real images of the vocal folds in action during speech production. It can be argued that this is a positive finding in that the vast majority of participants in the total sample and in the subgroup of children who provided stuttering-specific comments were not inclined to comment on the vocal fold segment. This suggests that the majority of children were appropriately prepared by the teachers who implemented the program. Instructions in *TAB* ask those delivering the program to "prepare the students to see real images of the vocal folds in action," which were included to "demonstrate the fascinating process of human sound production." However, future revisions of the video could include more preparatory footage and updated images of the vocal folds or animated footage of vocal fold vibration.

A limitation of this study is that the questions asked were broad, pertaining to the program in general. To gain a better understanding of aspects of the stuttering education unit that are more or less meaningful to students and to provide direction for future development, further research might well request comments that relate specifically to components of the stuttering education unit.

Conclusions

Results of this study provide further evidence that school-age children are open to and interested in learning about stuttering. Although few in number, children's stuttering-specific comments give direction for development of stuttering education resources for school-age children.

Chapter 21

Attitudes Toward Stuttering: An Annotated Bibliography

Stephanie Hughes

Introduction

This annotated bibliography includes 76 published studies on the topic of attitudes toward people who stutter and spans many decades of published research. It provides a comprehensive overview of the literature, though as readers can imagine, it is impractical to review each and every study published to date, however worthy that might be. Instead, this bibliography strives to provide readers with descriptions of (1) seminal studies in the field, (2) some little-known research gems that can inform current research, and (3) recent studies that may provide new directions for measuring attitudes and changing perceptions of people who stutter. Note that these summaries are not meant to include all the relevant details of each study, nor should they be used in place of reading the entire articles. Instead they are provided to assist readers in identifying relevant literature that relates to the content of this book.

The entries in the bibliography are numbered and arranged in a roughly chronological order, though entries are sometimes grouped according to thematic similarity, especially for follow-up studies or replicated studies. Each entry in the bibliography generally contains a description of participants, methods, and findings, and ends with implications for people who stutter or suggestions for future research. In some entries findings are related to other studies. In this case, readers will be directed to "see entry x" at the end of the citation for the related study. Some articles that are listed in the references do not have their own entries in this chapter. An author index for this annotated bioliography is provided at the end of the chapter.

1. Emerick, L. L. (1960). Extensional definition and attitude toward stuttering. *Journal of Speech and Hearing Research, 3,* 181–186.

   In one of the earliest studies of its kind, Emerick explored the relationship between elementary school teachers' ability to count or tally instances of stuttering and their attitudes toward stuttering. They filled out the *Iowa Scale of Attitude Toward Stuttering* as a measure of attitudes and tallied stuttering from an audiotaped recording of a male who stutters. Findings indicated a relationship between the frequency of disfluencies noted by participants and their attitudes toward people who stutter. Participants who had a more tolerant attitude toward stuttering tended to observe more disfluencies. This trend applied most particularly to those teachers who had taken at least one course in speech pathology as compared to teachers with no formal training. Emerick suggested that training in speech pathology might result in more tolerant attitudes toward stuttering while at the same time decreasing tolerance for speech nonfluencies (e.g., typically occurring disfluencies that are not generally considered to be core stuttering behaviors).

2. Bar, A. (1969). Effects of type of listeners and listening instructions on the attention to manner and content of a severe stutterer's speech. *Journal of Communication Disorders, 2,* 344–349.

   Bar investigated how listening instructions, severity of stuttering, and listener experiences with stuttering affect speech-language pathologists' (SLPs) and naive listeners' attitudes toward people who stutter. All participants listened to the same sample of a speaker who stutters, but the instructions that prefaced the listening activity varied. Participants in the "content" group were told only to focus on the content of the speech. Participants in the "manner" group were told to pay attention to the way the speaker spoke. Participants in the "biased" group were told that the speaker was a very severe stutterer. Participants in the "no instructions" group served as a control. After the listening task, participants estimated the speaker's stuttering and attempted to recall factual information from the speech. Both SLPs and naive listeners paid significantly more attention to the manner of the speech (stuttering) than they did its content, particularly when no listening instructions were given. SLPs were able to focus more on the content of the speech than naive listeners, and listening instructions did not significantly influence SLPs' perceptions of the speaker as they did for naive listeners. When stuttering was described as severe, all listeners, including SLPs, tended to be distracted and paid more attention to stuttering than the content of stuttered speech.

3. Yairi, E., & Williams, D. E. (1970). Speech clinicians' stereotypes of elementary-school boys who stutter. *Journal of Communication Disorders, 3*, 161–170.

Yairi and Williams asked all of the school-based speech clinicians in the state of Iowa to provide a written list of traits that describe elementary school-age boys who stutter. Participants most frequently provided a total of 26 traits to describe boys who stutter. Seventeen of these traits were judged by the researchers to be negative or undesirable, and only nine of the traits were judged to be positive or desirable. Most traits described the personality of boys who stutter rather than their physical traits or intelligence. The 10 most cited traits, in order of the most frequently occurring, were *nervous, shy, withdrawn, tense, anxious, self-conscious, insecure, sensitive, quiet,* and *intelligent.* As the clinicians' years of clinical experience increased, so too did the median number of adjectives used to describe boys who stutter. The provision of more adjectives was viewed as indicative of a stronger, more stereotypical belief system about boys who stutter.

4. Woods, C. L., & Williams, D. E. (1971). Speech clinicians' conceptions of boys and men who stutter. *Journal of Speech and Hearing Disorders, 36,* 225–234.

Woods and Williams asked speech clinicians to write adjectives that described adult men who stutter, replicating a similar study by Yairi and Williams (1970; see entry 3) in which clinicians described boys who stutter. The similarity of the adjectives used to describe both men and boys who stutter indicated that clinicians may stereotype people who stutter regard-less of individual differences. Thus, there may be a trend among clinicians to believe that "a stutterer is a stutterer is a stutterer" (Woods & Williams, 1971, p. 232).

5. Woods, C. L., & Williams, D. E. (1976). Traits attributed to stuttering and normally fluent males. *Journal of Speech and Hearing Research, 19,* 267–278.

Woods and Williams arranged adjectives that speech clinicians provided to describe boys and men who stutter (Woods & Williams, 1971; Yairi & Williams, 1970, see entries 4 and 3, respectively) as semantic differen-tial scales. These scales consisted of 25 paired items (e.g., open–guarded, friendly–unfriendly, fearful–fearless), and were administered to seven groups of respondents, including SLPs, students, and teachers. Participants used these scales to rate each of four hypothetical people, including a typical eight-year-old male, a typical eight-year-old male who stutters, a typical adult male, and a typical adult male who stutters. Results indicated that 95% of traits that were judged as negative were applied to males who stutter versus typical males who did not stutter. Significant differences in ratings were not found based on the age of the hypothetical person who stutters (child versus adult) or participant group (e.g., speech clinicians, students, teachers). These negative attitudes suggested the presence of a pervasive negative stereotype toward people who stutter by most groups of listeners.

6. Crowe, T. A., & Cooper, E. B. (1977). Parental attitudes toward and knowledge of stuttering. *Journal of Communication Disorders, 10,* 343–357.

   Crowe and Cooper compared the attitudes of parents of children who stutter (CWS) and children who do not stutter (CWNS) using the *Parental Attitudes Toward Stuttering (PATS) Inventory* and the *Alabama Stuttering Knowledge (ASK) Test.* The authors found that parents of CWNS seemed to have better attitudes toward stuttering and knew more about stuttering than did parents of CWS, though they cautioned that continued research was needed to validate the measures' clinical and research utility.

7. Fowlie, G. M., & Cooper, E. B. (1978). Traits attributed to stuttering and nonstuttering children by their mothers. *Journal of Fluency Disorders, 3,* 233–246.

   Fowlie and Cooper administered semantic differential scales (Woods & Williams, 1976; see entry 5) to mothers of children who stutter (CWS) and mothers of typically fluent children. Both types of mothers rated their child's traits, and group means on the scale items were compared. Results indicated that mothers of CWS tended to describe their child as significantly more anxious, introverted, fearful, sensitive, withdrawn, and insecure as compared to mothers who described their child who did not stutter. The study raised important questions about the temperament of children who stutter, but raised the equally important question of whether parents' stereotypical beliefs influence the traits of CWS.

8. Turnbaugh, K., Guitar, B., & Hoffman, P. (1979). Speech clinicians' attribution of personality traits as a function of stuttering severity. *Journal of Speech and Hearing Research, 22,* 37–45.

   Turnbaugh et al. used semantic differential scales (Woods & Williams, 1976; see entry 5) to measure the attitudes of SLPs toward people who stutter based upon stuttering severity. The 36 SLPs who served as participants were asked to rate a hypothetical "typical individual" who was (1) normally fluent, (2) stuttered mildly, (3) stuttered moderately, or (4) stuttered severely. Results confirmed that the SLPs perceived people who stutter more negatively as compared to fluent speakers. The severe stuttering condition resulted in more negative attitudes as compared to the mild stuttering condition. Only a weak negative correlation between years of experience as an SLP and ratings of stuttering people was found, leading the authors to conclude that there was not a linear relationship between SLPs' experiences with people who stutter and their attitudes toward people who stutter.

9. Crowe, T. A., & Walton, J. H. (1981). Teacher attitudes toward stuttering. *Journal of Fluency Disorders, 6,* 163–174.

    Crowe and Walton administered the *Teacher Attitudes Toward Stuttering (TATS) Inventory* to elementary school teachers. The *TATS* consisted of 36 attitude-based statements and nine general information questions about stuttering. The *TATS* had not been validated at the time of the study. Participants also completed the *Alabama Stuttering Knowledge (ASK) Test*, which consisted of 26 true/false statements about stuttering. Results indicated that teachers who had a greater knowledge of stuttering as measured on the *ASK Test* had more desirable attitudes toward stuttering. Teachers who indicated that they currently had a student who stuttered in their classroom had less desirable attitudes and scored lower on the *ASK Test* than did teachers who did not have a student who stuttered. These findings suggested that educators who teach students who stutter develop more negative attitudes toward stuttering and people who stutter as compared to educators who have not had a student who stutters in the classroom.

10. St. Louis, K. O., & Lass, N. J. (1981). A survey of communicative disorders students' attitudes toward stuttering. *Journal of Fluency Disorders, 6,* 49–79.

    St. Louis and Lass administered the *Clinician Attitude Toward Stuttering (CATS) Inventory* to nearly 2,000 SLP and audiology students. As a group, the students appeared to believe that people who stutter have psychosocial problems and that counseling stuttering individuals and their parents is an important component of stuttering therapy. Students who had more clinical training also seemed to hold these views, a finding that the authors attributed more to social acculturation in the United States than a by-product of clinician training. Participants also seemed to feel that stuttering was one of the hardest disorders to treat and indicated that most SLPs are neither competent nor comfortable when treating stuttering patients. The authors suggested that more research is needed to examine the effects of specific types of training on student clinicians' attitudes toward people who stutter.

11. Turnbaugh, K., Guitar, B., & Hoffman, P. (1981). The attribution of personality traits: The stutterer and nonstutterer. *Journal of Speech and Hearing Research, 24,* 288–291.

    Turnbaugh et al. examined the extent to which raters assign personality traits on the basis of audio versus audiovisual recordings; primary, secondary, or no stuttering behaviors; and stutterer label versus no label. Three videotapes were made in which a male simulated stuttering with various degrees of severity and primary versus secondary stuttering behaviors. One videotape consisted of fluent speech, another had a moderate amount of primary stuttering behaviors, and the third videotape consisted of a moderate amount of syllables stuttered in which secondary behaviors were present. Audiotapes were then made from each of the three videotapes, creating a total of six conditions. Participants were assigned to one condition and were told that they were listening to and/or watching an interview with a male who stutters. This procedure was then repeated with another group of additional participants who were told only that the tapes were of an interview with a male, thus allowing the researchers to identify differences in rater perceptions based on the label of stuttering. Participants' responses to a modified version of the Woods and Williams (1976; see entry 5) semantic differential scales revealed that the participants assigned similar personality traits to the speaker regardless of the presentation mode; presence or absence of primary, secondary, or no stuttering behaviors; or the presence or absence of a stutterer label. A second part of the study consisted of participants rating either a "hypothetical normal speaker" or a "hypothetical stutterer." Participants rated the hypothetical stutterer more negatively on several semantic differential items as compared to the hypothetical normal speaker. Ratings for the hypothetical stutterer were also similar to those provided by participants in the first part of the study, suggesting that the context in which fluent speakers watch, listen, or read about people who stutter makes little difference in their ratings of stuttering people.

12. Ragsdale, J. D., & Ashby, J. K. (1982). Speech-language pathologists' connotations of stuttering. *Journal of Speech and Hearing Research, 25,* 75–80.

    Ragsdale and Ashby administered a newly developed semantic differential scale that assessed SLPs' attitudes toward people who stutter on five dimensions, including evaluation (e.g., good/bad, successful/unsuccessful), potency (e.g., strong/weak, hard/soft), activity (e.g., tense/relaxed, active/passive), understandability (e.g., clear/confusing, usual/unusual), and anxiety (e.g., anxious/calm, disturbed/undisturbed). SLPs were found to

315

hold mostly negative views of people who stutter; however, SLPs who possessed the American Speech-Language-Hearing Association's Certificate of Clinical Competence showed more favorable responses to stuttered speech samples. Perhaps most surprising was the finding that SLPs' coursework or clinical experiences with people who stutter did not result in significantly more favorable ratings of stuttering people. In addition, the speech sample of a female who stuttered was rated more favorably on some dimensions than a male who stuttered. The authors suggested that this finding may be related to the fact that more males than females stutter, and that SLPs may have stronger preconceived notions or more actual clinical experiences with males who stutter than females who stutter.

13. Silverman, E. (1982). Speech-language clinicians' and university students' impressions of women and girls who stutter. *Journal of Fluency Disorders, 7,* 469–478.

Silverman investigated the perceptions of SLPs and university students regarding eight hypothetical individuals, including a girl, a girl who stutters, a boy, a boy who stutters, a woman, a woman who stutters, a man, and a man who stutters. The primary purpose of this study was to determine if perceptions of girls and women who stutter are different than the negative stereotype that has been reported for boys and men who stutter. A 47-scale semantic differential questionnaire (Silverman & Zimmer, 1979) was administered to participants, with approximately 20 participants each completing the scales for only one of the eight hypothetical individuals. Results indicated that SLPs view females who stutter as being significantly different on a variety of personality traits as compared to females in general and males who stutter. SLPs seemed to have a stronger negative stereotype for a female who stutters than for a male who stutters, a finding that conflicts with that of Ragsdale and Ashby (1982; see entry 12). The university students who participated in the study appeared to have a stronger stereotype for males than for females who stutter, suggesting that different groups of people (e.g., professionals versus laypeople) may hold different perceptions of people who stutter depending on the gender of the stuttering individual.

14. Hurst, M. A., & Cooper, E. B. (1983a). Employer attitudes toward stuttering. *Journal of Fluency Disorders, 8,* 1–12.

Hurst and Cooper administered the *Employer Attitudes Toward Stuttering (EATS) Inventory* to 644 employers. The *EATS Inventory* did not undergo validity or reliability assessment prior to being used in the study. It consisted of seven attitudinal statements about stuttering to which respondents indicated their agreement on a 5-point scale that ranged from "strongly agree" to "strongly disagree." Employers who participated in the study had a variety of experience with interviewing and employing people who stutter: 36% had interviewed between one and three stuttering applicants, and 40% reported employing between one and three people who stutter. Results indicated that most employers believed that stuttering interferes with employability, but does not necessarily impact job performance. Three out of five employers reported feeling uncomfortable when speaking with stuttering individuals, and the same ratio of employers rejected the idea of affirmative action programs for people who stutter. These findings suggested that stuttering may handicap people who stutter for employability purposes.

15. Hurst, M. A., & Cooper, E. B. (1983b). Vocational rehabilitation counselors' attitudes toward stuttering. *Journal of Fluency Disorders, 8,* 13–27.

Hurst and Cooper developed the *Alabama Rehabilitation Counselor's Attitudes Toward Stuttering (ARCATS) Inventory* to assess vocational rehabilitation counselors' attitudes toward and knowledge of stuttering. The *ARCATS Inventory* consisted of 25 true/false statements that assess knowledge of stuttering and 15 statements that assess attitudes toward stuttering. One hundred fifty-two vocational rehabilitation counselors in the state of Alabama completed the *ARCATS Inventory*. Results suggested that participants believed stuttering individuals have psychological problems and certain identifiable personality traits. On a positive note, the rehabilitation counselors' responses suggested that stuttering is perceived as amenable to therapy and that people who stutter are good candidates for vocational rehabilitation. Thus, vocational rehabilitation counselors may hold attitudes that are conducive to the rehabilitation of people who stutter.

16. Tatchell, R. H., van den Berg, S., & Lerman, J. W. (1983). Fluency and eye contact as factors influencing observers' perceptions of stutterers. *Journal of Fluency Disorders, 8,* 221–231.

Tatchell et al. examined the effects of eye contact and fluency on college students' perceptions of people who stutter. A videotape was shown in which one of four conditions was portrayed by an actor in conversation with another actor. These conditions were normal eye contact and normal fluency, normal eye contact and disfluency, low eye contact and normal fluency, and low eye contact and disfluency. Participants then completed semantic differential scales related to such variables such as trustworthiness, competence, and dynamism. Results indicated significant interaction effects for fluency and eye contact, leading the authors to conclude that increased eye contact by stuttering individuals can lead to improved listener attitudes toward people who stutter.

17. White, P. A., & Collins, S. R. C. (1984). Stereotype formation by inference: A possible explanation for the "stutterer" stereotype. *Journal of Speech and Hearing Research, 27,* 567–570.

White and Collins used semantic differential scales (Woods & Williams, 1976; see entry 5) to examine the origin of the stuttering personality stereotype. The authors hypothesized that student ratings of "a typical adult male stutterer" versus "a normally fluent adult male speaker who suddenly starts to stutter for a short period of time, after which he speaks fluently again" would be similar. The semantic differential scales were administered to 80 undergraduate students with 40 students in each condition. Student ratings of a typical adult male who stutters were indeed similar to those of a normally fluent male who stutters only temporarily. The authors proposed that listeners make inferences from their beliefs about the internal states of fluent speakers who exhibit disfluencies (i.e., fluent speakers who exhibit disfluencies do so because they are experiencing nervousness, shyness, etc.) and apply these inferences to people who stutter (e.g., people stutter because they are nervous, shy, etc.). Thus, stereotypically negative judgments of stuttering people may be made out of uncertainty rather than derived from motivational factors.

18. Weisel, A., & Spektor, G. (1998). Attitudes toward own communication and toward stutterers. *Journal of Fluency Disorders, 23,* 157–172.

Weisel and Spektor investigated the extent to which the stuttering formation by inference theory (White & Collins, 1984; see entry 17) applies to adolescents. The authors hypothesized that a relationship exists between feelings toward one's own communication and that of people who stutter (though unclear due to typographical errors in the study's title). They also investigated the extent to which males and females have different attitudes toward people who stutter. Data were collected via Woods and Williams's (1976; see entry 5) semantic differential scale (segmented into "Tenseness and Pleasantness scales" (as per Horsley & Fitzgibbon, 1987; see entry 26) and the *Erickson Modified 24 Scale.* These measures were administered to 164 Israeli adolescents, half of whom rated an adolescent girl who stuttered and the other half an adolescent boy who stuttered. No sex-based differences were found on the Erickson scale, though females had more positive attitudes than males toward stuttering people on the semantic differential scales. The sex of the hypothetical person who stutters did not affect participants' ratings. The authors did note that boys who had more positive views of their own communication tended to have more positive views of people who stutter on the Tenseness semantic differential scales. These authors were not able to come to definite conclusions on the relationship between self-attitudes toward communication and attitudes toward people who stutter, and observed only partial support for the stuttering formation by inference theory.

19. MacKinnon, S. P., Hall, S., & MacIntyre, P. D. (2007). Origins of the stuttering stereotype: Stereotype formation through anchoring–adjustment. *Journal of Fluency Disorders, 32,* 297–309.

    MacKinnon et al. elaborated on the "stereotype formation by inference hypothesis" (White & Collins, 1984; see entry 17). They proposed that stuttering stereotypes occur when typically fluent individuals first "anchor" their stereotypical impressions of people who stutter in personal experiences with speech disfluencies. Individuals may then slightly adjust their perceptions depending on the context in which judgments are made. The anchor effect is generally strong enough that individuals do not deviate very much from their initial anchoring thoughts. To test this theory, the authors developed a study in which they administered the Woods and Williams (1976; see entry 5) semantic differential scale to psychology majors at a university. Participants in one group rated "an adult male with an uncontrollable stutter" (i.e., the "trait stutterer" condition) and "a normally fluent adult male speaker who suddenly begins to stutter for a short period of time, after which he speaks fluently again" (i.e., the "state disfluent male" condition). A control group rated "a typical adult male." As a group, participants assigned more stereotypical characteristics to both the chronic or "trait stutterer" and the "state" or non-chronic stutterer as compared to the "typical male." Analyses of state versus trait ratings supported both the anchoring and adjustment parts of the hypothesis in that for most differences between the two hypothetical "stutterers," the "state" or non-chronic stutterer was regarded with more negative attitudes than the "trait" or chronic one. The authors suggested that fluent speakers use their feelings during their own temporary state disfluencies as their anchor. They then adjust these feelings when making evaluative judgments about individuals who stutter.

20. Cooper, E. B., & Cooper, C. S. (1985). Clinician attitudes toward stuttering: A decade of change (1973–1983). *Journal of Fluency Disorders, 10,* 19–33.

    Cooper and Cooper (1985) noted that it is important to investigate SLPs' attitudes toward stuttering and people who stutter as these attitudes will presumably influence therapeutic protocols and treatment outcomes. They examined the attitudes of 674 SLPs toward stuttering, stuttering people, and related issues by administering the *Clinician Attitude Toward Stuttering (CATS) Inventory* to SLPs who attended a workshop on stuttering over a 10-year period. The authors found that over this period there were some changes in SLPs' attitudes toward the personality of people who stutter. For example, as compared to the sample gathered in 1973–1974, significantly fewer SLPs agreed in 1983 that stuttering individuals have psychological problems and hold distorted perceptions of their own stuttering behavior and social relationships. Other attitudes toward the personality of people who stutter did not show a significant change over the course of the study. The majority of SLPs continued to believe that stuttering, as compared to other speech disorders, is the most psychologically devastating. They also believed that there are personality traits that are representative of stuttering people, and that those who stutter have feelings of inferiority. Cooper and Cooper (1996) continued to collect *CATS Inventory* data, but found that clinicians' attitudes about the personality of people who stutter had not changed significantly across two decades of research.

21. Cooper, E. B., & Rustin, L. (1985). Clinician attitudes toward stuttering in the United States and Great Britain: A cross-cultural study. *Journal of Fluency Disorders, 10,* 1–17.

    Cooper and Rustin utilized the *Clinician Attitude Toward Stuttering (CATS) Inventory* to assess cross-cultural attitudes toward stuttering and stuttering people. They administered the *CATS Inventory* to 371 American SLPs from six states and 331 SLPs from Great Britain. The results indicated that there were significant differences between British and American clinicians in terms of appropriate treatment strategies and perceptions of attitudes toward people who stutter. British clinicians were more likely to believe that stuttering people have psychological problems, but American clinicians were more likely to believe that clinicians should be more understanding of the feelings of their clients who stutter. American clinicians were also more likely to believe that the general public has a more negative response toward stuttering than do British clinicians. The authors indicated that the trend for both American and British clinicians to attribute certain personality traits to people who stutter is troubling, as there is little data to support these beliefs.

22. Crichton-Smith, I., Wright, J., & Stackhouse, J. (2003). Attitudes of speech and language therapists toward stammering: 1985 and 2000. *International Journal of Language and Communication Disorders, 38*, 213–234.

Crichton-Smith et al. noted that most studies about SLPs' attitudes toward stuttering have utilized American participants; further, studies that investigated attitudes of UK clinicians related to stuttering were perhaps out of date, given the increased number of stuttering specialists and the advent of the Lidcombe Programme for children who stutter. Accordingly, the authors administered a slightly modified version of the *Clinician Attitude Toward Stuttering (CATS) Inventory* to 260 SLPs in the UK and compared them to attitudes measured 15 years previously by Cooper and Rustin (1985; see entry 21). The results of the updated survey indicated that attitudes of SLPs in the UK had become more positive with respect to early intervention for stuttering, stereotypes of people who stutter, and parents' roles in stuttering and stuttering therapy. SLPs who were not stuttering specialists were still unsure about which stuttering treatments were most appropriate to employ when treating people who stutter. Crichton-Smith et al. recommended that all therapists who work with people who stutter seek continuing education opportunities, as well as support from colleagues and special interest groups.

23. Maviş, İ., St. Louis, K. O., Özdemir, S., & Toğram, B. (2013). Attitudes of Turkish speech and language therapists toward stuttering. *Journal of Fluency Disorders, 38*, 157–170.

Maviş et al. noted that while there were only 65 practicing SLPs in Turkey at the time of the study, these SLPs had caseloads with large numbers of clients who stutter. The authors administered the *Clinician Attitudes Toward Stuttering (CATS) Inventory* to 61 SLPs in Turkey and subsequently compared these results to data gathered from SLPs in the United States (see reference for Cooper & Cooper, 1985, in entry 20) and the United Kingdom (see entry 22 for Crichton-Smith et al., 2003). Turkish SLPs differed from their U.S. and UK counterparts in that they tended to believe that people who stutter have psychological problems and that school counselors rather than SLPs should take the lead role in counseling children who stutter. Differences among SLPs of all three countries were noted, however, and readers are directed to the article for more detail.

24. Burley, P. M., & Rinaldi, W. (1986). Effects of sex of listener and of stutterer on ratings of stuttering speakers. *Journal of Fluency Disorders, 17,* 329–333.

    Burley and Rinaldi asked 10 male and 10 female naive listeners who ranged in age from 15 to 35 years to rate recorded speech samples of both male and female people who stutter. Semantic differential scales were used to identify the extent to which participants assigned traits to stuttering people. There were significant differences between male and female listener ratings, with males tending to rate the speech samples of people who stutter more negatively than females. The sex of the person who stutters did not have an effect on the ratings by male or female listeners.

25. Patterson, J., & Pring, T. (1991). Listener attitudes to stuttering speakers: No evidence for a gender difference. *Journal of Fluency Disorders, 16,* 201–205.

    Patterson and Pring replicated Burley and Rinaldi's (1986; see entry 24) study, but included a control group of fluent speech samples for 20 male and 20 female naive listeners. Results indicated that male and female listeners did not provide significantly different ratings. In both the Burley and Rinaldi and the Patterson and Pring studies, there was no gender difference observed when respondents rated both male and female stuttered speech samples. Findings suggested that the gender of people who stutter and their fluent listeners may be irrelevant in the formation and maintenance of negative attitudes toward stuttering people.

26. Horsley, I. A., & FitzGibbon, C. T. (1987). Stuttering children: Investigation of a stereotype. *British Journal of Disorders of Communication, 22,* 19–35.

    Horsley and FitzGibbon investigated the attitudes of speech clinicians and student speech clinicians with various degrees of training toward children who stutter. For comparison purposes, primary school student teachers and secondary school teachers also served as participants. Participants completed semantic differential scales (Woods & Williams, 1976; see entry 5) for each of eight hypothetical "typical" children presented in random order, including a preschool girl, preschool boy, eight-year-old girl, eight-year-old boy, preschool girl stutterer, preschool boy stutterer, eight-year-old girl stutterer, and eight-year-old boy stutterer. Ratings of children who stutter were consistently negative, and for all but five traits a statistically significant difference was found between ratings of children who stutter and children who do not stutter. While student clinicians and student teachers knew the least number of stuttering individuals, the number of people who stutter known did not significantly affect participants' ratings of people who stutter. The authors suggested that stereotypes held by SLPs may have an effect on therapeutic interactions between clinicians and their clients who stutter, perhaps even to the extent that young children who stutter may learn to fulfill clinicians' negative expectations.

27. Silverman, F. H. (1988). Impact of a T-shirt message on stutterer stereotypes. *Journal of Fluency Disorders, 13,* 279–281.

Silverman asked college students who were enrolled in an introductory speech class to respond to an 81-item semantic differential questionnaire (Silverman, 1985) in which they rated either "a stutterer" or "a stutterer wearing a shirt on which is printed 'I stutter. So what!'" The person who wears a T-shirt that acknowledges the stuttering was rated more positively on 29 of the 81 traits; however, the trait "immature" was also associated with the T-shirt condition.

28. Lass, N. J., Ruscello, D. M., Pannbacker, M., Schmitt, J. F., & Everly-Myers, D. S. (1989). Speech-language pathologists' perceptions of child and adult female and male stutterers. *Journal of Fluency Disorders, 14,* 127–134.

Lass et al. asked SLPs to write adjectives that described four hypothetical people who stutter, including a female child, male child, female adult, and male adult. The inclusion of females (i.e., a female child and female adult) was lacking in previous studies that had used this methodology (Woods & Williams, 1970; Yairi & Williams, 1971; see entries 5 and 3, respectively). The SLPs provided a total of 529 adjectives to describe the four types of hypothetical people who stutter, of which 69.9% were negative, 24.2% were positive, and 5.9% were neutral. Traits that described personality were most often listed, suggesting that many SLPs have negative stereotypes of people who stutter. The authors suggested that these negative stereotypes may be alleviated if SLPs can learn to separate the person who stutters from his or her stuttering. Lass and colleagues replicated this study and found similar results for teachers (Lass, Ruscello, Schmitt, Pannbacker, Orlando, Dean, Ruziska, & Bradshaw, 1992), special educators (Ruscello, Lass, Schmitt, & Pannbacker, 1994), and school administrators (Lass, Ruscello, Pannbacker, Schmitt, Kiser, Mussa, & Lockhart, 1994).

29. Collins, C. R., & Blood, G. W. (1990). Acknowledgment and severity of stuttering as factors influencing nonstutterers' perceptions of stutterers. *Journal of Speech and Hearing Disorders, 55,* 75–81.

Collins and Blood examined the effects of stuttering severity and acknowledgment of stuttering in a positive and affirming manner as factors that may influence listeners' perceptions of people who stutter. Participants were 84 female college students who were given a cover story in which they were told that they would work with one of two men who stutter for a class project about the effects of working with people who stutter. Furthermore, in an effort to save time, students were to watch brief interviews with the men who stuttered in order to determine with whom they would prefer to work. Participants then watched one of four videotapes that consisted of two 2–4-minute interviews with males who stuttered mildly or severely and who did or did not acknowledge their stuttering. After watching each interview, participants completed a survey that consisted of a 14-item semantic differential questionnaire (Burley & Rinaldi, 1986; see entry 24) and a written open-ended survey that asked participants to explain how they felt the speaker would interact with strangers and how he would act in a noisy environment. Participants were also asked to discuss how they would act around the speaker. Finally, after having watched both interviews, participants were asked to state which speaker they would prefer to work with and why. Results indicated that people who stutter, particularly those who stuttered severely, were rated more favorably by participants when they acknowledged their stuttering. Ratings were more negative for people who stuttered severely (regardless of whether or not they acknowledged their stuttering) as compared to those who stuttered mildly. Findings suggested that helping clients who stutter to acknowledge their stuttering may facilitate improved interactions with others.

30. Ham, R. E. (1990). What is stuttering: Variations and stereotypes. *Journal of Fluency Disorders, 15*, 259–273.

Ham asked 536 people from Tallahassee, Florida, to provide their perceptions of people who stutter via semi-structured telephone interviews. These interviews were conducted by graduate and undergraduate students who each called 10 people randomly in the Tallahassee phone book. The age range of the participants varied from 11 to 85 years, and a wide variety of occupations were represented. Methodologically, some concerns exist regarding this study, particularly that the interviewers were described as "naïve" and did not seem to undergo training before conducting the interviews. In addition, the author reported that he was unable to verify the interviewees' responses, presumably because the interviews were not audio-recorded. Nevertheless, Ham found that participants provided a broad range of responses when asked to define stuttering, state whether they have known a stutterer or stuttered themselves, identify the sort of person they thought would be most likely to develop stuttering, and provide advice to people who stutter to help their stuttering. Results indicated that although many of the participants knew someone who stutters, there was confusion regarding the definition of stuttering. Adding to this confusion over the definition of stuttering is that approximately 21% of participants said that they had stuttered in their past, and 12% of the participants felt that they currently stuttered. This unusually high incidence and prevalence of stuttering suggested that laypeople consider stuttering to include disfluencies that are considered typical by SLPs (e.g., revisions or repetitions of phrases), or that laypeople who infrequently use part-word repetitions consider themselves to stutter on such occasions. More than one-third of the participants indicated that they felt stuttering speakers are psychologically different from fluent speakers, and described people who stutter as shy, frustrated, and anxious. Only 15% of the respondents indicated that speech therapy might be beneficial. These results suggested that stuttering is not well understood by the general public.

31. Silverman, F. H., & Paynter, K. K. (1990). Impact of stuttering on perception of occupational competence. *Journal of Fluency Disorders, 15*, 87–91.

Silverman and Paynter used an 81-item semantic differential questionnaire (Silverman, 1985) to assess college students' perceptions of the occupational competency of people who stutter as compared to fluent speakers in the same occupations. Four groups of 12 students rated one of four hypothetical employees, including a factory worker, a factory worker who stutters, a lawyer, and a lawyer who stutters. Students judged the factory worker who stutters to be more afraid, insecure, tense, cowardly, and weak than the factory worker who does not stutter. In addition, the factory worker who stutters was perceived as less talkative, sociable, coordinated, dominant, affluent, aggressive, and confident. As compared to a typical lawyer, a lawyer who stutters was judged to be more afraid, confused, tense, discontented, frightened, lazy, dependent, uncomfortable, naive, and disorganized, as well as less intelligent, employable, competent, educated, confident, talkative, mature, secure, natural, witty, stable, dominant, rich, sane, alert, and aggressive. These findings suggested that people who stutter may be perceived more negatively if they have careers in which communication is more highly valued.

32. Bebout, L., & Arthur, B. (1992). Cross-cultural attitudes toward speech disorders. *Journal of Speech and Hearing Research, 35*, 45–52.

Bebout and Arthur compared attitudes of foreign-born students toward communication disorders, including stuttering, to those of students born in North America. Participants were from various Asian countries, Latin America, the United States, and Canada. They responded to a 12-item questionnaire in which they were asked to respond to various statements on a 4-point scale that ranged from "probably no," to "probably yes." Items addressed characteristics of stuttering individuals, such as intelligence and emotional stability; whether people who stutter should seek professional help from doctors or other helping professionals; effects of stuttering on people who stutter; and how people should act toward stuttering people. Foreign-born students in general were more likely than North American–born students to think that people with communication disorders are emotionally disturbed. As compared to all other participants, students from Asian countries were more likely to think that people with communication disorders could speak better if they tried harder than any other group. The authors concluded that it is important for SLPs to be aware of listeners' culturally influenced beliefs and attitudes toward communication disorders in order to provide more effective treatment.

33. Yairi, E., & Carrico, D. M. (1992). Early childhood stuttering: Pediatricians' attitudes and practices. *American Journal of Speech-Language Pathology, 1,* 51–62.

    Pediatricians responded to a questionnaire that asked about their attitudes and practices toward young children who stutter. Results appeared to indicate that the majority of physicians believe that there is no difference between preschoolers who stutter and those who do not on the traits of emotional stability, intelligence, and maturity.

34. Doody, I., Kalinowski, J., Armson, J., & Stuart, A. (1993). Stereotypes of stutterers and nonstutterers in three rural communities in Newfoundland. *Journal of Fluency Disorders, 18,* 363–373.

    Doody et al. investigated attitudes toward adult males who stutter as compared to adult males who do not stutter and examined familiarity with people who stutter as a mediating factor in negative attitudes toward stuttering. Participants were members of the general public in three small rural communities in Newfoundland, Canada. They completed a 25-item semantic differential questionnaire (Woods & Williams, 1976; see entry 5). Eighty-five percent of participants knew at least one person who stutters and 39% reported a familial relationship with someone who stutters. There were no significant differences between members of the three rural communities or between respondents with a family member who stutters versus those who did not. People who stutter were perceived as significantly different from people who do not stutter on 20 of the 25 scale items; most of these were negative traits, but some were positive, including being friendly, cooperative, pleasant, and intelligent. Thus, the rural communities under investigation had mostly negative attitudes toward a hypothetical adult male who stutters as compared to a hypothetical typical normal adult male speaker. The authors suggested that the negative stereotype of people who stutter might persist despite familiarity or close relationships because (1) the stuttering behavior (e.g., tension, struggle) is particularly salient, or (2) people who stutter may actually have significantly different character traits as compared to fluent speakers.

35. Kalinowski, J., Armson, J., Stuart, A., & Lerman, J. W. (1993). Speech clinicians' and the general public's perceptions of self and stutterers. *Journal of Speech-Language Pathology and Audiology, 17*, 79–85.

    Kalinowski et al. compared self-perceptions of SLPs and members of the general public to their perceptions of people who stutter. Semantic differential scales adapted from Woods and Williams (1976; see entry 5) were administered to SLPs and members of the general public. Participants were asked to complete the scales for themselves and for "a hypothetical typical adult male stutterer." Findings indicated that SLPs' perceptions of people who stutter were more negative than their self-perceptions. The attitudes of SLPs were also similarly negative to those of the general public, despite the average of 10 years of clinical experience the SLPs possessed. The authors called for more research on the ways in which SLPs' negative stereotypes of stuttering people may affect clinical outcomes.

36. Hulit, L. M., & Wirtz, L. (1994). The association of attitudes toward stuttering with selected variables. *Journal of Fluency Disorders, 19*, 247–267.

    Hulit and Wirtz sought to determine how several variables impact attitudes toward people who stutter by administering the *Stuttering Inventory* to members of the general public, students in speech-language pathology classes, and professional staff at a school district. The *Stuttering Inventory* consisted of items on a Likert scale that assess knowledge of and attitudes toward stuttering. It was constructed from a variety of existing survey instruments, including the *Clinician Attitudes Toward Stuttering Inventory*, the *Parental Attitudes Toward Stuttering Inventory*, and the *Alabama Stuttering Knowledge Test*. Results indicated that gender, age, years of education, knowing people who stutter, knowledge of stuttering, completing a stuttering course, and holding a certificate of clinical competence in speech-language pathology were not good predictors of attitudes toward stuttering. The authors indicated that there was a narrow range in participants' attitude scores and suggested that the variables under investigation did not have an association with attitudes toward stuttering. They further suggested that the field was at a crossroads in attitude measurement and provided a list of the problems that are inherent with survey research about stuttering. One of these problems is that there is no universally accepted definition of stuttering. Researchers have typically assumed that stuttering has the same meaning for everyone when in fact it may not. Another issue is that the validity of the inventories used to measure attitudes toward stuttering has never been demonstrated, and it is very difficult to measure the validity of something as broad and inferential as an attitude. Finally, regardless of their methods, researchers have asked respondents to make judgments about people who stutter. The term "stuttering" may have negative implications and provides a signal to the respondent that the person that he or she is judging has a communication disorder.

37. Leahy, M. (1994). Attempting to ameliorate student therapists' negative stereotype of the stutterer. *International Journal of Language and Communication Disorders, 29,* 39–49.

Leahy investigated the extent to which undergraduate students in a speech-language pathology program would improve their attitudes toward people who stutter on the basis of their fluency coursework or clinical exposure to stuttering people. Semantic differential scales were administered to students before and after the experiment, in which they took the fluency course or worked with people who stutter. Learning about negative stereotypes of people who stutter and how stuttering individuals can be affected by these stereotypes in therapy did not improve attitudes. Some improvement in attitudes resulted from learning "alternative means of stuttering," various therapeutic approaches, and theories of change. Students who also experimented with personal change also demonstrated some improvement in attitudes. The author concluded that relevant clinical experiences with people who stutter helped to ameliorate some students' attitudes.

38. Kalinowski, J., Stuart, A., & Armson, J. (1996). Perceptions of stutterers and nonstutterers during speaking and nonspeaking situations. *American Journal of Speech-Language Pathology, 5,* 61–67.

Kalinowski et al. investigated whether the perceptions of people who stutter versus fluent speakers vary depending on speaking and non-speaking situations. Members of the general public were surveyed using semantic differential scales (Woods & Williams, 1976; see entry 5), and each participant received two questionnaires. Some received questionnaires that asked them to rate both "a typical normal adult male" and "a typical adult male stutterer when speaking in everyday situations." Other participants received questionnaires that asked them to rate both "a typical normal adult male" and "a typical adult male stutterer in everyday life when not involved in speaking situations." Statistical analysis revealed that a hypothetical person who stutters was perceived more negatively than a typical, normal adult male regardless of whether speaking situations were involved or not. The authors suggested that stereotypes about people who stutter develop and are maintained because the physical tension and effort associated with stuttering is so powerful. Thus, as Lass et al. (1989; see entry 28) have suggested, laypeople may not be able to separate the speech of the person who stutters from the person himself or herself.

39. McGee, L., Kalinowski, J., & Stuart, A. (1996). Effect of a videotape documentary on high school students' perceptions of a high school male who stutters. *Journal of Speech-Language Pathology and Audiology, 20,* 240–246.

McGee et al. examined whether watching a videotape about stuttering would change negative perceptions of high school students toward a hypothetical high school male who stutters. Thirty-six high school students completed semantic differential scales (Woods & Williams, 1976; see entry 5) for either a hypothetical "normal high school male" or a "high school male who stutters." Data analysis indicated that the high school students held strong negative stereotypes of a high school male who stutters. These stereotypes remained unchanged after participants watched the video *Voices to Remember* featuring stories of stuttering of several adults and an 11-year-old female narrator. The results of this study suggested that watching the video was not enough to change viewers' attitudes about people who stutter. It may also be that the video simply enhanced the negative stereotypes that the participants already possessed.

40. Snyder, G. J. (2001). Exploratory research in the measurement and modification of attitudes toward stuttering. *Journal of Fluency Disorders, 26,* 149–160.

Like McGee et al. (1996; see entry 39), Snyder investigated how attitudes toward people who stutter may be changed as a result of learning about stuttering via videotapes. Twenty-one graduate students in a speech-language pathology program were administered the *Clinician Attitudes Toward Stuttering (CATS) Inventory* prior to and after watching an emotionally charged, video that documented the life of a young girl who stutters, entitled *Speaking of Courage*. Another group of 34 graduate SLP students completed the *CATS Inventory* prior to and after watching a videotape that demonstrated immediate amelioration of stuttering via use of altered auditory feedback (AAF). A comparison of the two conditions indicated that only a few subtle changes in students' beliefs were noted after they viewed the videotapes, though more changes were noted for the AAF video. The extent to which these changes could be considered positive is debatable. For example, after watching the clinic video, students moderately agreed that it was easy to change stuttering behaviors whereas before the video they were undecided. It was difficult to provide a rationale for how the videos may have influenced students' beliefs; Snyder suggested that problems with the reliability of the *CATS Inventory* could be responsible for some of the findings rather than a true change in attitudes. Accordingly, Snyder indicated that it may be more beneficial to measure listeners' psychophysiological responses to stuttering rather than continue to administer paper-and-pencil questionnaires to measure attitudes toward people who stutter. Readers are directed to Guntupalli et al.'s 2006 study (entry 61) for an example of such psychophysiological measures, though it should be noted that attitudes toward people who stutter and not attitudinal change were measured in this study.

41. Flynn, T. W., & St. Louis, K. O. (2011). Changing adolescent attitudes toward stuttering. *Journal of Fluency Disorders, 36*, 110–121.

    Flynn and St. Louis examined the extent to which high school students' attitudes toward stuttering could be changed depending on the mechanism for change (i.e., oral presentation, video). Eighty-three high school students (average age of 16.4 years) participated in the study. All students completed the *Public Opinion Survey on Human Attributes–Stuttering* (*POSHA–S*) pre-experiment. Students in the "oral" condition then listened to a live presentation by the first author, a moderate–severe stutterer. Students in the "video" condition watched a 45-minute video (MTV *True Life*®: *I Stutter*) that featured the first author. Students in these conditions then took the *POSHA–S* questionnaire for a second time post-experiment. The first author then presented a 20-minute oral presentation to students in the "video" condition, creating a third "video + oral" condition. Students in this condition took the *POSHA–S* for a third time. Findings suggested that the live presentation in the "oral" condition was more effective in changing negative attitudes than the other conditions, although the "video" condition was also associated with considerable improvements in attitudes and the "video + oral" condition generated *POSHA–S* scores similar to those of the "oral" condition. The authors speculate that use of humor and the presenter's relatively young age may have influenced the positive change in attitudes. These considerations may partly explain why showing a video about stuttering in the McGee et al. (1996; see entry 39) and Snyder (2001; see entry 40) studies did not change attitudes toward stuttering and people who stutter.

42. Silverman, F. H., & Bongey, T. A. (1997). Nurses' attitudes toward physicians who stutter. *Journal of Fluency Disorders, 22*, 61–62.

Silverman and Bongey used a 20-item semantic differential questionnaire to assess nurses' attitudes toward physicians who stutter. Ten nurses received a questionnaire that asked them to rate "a physician" and 10 nurses received the same questionnaire that asked them to rate "a physician who stutters." A physician who stutters was rated as more afraid, tense, nervous, and aggravating in addition to being less mature, intelligent, secure, competent, confident, educated, and reputable than a physician who does not stutter. These results indicated that nurses, and perhaps others in the medical profession, hold negative stereotypes of professionals who stutter.

43. Manning, W. H., Burlison, A. E., & Thaxton, D. (1999). Listener response to stuttering modification techniques. *Journal of Fluency Disorders, 24*, 267–280.

Manning et al. conducted two independent investigations to evaluate listener responses to stuttering modification techniques. Participants in the first study consisted of 24 employees of a food-processing plant who viewed two videotaped speech samples of a male speaker who simulated stuttering. In one sample (the stuttering only video), the speaker simulated fluency breaks to a mild extent characterized by repetitions, sound prolongations, and blocks. In the other sample (the stuttering plus cancellation video), the speaker reiterated the first speech sample, but also utilized cancellations after fluency breaks. Participants in the second study consisted of 50 employees of a county school district. They also watched two videotaped speech samples of a man who simulated stuttering. One of these videos was the stuttering-only video from the first study. The other video consisted of the same speaker applying pullouts, a stuttering-modification strategy of intercepting and changing each stutter (the stuttering plus pullout video). After each video was presented, participants in both studies completed semantic differential scales (Woods & Williams, 1976; see entry 5) and a

5-point handicap scale, in which listeners indicated how much they felt the speaker was handicapped by his condition. They then responded to open-ended questions that elicited general reactions to the speaker, the degree to which they would interact socially with the speaker, and what it would be like to work with the speaker. The results of both studies indicated that participants felt that people who stutter who use pullouts or cancellations are more handicapped than those who do not employ these techniques. Participants also responded less favorably to 42 of 50 semantic differential items when the speaker used therapy techniques. Responses to the open-ended questions revealed that participants in both studies provided the same types of generally negative reactions to the speaker who used therapy techniques. Results suggested that listeners react more negatively to stuttering modification techniques than stuttering only; however, the ability to generalize these results is limited because responses to only one speaker were gathered.

44. St. Louis, K. O. (1999). Person-first labeling and stuttering. *Journal of Fluency Disorders, 24,* 1–24.

St. Louis conducted a preliminary investigation into the effects of using person-first labeling (i.e., "person who stutters") versus direct labels (i.e., "stutterer"). Survey respondents came from a wide variety of ages and backgrounds and included members of the general public; SLPs; graduate SLP students; speech, language, or hearing-impaired clients; and parents of these clients. Participants provided responses to various questions about 12 types of disorders (including stuttering) using Likert-type scales. Participants did not respond significantly differently to the term "stutterer" versus "person who stutters," indicating that person-first labeling does not lessen negative ratings related to stuttering and people who stutter.

45. Van Borsel, J., Verniers, I., & Bouvry, S. (1999). Public awareness of stuttering. *Folia Phoniatrica Et Logopaedica, 51,* 124–132.

Van Borsel et al. investigated the attitudes of laypeople toward stuttering in Flanders, Belgium. The authors approached people on a busy street and administered a 13-item questionnaire about stuttering to those who agreed to participate. The results indicated that the majority of participants knew someone who stutters and believed that (1) the prevalence of stuttering is greater than 5% of the population, (2) stuttering begins between the ages of two and five years, (3) stuttering is more prevalent in boys than girls, (4) stuttering occurs regardless of handedness or race, (5) the cause of stuttering is psychogenic, (6) stuttering can be treated, (7) there is no difference between the IQ of people who stutter and fluent speakers, (8) stuttering is not hereditary, (9) stuttering is a severe handicap, and (10) parents should take a child who stutters to an SLP. The authors concluded that public awareness campaigns about stuttering are warranted given some of the misinformation about stuttering that exists in Belgium.

46. Xing Ming, J., Jing, Z., Yi Wen, Z., & Van Borsel, J. (2001). Public awareness of stuttering in Shanghai, China. *Logopedics Phoniatrics Vocology, 26*, 145–150.

    Xing Ming et al. observed that there are an estimated 10 million people who stutter in China, yet there are few investigations of stuttering stereotypes in that country. Accordingly, the authors replicated a study by Van Borsel et al. (1999; see entry 45) with Chinese laypeople living in Shanghai. The results indicated that responses tended to differ significantly depending on age group (older participants aged 21–55 and younger participants < 21 years). For example, older people were acquainted with more people who stutter, believed that stuttering was more prevalent for boys than girls, and were more likely to think that stuttering has a psychogenic cause. More older people than younger people indicated that they would take their child who stutters to an SLP or family doctor. Some differences were observed for gender, with men less likely to believe that stuttering is hereditary and can be treated. Women were less likely to take their child who stutters to a family doctor or SLP as compared to men. The authors concluded that stuttering is known in China, but that the general public could benefit from more scientific information about stuttering to reduce stereotypes of people who stutter.

47. de Britto Pereira, M., Rossi, J., & Van Borsel, J. (2008). Public awareness and knowledge of stuttering in Rio de Janeiro. *Journal of Fluency Disorders, 33*, 24–31.

    de Britto Pereira et al. used on-the-street sampling to gather data on the general public's beliefs about stuttering. This study replicated a similar study involving Belgian public awareness of stuttering (Van Borsel et al., 1999; see entry 45). Data from over 600 participants in Rio de Janiero, Brazil, were analyzed on the basis of participants' gender, educational level, and age. In general, the results suggested that (1) women had more accurate beliefs than men in terms of prevalence of stuttering and the intelligence of people who stutter; (2) younger people were more optimistic about treatment for stuttering whereas older people were less likely to recommend speech therapy; and (3) more highly educated people were more accurate in their beliefs about the prevalence and gender distribution of stuttering, as well as the occurrence of stuttering in other cultures. The authors concluded by noting that the beliefs of their Brazilian participants were not generally different than the beliefs of other participants documented in the literature.

48. Dorsey, M., & Guenther, R. K. (2000). Attitudes of professors and students toward college students who stutter. *Journal of Fluency Disorders, 25*, 77–83.

Dorsey and Guenther conducted a survey in which 34 professors and 57 college students used a 7-point semantic differential scale to rate either an average college student or a college student who stutters on 20 personality traits. Four of the 20 traits (*guarded, perfectionist, reserved,* and *talkative*) were judged to be neutral traits by a separate group of college students and professors, and so participants' responses on these traits were not analyzed. The remaining items consisted of a number of positive traits (*open, intelligent, bold, calm, self-assured, competent,* and *bright*) and negative traits (*nervous, shy, self-conscious, passive, aggressive, dull, mediocre, reticent,* and *incompetent*). Results indicated that for all but one trait, i.e., *aggressiveness,* professors rated the college student who stutters as possessing more negative traits than the average college student. College students perceived the college student who stutters to hold more negative personality traits for 13 items as compared to the average college student. College student participants felt that a student who stutters was more likely to be less aggressive, less incompetent, and more intelligent as compared to the average college student. Overall, professors who participated in the study rated the college student who stutters more negatively than did the college students, though these ratings varied on individual items. The authors suggested that although college students and professors may be reluctant to engage in interactions with students who stutter, increased interaction opportunities and educational programs about stuttering may help to change negative attitudes toward people who stutter.

49. Ezrati-Vinacour, R., Platzky, R., & Yairi, E. (2001). The young child's awareness of stuttering-like disfluency. *Journal of Speech, Language, and Hearing Research, 44,* 368–380.

Ezrati-Vinacour et al. examined children's awareness of stuttering-like disfluencies in an attempt to (1) identify the age at which fluent children begin to recognize disfluencies, (2) investigate whether specific types of disfluencies influence the age at which children become aware of stuttering, and (3) determine if there is a relationship between children's attitudes toward stuttering-like disfluencies and their level of awareness. Eighty children ranging from ages three to seven years individually watched videotapes of two identical seal puppets that were positioned side by side. One puppet uttered six-word sentences using sound, syllable, and single-syllable-word repetitions for some of the sentences, and blocks and prolongations for the others. The other puppet uttered these same sentences fluently. The order of fluent and nonfluent sentences was counterbalanced. After the child watched the puppets say a pair of sentences, the experimenter paused the tape and asked the child if both puppets talked in the same way. The child was also asked to point to the puppet on the screen that talked like him or her. After all six pairs of sentences were viewed, the child was asked to label the talking (e.g., "What do we call this kind of talking?"). The child was also asked if that kind of talking was good or not good. The child then viewed another pair of fluent–disfluent utterances from the puppets and was asked which puppet she or he would like to play with and why. Results indicated that children as young as age three can discriminate between fluent speech and stuttering-like disfluencies, but that awareness of stuttering continues to rise as children reach four and five years of age. The majority of five-year-olds can discriminate fluent from stuttered speech. Children had a greater awareness of disfluencies that were characterized by repetitions versus blocks or prolongations. The word "stuttering" was rarely used by children to label the stuttering-like disfluencies, but as children became older, they were able to provide descriptions of stuttered speech. Children four years and older almost unanimously agreed that the stuttered speech was "not good" and that they would prefer to have a fluent speaker for a friend. These findings suggested that the development of negative stereotypes may occur very early in a child's development, and that age-appropriate educational programs may be beneficial to prevent negative attitudes toward people who stutter and others with disabilities.

50. Langevin, M., Packman, A., & Onslow, M. (2009). Peer responses to stuttering in the preschool setting. *American Journal of Speech-Language Pathology, 18*, 264–276.

    Langevin et al. videotaped four preschool children who stutter during play interactions with their peers. Instances of stuttering were documented, as were peer responses. Most responses were judged to be neutral or positive, but some negative responses emerged in reaction to long or complex stuttering episodes. These negative responses included mocking, ignoring, or interrupting the child who stuttered. Further, the children who stuttered experienced some difficulties in terms of their ability to be leaders, to engage in pretend play, and to resolve peer conflicts. These findings highlight the need for appropriate early intervention for children who stutter, including peer education from a young age.

51. Klassen, T. R. (2001). Perceptions of people who stutter: Re-assessing the negative stereotype. *Perceptual and Motor Skills, 92*, 551–559.

Klassen gave friends and colleagues of people who stutter a two-part written questionnaire. The first part assessed participants' attitudes toward stuttering people in general and consisted of semantic differential scales (Woods & Williams, 1976; see entry 5), portions of the *CATS Inventory*, and the *Parental Attitudes Toward Stuttering* inventory. The second part assessed participants' attitudes toward one person who stutters and with whom they were familiar. Participants in this study reported having less stereotypical beliefs about stuttering individuals in general as compared to previously reported results (e.g., Hulit & Wirtz, 1994; see entry 36). Results indicated that the increased social closeness of some people to people who stutter had a positive effect on their attitudes toward stuttering people in general.

52. Klassen, T. R. (2002). Social distance and the negative stereotype of people who stutter. *Journal of Speech-Language Pathology and Audiology, 26*, 90–99.

Using a similar methodology to his 2001 study (see entry 51), Klassen identified six people who stutter and surveyed their close acquaintances (including friends, family, teachers, fellow students, and colleagues) to see if these significant others held the same negative stereotypes toward stuttering people that have been pervasive throughout the stuttering literature. The six stuttering participants were also surveyed for comparison purposes. Results indicated that the participants who were personally acquainted with at least one person who stutters rated people who stutter more favorably on personality dimensions than had been reported for members of the general public (e.g., Hulit & Wirtz, 1994; see entry 36). These results are consistent with the findings of St. Louis, Kuhn, and Lytwak (this volume). In addition, the stuttering participants rated their speech as more abnormal than did their acquaintances. These findings suggested that different groups of people may hold different attitudes toward people who stutter depending on their level of social distance. As a whole, the Klassen (2001, 2002) studies suggested that ongoing contact with someone who stutters may lead to increased positive attitudes toward people who stutter; conversely, people who have little or no contact with someone who stutters may be more likely to hold negative stereotypes about stuttering people.

53. Susca, M., & Healey, E. C. (2001). Perceptions of simulated stuttering and fluency. *Journal of Speech, Language, and Hearing Research, 44,* 61–72.

Susca and Healey investigated listeners' perceptions of simulated stuttering and fluency. Individuals comprised of university staff, undergraduate students, and members of the general public served as participants. A speech sample from a 27-year-old male who stuttered while reading the Rainbow Passage was digitized and used as stimulus material. From this "core" sample containing 10% stuttered disfluencies, additional stimuli containing 0%, 5%, and 15% stuttered disfluencies were created from a computer program. A normal sample was developed that consisted of a 24-year-old male reading the Rainbow Passage with a normal rate and manner. Each participant was randomly assigned to one of the six conditions. After listening to the sample, participants were asked to verbally describe the speaker's speech, rate the perceptual features associated with the speaker using Likert scales, and answer three open-ended questions. To interpret the data, the authors quantified the qualitative data, and counted the number of participants' positive versus negative comments. Results indicated that as the percentage of stuttered disfluencies increased, so too did the number of negative comments provided by participants. Likert data suggested that as the speaker's disfluencies increased, the participants' comfort level decreased, and the speaker who stuttered was perceived as having less speech competency and fluency than the typical speaker.

54. Susca, M., & Healey, E. C. (2002). Listener perceptions along a fluency–disfluency continuum: A phenomenological analysis. *Journal of Fluency Disorders, 27,* 135–161.

Susca and Healey performed a phenomenological (qualitative) analysis of listeners' comments gathered in a previous study (Susca & Healey, 2001; see entry 53) investigating listeners' perceptions of stuttering based on speech stimuli with different fluency levels. Listeners' responses were organized into three categories that included comments about the speaker, comments about the listener, and comments about the story (e.g., the Rainbow Passage). Results indicated that listeners tend to hold more negative attitudes toward a speaker when increased stuttering is present in the speech sample; however, listeners also judge a person's speech on a variety of parameters other than stuttering. Furthermore, listener attributes as well as speaker attributes appear to be influential in perceptions of people who stutter, suggesting that therapeutic techniques should focus on helping clients who stutter be more effective communicators in addition to reducing the frequency of stuttering.

55. Daniels, D. E., & Gabel, R. M. (2004). The impact of stuttering on identity construction. *Topics in Language Disorders, 24,* 200–215.

Daniels and Gabel provided an in-depth examination of the concept of identity. They discussed how the identity of people who stutter can be shaped by societal attitudes and listener reactions toward stuttering. A case study at the end of the literature review demonstrated how identity can be influenced by assessment and treatment protocols during fluency therapy. For example, "John" described how his identity as more than "just" a person who stutters was validated by his clinicians. The authors indicated that SLPs who treat their clients holistically, as if they are more than simply a diagnostic label, can positively influence their clients' sense of identity and clinical outcomes. Implications for stuttering intervention, especially the need for positive communicative experiences in childhood, were presented.

56. Gabel, R. M., Blood, G. W., Tellis, G. M., & Althouse, M. T. (2004). Measuring role entrapment of people who stutter. *Journal of Fluency Disorders, 29,* 27–49.

Gabel et al. developed and administered the *Vocational Advice Scale* (*VAS*) to investigate college students' perceptions of appropriate career choices for people who stutter. The *VAS* is a written questionnaire that asks respondents to indicate the degree (on a 5-point Likert-type scale) to which they would advise someone to train for 43 jobs. The *VAS* was administered to 385 university students. One group of students was asked to provide career advice to an adult male who stuttered, and the other group of students was asked to give advice to an adult male who did not stutter. Statistical analysis indicated that 20 of 43 careers were judged to be significantly less advisable for an adult male who stuttered than a typical adult male. The authors noted that there appeared to be some similarities among the careers that were judged as being less acceptable for people who stutter. Some such careers (e.g., psychologist, physician, speech-language pathologist, etc.) may have been perceived as requiring high levels of communicative competence or the ability to help others by speaking well. This perception may limit the career choices of people who stutter due to occupational stereotyping.

57. Irani, F., Gabel, R., Hughes, S., Swartz, E. R., & Palasik, S. T. (2009). Role entrapment of people who stutter reported by K–12 teachers. *Contemporary Issues in Communication Science and Disorders, 36,* 48–56.

Irani et al. conducted an occupational stereotyping survey of over 200 kindergarten through Grade 12 (K–12) teachers from across the United

States. The *Vocational Advice Scale* (*VAS*) (Gabel et al., 2004; see entry 56) was administered to teachers to determine the extent to which teachers engage in occupational stereotyping of people who stutter. Teachers were randomly assigned to one of two survey conditions in which they completed the *VAS* in reaction to: (1) a person who stuttered and had no other communication disorder, and (2) a person who did not stutter and had no other communication disorder. Results indicated that people who stutter were less likely to be advised to pursue 10 out of the 43 careers on the *VAS*, including judge, attorney, SLP, minister, parole officer, guidance/employment counselor, psychologist, physician, hospital administrator, and pharmacist. K–12 teachers recommended more careers as appropriate for people who stutter as compared to university students in Gabel et al.'s (2004) original *VAS* study. The authors concluded that teachers did not engage in role entrapment of stuttering people to the extent reported for the university students in Gabel et al.'s study.

58. Swartz, E., Gabel, R., Hughes, S., & Irani, F. (2009). Speech-language pathologists' responses on surveys on vocational stereotyping (role entrapment) regarding people who stutter. *Contemporary Issues in Communication Science and Disorders, 36,* 157–165.

Swartz et al. administered the *Vocational Advice Scale* (*VAS*) (Gabel et al., 2004; see entry 56) to 158 SLPs recruited from the American Speech-Language-Hearing Association membership directory. Participants were assigned to one of two conditions in which they completed the *VAS* in reaction to either (1) a male individual who stuttered and had no other communication disorder, or (2) a male who did not stutter and had no other communication disorder. Mean scores on the *VAS* were not significantly different for SLPs in the two conditions, and indicated relatively positive attitudes overall. Participants were less likely to advise an individual who stutters to pursue a career as an attorney or SLP. Participants who reported completing professional readings in stuttering were more likely to advise people who stutter to become a judge, attorney, hospital administrator, guidance/employment counselor, or physician.

59. Panico, J., Healey, E. C., Brouwer, K., & Susca, M. (2005). Listener perceptions of stuttering across two presentation modes: A quantitative and qualitative approach. *Journal of Fluency Disorders, 30,* 65–85.

Panico et al. used a mixed methods approach to examine the impact of presentation mode (audio versus audiovisual) and stuttering severity (0, 5,

10, or 15% disfluent) on raters' attitudes toward people who stutter. Participants watched or listened to one of the samples and then completed a Likert-type scale and four open-ended questions. Data analysis involved (1) frequency counts of positive versus negative statements made by the raters and (2) the development of theme clusters. The authors concluded that there were no significant differences between audio and audiovisual stuttered speech samples. In addition, as the level of stuttering severity increased, so did the raters' negative comments. This finding is consistent with a similar study by Susca and Healey (2001; see entry 53) in which Likert-scale data and written comments suggested that negative ratings and comments about people who stutter increase as level of stuttering severity increases.

60. Gabel, R. M. (2006). Effects of stuttering severity and therapy involvement on attitudes towards people who stutter. *Journal of Fluency Disorders, 31*, 216–227.

Gabel investigated university students' attitudes toward people who stutter based on stuttering severity and level of therapy involvement. Participants were given a 25-item semantic differential questionnaire (Woods & Williams, 1976; see entry 5) and were asked to rate one of four hypothetical conditions in which a man who stuttered severely or mildly chose or did not choose to attend therapy to improve his stuttering. Results indicated that participants reported more positive traits for the male who stuttered mildly than the male who stuttered severely. Attending therapy to improve stuttering was also perceived more positively than not attending therapy. There was no interaction between the stuttering and therapy variables, so that a person who stutters severely was not regarded more positively for attending therapy than someone who stutters mildly. The author suggested that most participants felt mildly positive or mildly negative toward stuttering people based on their semantic differential scores, indicating that people in general may feel mostly neutral or ambivalent toward those who stutter.

61. Guntupalli, V. K., Kalinowski, J., Nanjundeswaran, C., Saltuklaroglu, T., & Everhart, D. E. (2006). Psychophysiological responses of adults who do not stutter while listening to stuttering. *International Journal of Psychophysiology, 62*, 1–8.

Guntupalli et al. examined the psychophysiological responses of fluent speakers to people who stutter. Fifteen fluent speakers, including university students and other laypeople, watched one-minute video samples of stuttering and fluent speakers. Data about participants' emotional and physiological reactions were gathered via measurements of heart rate and skin conductance. Participants tended to have a slower heart rate when listening to people who stutter, indicating that listeners pay more attention to the speech of stuttering than fluent speakers. Increased skin conductance was noted as participants watched videos of people who stutter, suggesting that listeners experience unpleasant emotional arousal when listening to stuttering. This study did not pair heart rate and skin conductance measures with participants' self-reports about their experiences while watching people who stutter speak. Future research could combine psychophysiological and self-report data in order to provide a more complete understanding of attitudes toward people who stutter.

62. Healey, E. C., Gabel, R. M., Daniels, D. E., & Kawai, N. (2007). The effects of self-disclosure and non self-disclosure of stuttering on listeners' perceptions of a person who stutters. *Journal of Fluency Disorders, 32*, 51–69.

Healey et al. examined laypeople's perceptions of videotaped samples of a male speaker who stuttered severely. Participants were randomly assigned to one of three groups for a total of 30 participants in each group. In each of the three videos, the male speaker who stuttered was asked the same question by the interviewer: "Can you tell me about a job you have had?" In one video, the male speaker who stuttered disclosed that he stuttered at the beginning of his monologue. In another video, the disclosure came at the end of the monologue. The third video consisted of the monologue only, and no reference to the speaker's stuttering was made. To assess participants' reactions to each of these conditions, a six-item Likert scale questionnaire was administered. These items included the following statements: (1) "This person seems sincere." (2) "This person is likeable." (3) "This person is trustworthy." (4) "This person is friendly." (5) "This person shows character." (6) "This person is emotionally well adjusted." After completing the Likert scale, all participants were asked open-ended questions about their comfort level while listening to the speaker and whether disclosure of stuttering impacted their perceptions of the speaker. Results from the Likert scale data indicated that disclosing versus not disclosing stuttering did not result in an overall difference in listeners' ratings of the speaker. The time of disclosure was not significant on five of the six Likert scales, though listeners perceived the speaker who disclosed his stuttering at the end to be more friendly. Data from the open-ended questions indicated that participants felt comfortable listening to the speaker whether or not he disclosed his stuttering. Some participants who were in the disclosure groups seemed to perceive benefits to disclosing stuttering, particularly at the beginning of a speech, but the majority of participants in the nondisclosure group did not report any perceived benefits of disclosure. The authors indicated that listeners may be comfortable with stuttering, regardless of its severity, though more research is needed to determine whether society in general has become more accepting of people who stutter and stuttering.

63. Gabel, R., Hughes, S., & Daniels, D. (2008). Effects of stuttering severity and therapy involvement on role entrapment of people who stutter. *Journal of Communication Disorders, 41*, 146–158.

Gabel et al. surveyed university students to determine if stuttering severity level or engagement in therapy affects reports of role entrapment (i.e., occupational stereotyping) for people who stutter. Participants were assigned to one of four conditions: (1) a male who stuttered severely and chose to attend therapy to improve his stuttering, (2) a male who stuttered mildly and chose to attend therapy, (3) a male who stuttered severely and chose not to attend therapy, and (4) a male who stuttered mildly and chose not to attend therapy. After reading the vignette, participants completed the *Vocational Advice Scale* (Gabel et al., 2004; see entry 56). Results indicated that stuttering severity and therapy status did not affect participants' perceptions of appropriate careers in general; however, participants were more likely to recommend that the hypothetical male who stuttered pursue a career as a speech therapist if he was receiving therapy.

64. Boyle, M. P., Blood, G. W., & Blood, I. M. (2009). Effects of perceived causality on perceptions of persons who stutter. *Journal of Fluency Disorders, 34*, 201–218.

Boyle et al. administered a variety of scales (social distance, adjective pair, and visual analogue scales) to university students to determine how the perceived cause of stuttering influences attitudes toward people who stutter. Participants were sorted randomly into one of four groups that varied depending on the cause that was attributed to a hypothetical person who stutters. All participants were given a vignette in which they were told to imagine a single, 25-year-old white man named Chris. In three of the four vignettes, Chris was described as a person who stuttered due to psychological factors, genetic factors, or idiopathic (unknown) factors. In the fourth (control) vignette, Chris was described as a person who did not stutter and was normally fluent. Results indicated that participants in the psychological-cause condition wanted increased social distance from people who stutter and described stuttering people more negatively as compared to participants in all other conditions. Findings suggest that people who stutter feel more stigma when interacting with those who believe stuttering has a psychological cause, and less stigma when interacting with people who believe stuttering to have a genetic or unknown cause.

65. Langevin, M. (2009). The *Peer Attitudes Toward Children Who Stutter* scale: Reliability, known groups validity, and negativity of elementary school-age children's attitudes. *Journal of Fluency Disorders, 34,* 72–86.

Langevin, having created the *Teasing and Bullying: Unacceptable Behaviour (TAB)* program (Langevin, 2000), developed a scale to assess the extent to which this program changed children's attitudes toward stuttering. This scale, the *Peer Attitudes toward Children Who Stutter (PATCS)* underwent a series of pre-testing, pilot studies, and revisions, which readers may find in additional articles not discussed here (i.e., Langevin, Bortnick, Hammer, & Wiebe, 1998; Langevin & Hagler, 2004; Langevin, Kleitman, Packman, & Onslow, 2009). The study under discussion attempted to further investigate the psychometric properties of the scale, and to replicate preliminary findings about peer attitudes toward stuttering. Results indicated generally good internal consistency with previous iterations of the *PATCS*, and indicated the *TAB* program improved peer attitudes toward stuttering. Findings were not significant for grade level and gender, leading the author to conclude that these factors may not be robust predictors of peer attitudes toward stuttering.

66. Schlagheck, A., Gabel, R., & Hughes, S. (2009). A mixed method study of stereotypes of people who stutter. *Contemporary Issues in Communication Science and Disorders, 36,* 108–117.

Schlagheck et al. administered an open-ended questionnaire to university students to assess how gender and familiarity with people who stutter may influence perceptions of (1) appropriate careers for stuttering people, and (2) characteristics associated with people who stutter. This mixed methods study found that participants who were female and participants who knew stuttering individuals made more positive comments and fewer negative comments about the characteristics of people who stutter. Most participants (82%) believed that stuttering people have employment difficulties, though gender and familiarity once again influenced participants' responses. Qualitative analysis of responses indicated that participants felt stuttering individuals have employment difficulties because they would have disabled communication, endure too much stress in the workplace, face difficulty with certain tasks, and avoid certain careers.

67. Hughes, S., Gabel, R., Irani, F., & Schlagheck, A. (2010a). University students' explanations for their descriptions of people who stutter: An exploratory mixed model study. *Journal of Fluency Disorders, 35,* 280–298.

Hughes et al. used a mixed (qualitative and quantitative) research design to investigate stereotypes of people who stutter. The authors' intent was to avoid the biases and limited explanatory power of semantic differential scales by asking participants open-ended questions about the characteristics of stuttering people. An electronic questionnaire was administered to 150 university students. Two open-ended questions ("How would you describe someone who stutters?" and "Why did you choose these words?") sought participants' views on characteristics of people who stutter. Responses to these questions were analyzed thematically. The number of responses noted for each theme was calculated and expressed in percentage of total responses. In addition, the effects of the demographic variables of gender and level of familiarity with stuttering people on participants' thematic responses were determined. Qualitative results indicated two descriptive themes, i.e., personal characteristics of people who stutter and stuttering-related communication difficulties. Three explanatory themes within participants' descriptions of people who stutter were also noted: (1) perceived emotional effects of stuttering on people who stutter, (2) listener difficulties when communicating with stuttering individuals, and (3) observations of people who stutter and self. Quantitative analysis indicated no significant differences in participants' responses on the basis of gender, familiarity with people who stutter, or the interaction between gender and familiarity. The authors concluded that people who stutter are perceived as warm and friendly people who are poor communicators, a combination of feelings that could lead to pity and paternalism. These results may challenge the long-standing notion that people perceive stuttering people as having inherently undesirable personality traits; more mixed methods (open-ended) research is necessary to confirm this interpretation of participants' responses.

68. Hughes, S., Gabel, R., Irani, F., & Schlagheck, A. (2010b). University students' perceptions of the life effects of stuttering. *Journal of Communication Disorders, 43,* 45–60.

Hughes et al. focused on how university students perceived the effects of stuttering on people who stutter by asking university students to answer the open-ended questions "How do you think people who stutter are affected by their stuttering" and "If you were a person who stutters, how would your life be different?" The authors used the same methodology as Hughes et al. 2010a (see entry 67). Four themes emerged from the analysis of both questions, including (1) difficulty communicating can have emotional and behavioral consequences for stuttering people; (2) people who stutter can be negatively affected by the actual or anticipated reactions of their listeners; (3) life effects of stuttering are broad and encompass social, academic, and occupational opportunities; and (4) individual differences among people who stutter result in variations in the life effects of stuttering. Quantitative analyses showed few differences in the number of responses for each theme on the basis of gender and familiarity with people who stutter. The findings supported the stuttering stereotype formation by inference hypothesis (White & Collins, 1984; see entry 17) and the anchoring-adjustment hypothesis (MacKinnon et al., 2007; see entry 19).

69. Von Tiling, J. (2011). Listener perceptions of stuttering, prolonged speech, and verbal avoidance behaviors. *Journal of Communication Disorders, 44*, 161–172.

Von Tiling investigated whether types of stuttered speech influenced listeners' perceptions of stuttering. The 115 listeners (German university students and members of the general public) were assigned to one of four groups and watched a vignette between three young men, one of whom, Marcus, stuttered. The four speech conditions included (1) stuttered speech that contained repetitions, prolongations, and blocks; (2) hesitant speech that contained avoidance behaviors such as interjections and revisions; (3) a combination of conditions one and two; and (4) the kind of prolonged speech learned in fluency-shaping therapy. After watching the vignette, listeners completed a questionnaire. The results indicated that listeners deemed the hesitant speech condition the least pleasant, intelligent, and communicatively competent as compared to all other ways of speaking. When Marcus used stuttered speech or prolonged speech, listener ratings of his self-confidence were higher (especially for male listeners) than when he used hesitant or stuttered/hesitant speech. Von Tiling discussed these results in the context of implicit theory (that is, whether listeners perceived stuttering to be a chronic or more temporary problem for the speaker). This research complements the work of MacKinnon et al. (2007; see entry 19) as well as White and Collins (1984; see entry 17).

70. St. Louis, K. O. (2012c). Research and development on a public attitude instrument for stuttering. *Journal of Communication Disorders, 45*, 129–146.

St. Louis described research studies that contributed to the development and psychometric evaluation of the *Public Opinion Survey of Human Attributes Stuttering* (*POSHA–S*). The author summarized numerous pilot studies that utilized early experimental versions of the *POSHA–S*, known as the *POSHA–E1* and *POSHA–E2*. Issues relating to translation of the *POSHA*, internal consistency, types of sampling and sampling size, definition of stuttering, manner of administration, and more were discussed. Future uses of the *POSHA–S* were presented, including a database and making the survey available to stakeholders. Numerous international studies using the *POSHA–S* have been conducted to date, and readers who would like more information about the results of these studies should review the works of Özdemir et al. (2011b), Abdalla & St. Louis (2012), St. Louis (2012a), Ip et al. (2012), and St. Louis et al. (2014) (see entries 71–75, respectively), and should also consult St. Louis's (2012a) reference list, as over 25 studies, papers, and presentations related to the *POSHA–S* are provided there.

71. Özdemir, R., St. Louis, K. O., & Topbaş, S. (2011b). Stuttering attitudes among Turkish family generations and neighbors from representative samples. *Journal of Fluency Disorders, 36*, 318–333.

Özdemir et al. utilized probability sampling to administer the *POSHA–S* (see St. Louis, 2012c, entry 70) for more information about the *POSHA–S*) to Grade 6 students who each distributed the *POSHA–S* to a parent, grandparent or other adult relative, and neighbor. Survey data were collected in 2008 and replicated in 2009. Few differences in attitudes toward stuttering in general were found when the two data sets were compared. Children, parents, grandparents/adult relatives, and neighbors held similar views toward stuttering within and between each data set; these attitudes were generally less positive compared to *POSHA–S* data gathered from other countries. The authors note that cultural and religious factors could contribute to Turkish perceptions of stuttering, but caution that percentile rankings comparing Turkish peoples to other world populations would probably change as more data are added to the *POSHA–S* database.

72. Abdalla, F. A., & St. Louis, K. O. (2012). Arab school teachers' knowledge, beliefs, and reactions regarding stuttering. *Journal of Fluency Disorders, 37*, 54–69.

Abdalla and St. Louis explored Arab educators' perceptions of stuttering by surveying in-service teachers and pre-service (student) teachers in Kuwait. An adapted version of the *POSHA–S*, translated into Arabic, was administered to participants. (See St. Louis, 2012, entry 70 for more information about the development of the *POSHA–S*.) The results of the study suggested that both pre-service and in-service teachers held generally similar views toward people who stutter, characterized by sensitivity to stuttering when interacting with stuttering individuals, but also stereotypical and misinformed views about stuttering and people who stutter. The study illustrated the importance of considering cultural factors when assessing and interpreting beliefs about people who stutter, the need for public awareness campaigns for teachers, and the importance of surveying a wider population of Arab peoples.

73. St. Louis, K. O. (2012a). Male versus female attitudes toward stuttering. *Journal of Communication Disorders, 45*, 246–253.

St. Louis analyzed the data obtained from 50 men and 50 women who had previously taken the *POSHA–S* (see St. Louis, 2012c, entry 70, for more information about the development of the *POSHA–S*) to determine the extent to which males and females differ in their attitudes toward stuttering and people who stutter. The data were obtained via random selection from diverse samples of people in many countries. Results indicated that there were no statistically significant or otherwise important differences in the attitudes of men and women. The author cautioned that subgroups of populations (e.g., people in certain professions) may still hold sex-based stereotypes of stuttering and people who stutter.

74. Ip, M., St. Louis, K. O., Myers, F. L., & An Xue, S. (2012). Stuttering attitudes in Hong Kong and adjacent mainland China. *International Journal of Speech-Language Pathology, 14*, 543–556.

Ip et al. noted that people in China and Hong Kong make up one-fifth of the world's population, yet few studies have examined people's attitudes toward stuttering in this part of the world. (See Xing Ming et al., 2001, entry 46 for a notable exception.) The authors administered the *POSHA–S* (see St. Louis, 2012c, entry 70, for more information about the development of the *POSHA–S*) to people in Hong Kong and adjacent mainland China to determine (1) whether there is a difference in people's attitudes toward stuttering in these two locales, and (2) whether people's attitudes toward stuttering in Hong Kong and China are different from people in other parts of the world. While there were few differences among the Hong Kong and mainland China respondents, there were distinct and often idiosyncratic differences when these data were compared to a database of *POSHA–S* scores from around the world. For example, respondents in the Chinese/Hong Kong sample were more likely to indicate that they would both try to ignore stuttering and help people who stutter; conversely, they were about as likely as the rest of the world to make jokes about stuttering. The authors hypothesized that Chinese attitudes toward stuttering could be similar for cultures within and outside of China (such as people living in Singapore), and that Western attitudes could impact Chinese attitudes toward stuttering.

75. St. Louis, K. O., Przepiórka, A. M., Beste-Guldborg, A., Williams, M. J., Błachnio, A., Guendouzi, J., Reichel, I. K., & Ware, M. B. (2014). Stuttering attitudes of students: Professional, intracultural, and international comparisons. *Journal of Fluency Disorders, 39*, 34–50.

St. Louis et al. administered the *POSHA–S* to university students in Poland and the United States. (See St. Louis, 2012c, entry 70, for more information about the development of the *POSHA–S*.) Subgroups of respondents included Native American (Plains Indian) students, graduate and undergraduate students, and speech-language pathology (SLP) and non-SLP majors. The results of the study indicated that (1) U.S. graduate students had more positive attitudes overall toward stuttering than undergraduates; (2) few statistically significant differences emerged for comparisons of U.S. graduate students who were non-SLP majors and U.S. undergraduate SLP majors; (3) SLP undergraduate majors in Poland had more overall positive scores than Polish students with other majors (e.g., psychology majors and a control group); (4) comparisons of Polish SLP majors and non-majors to U.S. SLP majors and non-majors resulted in significant differences that ranged from 22% to 33% of *POSHA–S* items, with U.S. students' attitudes being more positive on many but not all items; and (5) Native American students' scores were similar to those of U.S. non-SLP majors, though fewer significant differences between Native American students and Polish students were observed. The authors note that SLP students may have more favorable attitudes toward stuttering due to the halo effect, and that graduate SLP students may have more positive attitudes due to increased training. International differences were more pronounced than intercultural ones (i.e., Native American versus non-Native American students).

76. Boyle, M. P. (2013a). Assessment of stigma associated with stuttering: Development and evaluation of the *Self-Stigma of Stuttering Scale (4S)*. *Journal of Speech and Hearing Research, 56*, 1517–1529.

Boyle explained how people may internalize stigma based on negative attitudes from society. Levels of self-stigma were reviewed, including stigma awareness, stereotype agreement, and self-concurrence. Using this framework, the 4S scale was adapted from a self-stigma scale developed by researchers in the mental health profession. Nearly 300 adults who stutter (AWS), recruited from the National Stuttering Association and from Board Recognized Specialists in Fluency Disorders, took the experimental version of the 4S as well as scales measuring self-esteem, self-efficacy, and satisfaction with life. Psychometric properties of the 4S were judged to have adequate reliability and validity. The author concluded that SLPs may find the scale to be an easily administered way to assess the presence of self-stigma in adult clients who stutter.

Annotated Bibliography Author Index by Entry Number

Parenthetical numbers indicate that the author was cited in an entry but was not an author for that entry.

References

Abdalla, F., & Al-Saddah, A. (2009). *Stuttering and teachers in Kuwait: The story so far.* Paper presented at the 12th International Stuttering Awareness Day (ISAD) Online Conference. Retrieved from http://www.mnsu.edu/comdis/isad12/papers/abdalla12.html

Abdalla, F. A., & St. Louis, K. O. (2012). Arab school teachers' knowledge, beliefs, and reactions regarding stuttering. *Journal of Fluency Disorders, 37,* 54–69.

Abdalla, F., & St. Louis, K. O. (2014). Modifying attitudes of Arab school teachers toward stuttering. *Language, Speech, and Hearing Services in the Schools, 45,* 14–25.

Action for Stammering Children. (2014, September). Retrieved from http://www.stammeringcentre.org

Akehurst, L., Kohnken, G., Vrij, A., & Bull, R. (1996). Lay persons' and police officers' beliefs regarding deceptive behavior. *Applied Cognitive Psychology, 10,* 461–471.

Alghazo, E., & Gaad, E. (2004). General education teachers in the United Arab Emirates and their acceptance of students with disabilities. *British Journal of Special Education, 31,* 94–99.

Al-Khaledi, M., Lincoln, M., McCabe, P., Packman, A., & Alshatti, T. (2009). The attitudes, knowledge, and beliefs of Arab parents in Kuwait about stuttering. *Journal of Fluency Disorders, 34,* 44–59.

Allard, E. R., & Williams, D. F. (2008). Listeners' perceptions of speech and language disorders. *Journal of Communication Disorders, 41,* 108–123.

Allport, G.W. (1986). *The nature of prejudice* (25th anniversary ed.). Reading, MA: Addison-Wesley.

Altholz, S. (1991). *A study on the attitudes and knowledge social workers have in relation to people who stutter.* Unpublished manuscript, Grand Valley State University, Grand Rapids, MI.

Altholz, S., & Golensky, M. (2004). Counseling, support, and advocacy for clients who stutter. *Health and Social Work, 29,* 197–205.

American Psychiatric Association. (2013). *Diagnostic and statistical manual of mental disorders* (rev. 5th ed.). Washington, DC: American Psychiatric Association.

American Speech-Language-Hearing Association. (2014a). *Issues in ethics: Cultural and linguistic competence.* Retrieved from http://www.asha.org/Practice/ethics/Cultural-and-Linguistic-Competence/

American Speech-Language-Hearing Association. (2014b, September). *Scope of practice in speech-language pathology [Scope of Practice].* Retrieved from http://www.asha.org/policy/SP2007-00283/

Andreou, E., Didaskalou, E., & Vlachou, A. (2008). Outcomes of a curriculum-based anti-bullying intervention program on students' attitudes and behavior. *Emotional and Behavioural Difficulties, 13*, 235–248.

Andrews, G., & Cutler, J. (1974). Stuttering therapy: The relation between changes in symptom level and attitudes. *Journal of Speech and Hearing Research, 34*, 312–319.

Arnold, H., & Goltl, K. (2013, September). *Attitudes of teachers versus non-teachers towards people who stutter.* Poster and paper presented at the Stuttering Attitudes Research Symposium, Morgantown, WV.

Arora, C. M. J. (1994). Is there any point in trying to reduce bullying in secondary schools? *Educational Psychology in Practice, 10*, 155–162.

Ashurst, J. V., & Wasson, M. N. (2011). Developmental and persistent developmental stuttering: An overview for primary care physicians. *Journal of the American Osteopath Association, 111*, 576–580.

Baldry, A. C., & Farrington, D. P. (2005). Protective factors as moderators of risk factors in adolescence bullying. *School Psychology of Education, 8*, 263–284.

Ball, H. A., Arseneault, L., Taylor, A., Maughan, B., Caspi, A., & Moffitt, T. E. (2008). Genetic and environmental influences on victims, bullies, and bully-victims in childhood. *Journal of Child Psychology and Psychiatry, 49*, 104–112.

Baly, M., & Cornell, D. (2011). Effects of an educational video on student reports of bullying. *Journal of School Violence, 10*, 221–228.

Bandura, A. (1994). *Self-efficacy.* New York, NY: John Wiley & Sons.

Bandyopadhyay, S., Cornell, D. G., & Konold, T. R. (2009). Validity of three school climate scales to assess bullying, aggressive attitudes, and help seeking. *School Psychology Review, 38*, 338–355.

Bar, A. (1969). Effects of type of listeners and listening instructions on the attention to manner and content of a severe stutterer's speech. *Journal of Communication Disorders, 2*, 344–349.

Barreto, M., & Ellemers, N. (2010). Current issues in the study of social stigma: Some controversies and unresolved issues. *Journal of Social Issues, 66*, 431–445.

Beals, K. P., Peplau, L. A., & Gable, S. L. (2009). Stigma management and well-being: The role of perceived social support, emotional processing, and suppression. *Personality and Social Psychology Bulletin, 35*, 867–879.

Bebout, L., & Arthur, B. (1992). Cross-cultural attitudes toward speech disorders. *Journal of Speech and Hearing Research, 35*, 45–52.

Beilby, J. M., Byrnes, M. L., & Yaruss, J. S. (2012). Acceptance and commitment therapy for adults who stutter: Psychosocial adjustment and speech fluency. *Journal of Fluency Disorders, 37*, 289–299.

Benecken, J., & Spindler, C. (2004). Zur psychosozialen Situation stotternder Schulkinder in Allgemeinschulen [On the sociopsychological situation of stuttering pupils in regular classes]. *Die Sprachheilarbeit, 49*, 61–70.

Bengston, V. L., Biblarz, T. J., & Roberts, R. E. I. (2002). *How families still matter: A longitudinal study of youth in two generations.* Cambridge, UK: Cambridge University Press.

Berger, B. E., Ferrans, C. E., & Lashley, F. R. (2001). Measuring stigma in people with HIV: Psychometric assessment of the HIV Stigma Scale. *Research in Nursing and Health, 24*, 518–529.

Betz, I. R., Blood, G. W., & Blood, I. M. (2008). University students' perceptions of pre-school and kindergarten children who stutter. *Journal of Communication Disorders, 41*, 259–273.

Bingham, R. D., Haubrich, P. A., White, S. B., & Zipp, J. F. (1990). Dual standards among teachers: This school is good enough for other kids but not my child. *Urban Education, 25*, 274–288.

Blair, J., & Kooi, B. (2004). The gap between training and research in the detection of decep-tion. *International Journal of Police Science and Management, 6*, 77–83.

Blood, G. W. (1995a). POWER2: Relapse management with adolescents who stutter. *Lan-guage, Speech, and Hearing Services in Schools, 26*, 169–179.

Blood, G. W. (1995b). A behavioral-cognitive therapy program for adults who stutter: Com-puters and counseling. *Journal of Communication Disorders, 28*, 165–180.

Blood, G. W. (1999, November). *The stigma of stuttering: Centuries of negative percep-tions and stereotypes.* Paper presented at the annual meeting of the American Speech-Language-Hearing Association, San Francisco, CA.

Blood, G. W. (2003). *The POWERR game: Managing stuttering: A practical program for helping those who stutter make changes in their lives.* Memphis, TN: The Stuttering Foundation.

Blood, G. W., & Blood, I. M. (2004). Bullying in adolescents who stutter: Communicative competence and self-esteem. *Contemporary Issues in Communication Science and Dis-orders, 31*, 69–79.

Blood, G. W., & Blood, I. M. (2007). Preliminary study of self-reported experience of physical aggression and bullying of boys who stutter: Relation to increased anxiety. *Per-ceptual and Motor Skills, 104*, 1060–1066.

Blood, G. W., Blood, I. M., Dorward, S., Boyle, M. P., & Tramontana, G. M. (2011). Coping strategies and adolescents: Learning to take care of self and stuttering during treatment. *Perspectives on Fluency and Fluency Disorders, 21*, 68–77.

Blood, G. W., Blood, I. M., Tellis, G. M., & Gabel, R. M. (2003). A preliminary study of self-esteem, stigma, and self-disclosure in adolescents who stutter. *Journal of Fluency Disorders, 28*, 143–159.

Blood, G. W., Blood, I. M., Tramontana, G. M., Sylvia, A. J., Boyle, M. P., & Motzko, G. R. (2011). Self-reported experience of bullying of students who stutter: Relations with life satisfaction, life orientation, and self-esteem. *Perceptual and Motor Skills, 113*, 353–364.

Blood, G., Blood, I., Wertz, H., Wade, J., & Mapp, C. (1997). Coping with stuttering during adolescence. *Journal of Fluency Disorders, 22*, 114.

Blood, G. W., Boyle, M. P., Blood, I. M., & Nalesnik, G. R. (2010). Bullying in children who stutter: Speech-language pathologists' perceptions and intervention strategies. *Journal of Fluency Disorders, 35*, 92–109.

Blood, G. W., & Conture, E. G. (1998). Outcomes measurement issues in fluency disorders. In C. Frattali (Ed.), *Outcome measurement in speech–language pathology* (pp. 387–405). New York, NY: Thieme Medical.

Blood, G. W., Robins, L. A., Blood, I. M., Boyle, M. P., & Finke, E. H. (2011). Bul-lying, school-based speech-language pathologists, and English language learners:

Seriousness, intervention, and strategy selection. *Perspectives on School-Based Issues, 12*, 128–138.

Bloodstein, O. (1995). *A handbook on stuttering (5th ed.)*. San Diego, CA: Singular.

Bloodstein, O., & Bernstein Ratner, N. (2008). *A handbook on stuttering* (6th ed.). Clifton Park, NY: Thomson Delmar.

Blumgart, E., Tran, Y., & Craig, A. (2010). An investigation into the personal and financial costs associated with stuttering. *Journal of Fluency Disorders, 35*, 203–215.

Bockting, W. O., Miner, M. H., Swinburne , R. E., Hamilton, A., & Coleman, E. (2013). Stigma, mental health, and resilience in an online sample of the U.S. transgender population. *American Journal of Public Health, 103*, 943–951.

Bohan, J. S. (1996). *Psychology and sexual orientation: Coming to terms*. New York, NY: Routledge.

Bohner, G., & Dickel, N. (2011). Attitudes and attitude change. *Annual Review of Psychology, 62*, 391–417.

Bollmer, J. M., Milich, R., Harris, M. J., & Maras, M. A. (2005). A friend in need: The role of friendship quality as a protective factor in peer victimization and bullying. *Journal of Interpersonal Violence, 20*, 701–712.

Boltužić, M., Jelčić Jakšić, S., & St. Louis, K. O. (2013, June). *Attitudes toward stuttering of speech-language pathologists and special educators in primary schools in Croatia*. Paper presented at the 10th World Congress of the International Stuttering Association, Lunteren, Netherlands.

Bondarenko, V. (1992a). *Speaking of courage*. Oakville, ON: Magic Lantern Communication.

Bondarenko, V. (1992b). *Voices to remember*. Oakville, ON: Magic Lantern Communication.

Botterill, W. (2011). Developing the therapeutic relationship: From "expert" professional to "expert" person who stutters. *Journal of Fluency Disorders, 36*, 158–173.

Boulton, M. J., Trueman, M., Chau, C., Whitehand, C., & Amatya, K. (1999). Concurrent and longitudinal links between friendship and peer victimization: Implications for befriending interventions. *Journal of Adolescence, 22*, 461–466.

Boyle, M. P. (2011). Mindfulness training in stuttering therapy: A tutorial for speech-language pathologists. *Journal of Fluency Disorders, 36*, 122–129.

Boyle, M. P. (2012). *Self-stigma of stuttering: Implications for self-esteem, self-efficacy, and life satisfaction*. Unpublished doctoral dissertation, Pennsylvania State University.

Boyle, M. P. (2013a). Assessment of stigma associated with stuttering: Development and evaluation of the Self-Stigma of Stuttering Scale (4S). *Journal of Speech, Language, and Hearing Research, 56*, 1517–1529.

Boyle, M. P. (2013b). Psychological characteristics and perceptions of stuttering of adults who stutter with and without support group experience. *Journal of Fluency Disorders, 38*, 368.

Boyle, M. P., Blood, G. W., & Blood, I. M. (2009). Effects of perceived causality on perceptions of persons who stutter. *Journal of Fluency Disorders, 34*, 201–218.

Brant, C. (1990). Native ethics and rules of behavior. *Canadian Journal of Psychiatry, 35*, 534–539.

Brekhus, W. (2003). *Peacocks, chameleons, centaurs: Gay suburbia and the grammar of social identity*. Chicago: University of Chicago Press.

Brendgen, M., Boivin, M., Vitaro, F., Girard, A., Dionne, G., & Pérusse, D. (2008). Gene-environment interaction between peer victimization and child aggression. *Development and Psychopathology, 20*, 455–471.

Bricker-Katz, G., Lincoln, M., & Cumming, S. (2013). Stuttering and work life: An interpretative phenomenological analysis. *Journal of Fluency Disorders, 38*, 342–355.

Bricker-Katz, G., Lincoln, M., & McCabe, P. (2009). A life-time of stuttering: How emotional reactions to stuttering impact activities and participation in older people. *Disability and Rehabilitation: An International, Multidisciplinary Journal, 31*, 1742–1752.

Bricker-Katz, G., Lincoln, M., & McCabe, P. (2010). Older people who stutter: Barriers to communication and perceptions of treatment needs. *International Journal of Communication Disorders, 45*, 15–30.

Brisk, D. J., Healey, E. C., & Hux, K. A. (1997). Clinician's training and confidence associated with treating school-age children who stutter. *Language, Speech, and Hearing Services in Schools, 28*, 164–176.

British Stammering Association. (2014, September). *Basic information on stammering.* Retrieved from http://www.stammering.org/help-information/topics/what-stammering/basic-information-stammering

Bronfenbrenner, U., & Ceci, S. J., (1994). Nature-nurture reconceptualized in developmental perspective: A bioecological model. *Psychological Review, 101*, 568–586.

Brown, M. R. (2001). *Criminal investigation: Law and practice* (2nd ed.). Boston: Butterworth Heinemann.

Burley, P. M., & Rinaldi, W. (1986). Effects of sex of listener and of stutterer on ratings of stuttering speakers. *Journal of Fluency Disorders, 17*, 329–333.

Butler, C. (2013). Identity and stammering: Negotiating hesitation, side-stepping repetition, and sometimes avoiding deviation. *Sociology of Health & Illness, 35*, 1113–1127.

Camodeca, M., & Goossens, F. A. (2005). Children's opinions on effective strategies to cope with bullying: The importance of bullying role and perspective. *Educational Research, 47*, 93–105.

Card, N. A., & Hodges, E. V. E. (2008). Peer victimization among schoolchildren: Correlations, causes, consequences, and considerations in assessment and intervention. *School Psychology Quarterly, 23*, 451–461.

Causey, D. L., & Dubow, E. F. (1992). Development of a self-report coping measure for elementary school children. *Journal of Clinical Child Psychology, 21*, 47–59.

Central Intelligence Agency. (2014, September). *World Fact Book.* Retrieved from https://www.cia.gov/library/publications/the-world-factbook/geos/su.html

Chaudoir, S. R., Earnshaw, V. A., & Andel, S. (2013). "Discredited" versus "discreditable": Understanding how shared and unique stigma mechanisms affect psychological and physical health disparities. *Basic and Applied Social Psychology, 35*, 75–87.

Cheng, L. (1989). Service delivery to Asian/Pacific LEP children: A cross-cultural framework. *Topics in Language Disorders, 9*, 1–14.

Chevigny, P. (1995). *Edge of the knife: Police violence in the Americas.* New York, NY: New Press.

Chou, C. C., Robb, J. L., Clay, M. C., & Chronister, J. A. (2013). Social support as a mediator between internalized stigma and coping behaviors of individuals with substance abuse issues. *Rehabilitation Research, Policy, and Education, 27*, 104–107.

Clair, J. A., Beatty, J. E., & MacLean, T. L. (2005). Out of sight but not out of mind: Managing invisible social identities in the workplace. *Academy of Management Review, 30*, 78–95.

Clay, J. A. (1992). Native American independent living. *Rural Special Education Quarterly, 11*, 41–50.

Cohen, J. (1988). *Statistical power for the behavioral sciences* (2nd ed.). Hillsdale, NJ: Erlbaum.

Coleman, C., Weidner, M., Barney, E., Scott, N., Baker, J., Stephens, L., & Donsbach, C. (2013, September). *Changing peer perceptions of children who stutter.* Poster presented at the Stuttering Attitudes Research Symposium, Morgantown, WV.

Collins, C. R., & Blood, G. W. (1990). Acknowledgment and severity of stuttering as factors influencing nonstutterers' perceptions of stutterers. *Journal of Speech and Hearing Disorders, 55*, 75–81.

Constantino, D. P., Eger, S., & Matthies, M. (2013). Clinical use of self-reports to measure CBT program outcomes. *Perspectives on Fluency and Fluency Disorders, 23*, 15–20.

Cook, C. R., Williams, K. R., Guerra, N. G., Kim, T. E., & Sadek, S. (2010). Predictors of bullying and victimization in childhood and adolescence: A meta-analytic investigation. *School Psychology Quarterly, 25*, 65–83.

Cook, S. (2013). Development of a questionnaire to determine psychosocial impact of stuttering for children and adolescents. *Logos, 21*, 79–105.

Cook, S., Donlan, C., & Howell, P. (2013). Stuttering severity, psychosocial impact, and lexical diversity as predictors of outcome for treatment of stuttering. *Journal of Fluency Disorders, 38*, 124–133.

Cook, S. & Howell, P. (2014). Bullying in children and teenagers who stutter and the relation to self-seteem, social acceptance, and anxiety. *SIG 4 Perspectives on Fluency and Fluency Disorders, 24*, 46–57.

Cooper, E. B. (1975). *Clinician attitudes toward stutterers: A study of bigotry?* Paper presented at the Annual Convention of the American Speech-Language-Hearing Association, Washington, DC.

Cooper, E. B. (1993). Second opinion. Chronic perseverative stuttering syndrome: A harmful or helpful construct. *American Journal of Speech-Language Pathology, 2*, 11–15.

Cooper, E. B., & Cooper, C. S. (1985). Clinician attitudes toward stuttering: A decade of change. *Journal of Fluency Disorders, 10*, 19–33.

Cooper, E. B., & Cooper, C. S. (1996). Clinician attitudes towards stuttering: Two decades of change. *Journal of Fluency Disorders, 21*, 119–135.

Cooper, E. B., & Rustin, L. (1985). Clinician attitudes toward stuttering in the United States and Great Britain: A cross-cultural study. *Journal of Fluency Disorders, 10*, 1–17.

Corcoran, J. A., & Stewart, M. (1998). Stories of stuttering: A qualitative analysis of interview narratives. *Journal of Fluency Disorders, 23*, 247–264.

Cornell, D., Gregory, A., Huang, F., & Fan, X. (2013). Perceived prevalence of teasing and bullying predicts high school dropout rates. *Journal of Educational Psychology, 105*, 138–149.

Corrigan, P. W. (2004). How stigma interferes with mental health care. *American Psychologist, 59*, 614–625.

Corrigan, P. W., & Kosyluk, K. A. (2013). Erasing the stigma: Where science meets advocacy. *Basic and Applied Social Psychology, 35*, 131–140.

Corrigan, P. W., Larson, J. E., & Kuwabara, S. A. (2010). Social psychology of the stigma of mental illness: Public and self-stigma models. In J. E. Maddux & J. P. Tangey (Eds.), *Social psychological foundations of clinical psychology* (pp. 51–68). New York, NY: Guilford Press.

Corrigan, P. W., Larson, J. E., & Rüsch, N. (2009). Self-stigma and the "why try" effect: Impact on life goals and evidence-based practices. *World Psychiatry, 8*, 75–81.

Corrigan, P. W., & Lundin, R. (2001). *Don't call me nuts! Coping with the stigma of mental illness.* Tinley Park, IL: Recovery Press.

Corrigan, P., & Matthews, A. (2003). Stigma and disclosure: Implications for coming out of the closet. *Journal of Mental Health, 12*, 235–248.

Corrigan, P. W., Morris, S. B., Michaels, P. J., Rafacz, J. D., Rüsch, N. (2012). Challenging the public stigma of mental illness: A meta-analysis of outcome studies. *Psychiatric Services, 63*, 963–973.

Corrigan, P. W., & O'Shaughnessy, J. R. (2007). Changing mental illness stigma as it exists in the real world. *Australian Psychologist, 42*, 90–97.

Corrigan, P. W., Rafacz, J., & Rüsch, N. (2011). Examining a progressive model of self-stigma and its impact on people with serious mental illness. *Psychiatry Research, 189*, 339–343.

Corrigan, P. W., & Shapiro, J. R. (2010). Measuring the impact of programs that challenge the public stigma of mental illness. *Clinical Psychology Review, 30*, 907–922.

Corrigan, P. W., Sokol, K. A., & Rüsch, N. (2013). The impact of self-stigma and mutual help programs on the quality of life of people with serious mental illnesses. *Community Mental Health Journal, 49*, 1–6.

Corrigan, P. W., & Watson, A. C. (2002). The paradox of self-stigma and mental illness. *Clinical Psychology: Science and Practice, 9*, 35–53.

Corrigan, P. W., Watson, A. C., & Barr, L. (2006). The self-stigma of mental illness: Implications for self-esteem and self-efficacy. *Journal of Social and Clinical Psychology, 25*, 875–884.

Costa, D., & Kroll, R. (2000). Stuttering: an update for physicians. *Canadian Medical Association Journal, 162*, 1849–1855.

Craig, A. (2010). The association between quality of life and stuttering. *Journal of Fluency Disorders, 35*, 159–160.

Craig, A., Blumgart, E., & Tran, Y. (2009). The impact of stuttering on the quality of life in adults who stutter. *Journal of Fluency Disorders, 34*, 61–71.

Craig, A., Blumgart, E., & Tran, Y. (2011). Resilience and stuttering: Factors that protect people from the adversity of chronic stuttering. *Journal of Speech, Language, and Hearing Research, 54*, 1485–1496.

Craig, A. R., & Calver, P. (1991). Following up on treated stutterers: Studies of perceptions of fluency and job status. *Journal of Speech and Hearing Research, 34*, 279–284.

Craig, A., Hancock, K., Tran, Y., Craig, M., & Peters, K. (2003). Anxiety levels in people who stutter: A randomized people study. *Journal of Speech, Language, and Hearing Research, 46*, 1197–1206.

Craig, A., & Tran, Y. (2006). Chronic and social anxiety in people who stutter. *Advances in Psychiatric Treatment, 12*, 63–68.

Craig, A., Tran, Y., & Craig, M. (2003). Stereotypes toward stuttering for those who have never had direct contact with people who stutter: A randomized and stratified study. *Perceptual and Motor Skills, 97*, 235–245.

Craig, W. M. (1998). The relationship among bullying, victimization, depression, anxiety, and aggression in elementary school children. *Personality and Individual Differences, 24*, 123–130.

Craig, W. M., & Pepler, D. J. (1998). Observations of bullying and victimization in the school yard. *Canadian Journal of School Psychology, 13*, 41–60.

Craig, W. M., & Pepler, D. J. (2007). Understanding bullying: From research to practice. *Canadian Psychology, 48*, 86–93.

Craig, W., & Pepler, D. (2008). Understanding and addressing bullying: An international perspective. In D. Pepler & W. Craig (Eds.), *Understanding and addressing bullying: An international perspective* (pp. xix–xxvi). Bloomington, IN: AuthorHouse.

Craig, W., Pepler, D., & Blais, J. (2007). Responding to bullying: What works? *School Psychology International, 28*, 465–477.

Cream, A., Packman, A., & Llewellyn, G. (2004). The playground rocker: A metaphor for communication after treatment for adults who stutter. *Advances in Speech-Language Pathology, 6*, 182–187.

Cresswell, J. W. (1998). *Qualitative inquiry and research design: Choosing among five traditions.* Thousand Oaks, CA: Sage.

Crichton-Smith, I. (2002). Communicating in the real world: Accounts from people who stammer. *Journal of Fluency Disorders, 27*, 333–352.

Crichton-Smith, I., Wright, J., & Stackhouse, J. (2003). Attitudes of speech and language therapists toward stammering: 1985 and 2000. *International Journal of Language and Communication Disorders, 38*, 213–234.

Crocker, J., & Major, B. (1989). Social stigma and self-esteem: The self-protective properties of stigma. *Psychological Review, 96*, 608–630.

Crocker, J., Major, B., & Steele, C. (1998). Social stigma. In D. T. Gilbert, S. T. Fiske, & G. Lindzey (Eds.), *The handbook of social psychology* (4th ed.) (pp. 504–553). Oxford, UK: Oxford University Press.

Crowe, T. A., & Cooper, E. B. (1977). Parental attitudes toward and knowledge of stuttering. *Journal of Communication Disorders, 10*, 343–357.

Crowe, T. A., & Walton, J. H. (1981). Teacher attitudes toward stuttering. *Journal of Fluency Disorders, 6*, 163–174.

Cuddy, A. J. C., Fiske, S. T., & Glick, P. (2008). Warmth and competence as universal dimensions of social perception: The stereotype content model and the BIAS map. *Advances in Experimental Social Psychology, 40*, 61–150.

Cummins, R. A. (2010). Fluency disorders and life quality: Subjective wellbeing vs. health-related quality of life. *Journal of Fluency Disorders, 35*, 161–172.

Czopp, A. M. (2008). When is a compliment not a compliment? Evaluating expressions of positive stereotypes. *Journal of Experimental Social Psychology, 44,* 413–420.

Daniels, D. E., & Gabel, R. M. (2004). The impact of stuttering on identity construction. *Topics in Language Disorders, 24,* 200–215.

Daniels, D. E., Gabel, R. M., & Hughes, S. (2012). Recounting the K-12 school experiences of adults who stutter: A qualitative analysis. *Journal of Fluency Disorders, 37,* 71–82.

Daniels, D. E., Hagstrom, F., & Gabel, R. M. (2006). A qualitative study of how African American men who stutter attribute meaning to identity and life choices. *Journal of Fluency Disorders, 31,* 200–215.

Daniels, D. E., & Hughes, S. (2011, November). *Parents of children who stutter: A mixed-methods investigation.* Poster presented at the Annual Convention of the American Speech-Language-Hearing Association, San Diego, CA.

Davis, L. J. (2010). *The disability studies reader* (3rd ed.). New York, NY: Routledge.

Davis, S., Howell, P., & Cooke, F. (2002). Sociodynamic relationships between children who stutter and their nonstuttering classmates. *Journal of Child Psychology and Psychiatry, 43,* 939–947.

de Britto Pereira, M. M., Rossi, J. P., & Van Borsel, J. (2008). Public awareness and knowledge of stuttering in Rio de Janeiro. *Journal of Fluency Disorders, 33,* 24–31.

Decaro, J., Evans, L., & Dowaliby, F. (1982). Advising deaf youth to train for various occupations: Attitudes of significant others. *British Journal of Educational Psychology, 52,* 220–227.

Delaney, C. (2001). Modification of the negative stutterer stereotype. In G. Bosshardt, H. J. S. Yaruss, & H. F. Peters (Eds.), *Proceedings of World Congress of Fluency Disorders: Theory, Research, Treatment & Self-help* (pp. 614–618). Nijmegen, The Netherlands: Nijmegen University Press.

Deloria, V., Jr. (1988). *Custer died for your sins: An Indian manifesto.* Norman: University of Oklahoma Press.

Demissie, M., Getahun, H., & Lindtjørn, B. (2003). Community tuberculosis care through "TB clubs" in rural North Ethiopia. *Social Science & Medicine, 56,* 2009–2018.

De Nil, L. F., & Brutten, G. J. (1991). Speech-associated attitudes of stuttering and nonstuttering children. *Journal of Speech and Hearing Research, 34,* 60–66.

de Veer, S., Brouwers, A., Evers, W., & Tomic, W. (2009). A pilot study of the psychological impact of the Mindfulness-Based Stress Reduction Program on persons who stutter. *European Psychotherapy, 9,* 39–56.

Dewey, J. (1933). *How we think.* Boston: D. C. Heath.

DiLollo, A., & Manning, W. H. (2007). Counseling children who stutter and their parents. In E. G. Conture & R. F. Curlee (Eds.), *Stuttering and related disorders of fluency* (3rd ed.) (pp. 115–130). New York, NY: Thieme.

Doody, I., Kalinowski, J., Armson, J., & Stuart, A. (1993). Stereotypes of stutterers and nonstutterers in three rural communities in Newfoundland. *Journal of Fluency Disorders, 18,* 363–373.

Dooley, J. J., Pyzalski, J., & Cross, D. (2009). Cyberbullying versus face-to-face bullying: A theoretical and conceptual review. *Journal of Psychology, 217,* 182–188.

Dorsey, M., & Guenther, R. K. (2000). Attitudes of professors and students toward college students who stutter. *Journal of Fluency Disorders, 25,* 77–83.

Douglass, E., & Quarrington, B. (1952). The differentiation of interiorized and exteriorized secondary stuttering. *Journal of Speech and Hearing Disorders, 17,* 377–385.

Douglass, J. (2011). *An investigation of the transition process from covert stuttering to overt stuttering: An interpretive phenomenological analysis of individuals who stutter.* Unpublished dissertation, University of Louisiana at Lafayette, Lafayette, LA.

Dovidio, J. F., Gluszek, A., John, M. S., Ditlmann, R., & Lagunes, P. (2010). Understanding bias toward Latinos: Discrimination, dimensions of difference, and experience of exclusion. *Journal of Social Issues, 66,* 59–78.

Earnshaw, V. A., & Quinn, D. M. (2012). The impact of stigma in healthcare on people living with chronic illnesses. *Journal of Health Psychology, 17,* 157–168.

Eisenhart, M. A., Shrum, J. L., Harding, J. R., & Cuthbert, A. M. (1988). Teacher beliefs: Definitions, findings, and directions. *Educational Policy, 2,* 51–70.

Elafros, M. A., Mulenga, J., Mbewe, E., Haworth, A., Chomba, E., Atadzhanov, M., & Birbeck, G. L. (2013). Peer support groups as an intervention to decrease epilepsy-associated stigma. *Epilepsy & Behavior, 27,* 188–192.

Emerick, L. L. (1960). Extensional definition and attitude toward stuttering. *Journal of Speech and Hearing Research, 3,* 181–186.

Eribon, D. (2004). *Insult and the making of the gay self* (M. Lucey, Trans.). Durham, NC: Duke University Press.

Erickson, S., & Block, S. (2013). The social and communication impact of stuttering on adolescents and their families. *Journal of Fluency Disorders, 38,* 311–324.

Evans, D., Healey, E. C., Kawai, N., & Rowland, S. (2008). Middle school students' perceptions of a peer who stutters. *Journal of Fluency Disorders, 33,* 203–219.

Ezrati-Vinacour, R., & Levin, I. (2004). The relationship between anxiety and stuttering: A multidimensional approach. *Journal of Fluency Disorders, 29,* 135–148.

Ezrati-Vinacour, R., Platzky, R., & Yairi, E. (2001). The young child's awareness of stuttering-like disfluency. *Journal of Speech, Language, and Hearing Research, 44,* 368–380.

Fagerland, M. W. (2012). T-tests, nonparametric tests, and large studies—A paradox of statistical practice? *BMC Medical Research Methodology, 12,* 78–84.

Field, A. (2009). *Discovering Statistics using SPSS* (3rd ed.). London: Sage Publications.

Field, A. & Hole, G. (2003). *How to design and report experiments.* Sage Publications: London, England.

Finn, P., & Felsenfeld, S. (2004). Recovery from stuttering: The contributions of the qualitative research approach. *Advances in Speech-Language Pathology, 6,* 159–166.

Fish, J. (2000). What anthropology can do for psychology? Facing physics envy, ethnocentrism, and a belief in "race." *American Anthropologist, 102,* 552–563.

Fletcher, C. (1990). *What cops know: Cops talk about what they do, how they do it, and what it does to them.* New York, NY: Random House.

Flynn, T. W., & St. Louis, K. O. (2011). Changing adolescent attitudes toward stuttering. *Journal of Fluency Disorders, 36,* 110–121.

Forero, R., McLellan, L., Rissel, C., & Bauman, A. (1999). Bullying behaviour and psychosocial health among school students in New South Wales, Australia: Cross sectional survey. *British Medical Journal, 319*, 344–348.

Fowlie, G. M., & Cooper, E. B. (1978). Traits attributed to stuttering and nonstuttering children by their mothers. *Journal of Fluency Disorders, 3*, 233–246.

Frable, D. E. S., Hoey, S., & Platt, L. (1998). Concealable stigmas and positive self-perceptions: Feeling better around similar others. *Journal of Personality and Social Psychology, 74*, 909–922.

Gabel, R. M. (2006). Effects of stuttering severity and therapy involvement on attitudes towards people who stutter. *Journal of Fluency Disorders, 31*, 216–227.

Gabel, R., Althouse, M. T., & Tellis, G. (2002, November). *Effects of familiarity on occupational stereotyping of people who stutter.* Paper presented at the Annual Convention of the American Speech-Language-Hearing Association, Atlanta, GA.

Gabel, R. M., Blood, G. W., Tellis, G. M., & Althouse, M. T. (2004). Measuring role entrapment of people who stutter. *Journal of Fluency Disorders, 29*, 27–49.

Gabel, R. M., Brackenbury, T., & Irani, F. (2010). Access to information about stuttering and societal knowledge of stuttering. *Perspectives on Fluency and Fluency Disorders, 20*, 51–57.

Gabel, R. M., Hughes, S., & Daniels, D. (2008). Effects of stuttering severity and therapy involvement on role entrapment of people who stutter. *Journal of Communication Disorders, 41*, 146–158.

Gabel, R. M., Hughes, S., Forney, A. (2011, November). *Do gender and familiarity impact attitudes towards people who stutter?* Paper presented at the Annual Convention of the American Speech-Language-Hearing Association, San Diego, CA.

Gabel, R. M., Schlagheck, A., Eyestone, D., & Emch, J. (2006). *Fluency: A quantitative study of attitudes towards people who stutter.* Paper presented at the Annual Convention of the American Speech-Language-Hearing Association, Miami, FL.

Gallup Politics. (2014, September). Retrieved from http://www.gallup.com/poll/politics.aspx?ref=b

Garrett, J. E., & Garrett, M. T. (1994). The path of good medicine: Understanding and counseling Native Americans. *Journal of Multicultural Counseling and Development, 22*, 134–144.

Garrett, J. E., & Garrett, M. T. (1996). *Medicine of the Cherokee: The way of right relationship.* Santa Fe, NM: Bear & Company.

Garrett, M. T. (1996). Reflection by the riverside: The traditional education of Native American children. *Journal of Humanistic Education and Development, 35*, 12–28.

Garrett, M. T., & Myers, J. E. (1996). The rule of opposites: A paradigm for counseling Native Americans. Journal of Multicultural Counseling and Development, 24, 89–104.

Garrett, M. T., & Pichette, E. F. (2000). Red as an apple: Native American acculturation and counseling with or without reservation. *Journal of Counseling and Development, 78*, 3–13.

Gawronski, B., & Bodenhausen, G. V. (2006). Associative and propositional processes in evaluation: An integrative review of implicit and explicit attitude change. *Psychological Bulletin, 132*, 692–731.

Giddens, A. (2006). *Sociology* (5th ed.). Malden, MA: Polity Press.

Ginsberg, A. P. (2000). Shame, self-consciousness, and locus of control in people who stutter. *The Journal of Genetic Psychology, 161*, 389–399.

Ginsberg, A. P., & Wexler, K. B. (2000). Understanding stuttering and counseling clients who stutter. *Journal of Mental Health Counseling, 22*, 228–239.

Glew, G. M., Fan, M., Katon, W., Rivara, F. P., & Kernic, M. A. (2005). Bullying, psychosocial adjustment, and academic performance in elementary school. *Archives of Pediatric Adolescent Medicine, 159*, 1026–1031.

Goffman, E. (1959). *The presentation of self in everyday life.* Garden City, NY: Doubleday.

Goffman, E. (1963). *Stigma: Notes on management of a spoiled identity.* Englewood Cliff, NJ: Prentice-Hall.

Goldberg, A. E., Kinkler, L. A., & Hines, D. A. (2011). Perception and internalization of adoption stigma among gay, lesbian, and heterosexual adoptive parents. *Journal of GLBT Family Studies, 7*, 132–154.

Gottwald, S., Kent, L., St. Louis, K. O., & Hartley, J. (2014, November). *Altering attitudes towards stuttering through the use of oral histories.* Poster presented at the Annual Convention of the American Speech-Language-Hearing Association. Orlando, FL.

Gottwald, S. L., Warner, R., Hartley, J., Fraas, M., Hawver, K., & St. Louis, K. O. (2011, November). *Altering attitudes towards stuttering through the use of oral histories.* Poster presented at the Annual Convention of the American Speech-Language-Hearing Association, San Diego, CA.

Government of Sudan, Ministry of Social Development. (2013). *Sudanese Ministry of Social Development Annual Report.* Khartoum, Sudan: Author.

Green, G. (2009). *The end of stigma? Changes in the social experience of long-term illness.* London: Routledge.

Greene, K., & Banerjee, S. C. (2006). Disease-related stigma: Comparing predictors of AIDS and cancer stigma. *Journal of Homosexuality, 50*, 185–209.

Greenwald, A. G., McGhee, D. B., & Schwartz, J. K. L. (1998). Measuring individual differences in implicit cognition: The Implicit Association Test. *Journal of Personality and Social Psychology, 74*, 1464–1480.

Griffith, K. H., & Hebl, M. R. (2002). The disclosure dilemma for gay men and lesbians: "Coming out" at work. *Journal of Applied Psychology, 87*, 1191–1199.

Grytten, N., & Måseide, P. (2005). What is expressed is not always what is felt: Coping with stigma and the embodiment of perceived illegitimacy of multiple sclerosis. *Chronic Illness, 1*, 231–243.

Guerin, S., & Hennessy, E. (2002). Pupils' definitions of bullying. *European Journal of Psychology of Education, 17*, 249–261.

Guerra, N. G., Williams, K. R., & Sadek, S. (2011). Understanding bullying and victimization during childhood and adolescence: A mixed methods study. *Child Development, 82*, 295–310.

Guitar, B. (2005). *Stuttering: An integrated approach to its nature and treatment* (3rd ed.). Baltimore, MD: Williams & Wilkins.

Guitar, B. (2013). *Stuttering: An integrated approach to its nature and treatment* (4th ed.). Baltimore, MD: Williams & Wilkins.

Guitar, B., & Bass, C. (1978). Stuttering therapy: The relation between attitude change and long term outcome. *Journal of Speech and Hearing Disorders, 43*, 392–400.

Guntupalli, V. K., Everhart, D. E., Kalinowski, J., Nanjundeswaran, C., & Saltuklaroglu, T. (2007). Emotional and physiological responses of fluent listeners while watching the speech of adults who stutter. *International Journal of Language and Communication Disorders, 42*, 113–119.

Guntupalli, V. K., Kalinowski, J., Nanjundeswaran, C., Saltuklaroglu, T., & Everhart, D. E. (2006). Psychophysiological responses of adults who do not stutter while listening to stuttering. *International Journal of Psychophysiology, 62*, 1–8.

Guntupalli, V. K., Nanjundeswaran, C., Dayalu, V., & Kalinowski, J. (2012). Autonomic and emotional responses of graduate student clinicians in speech-language pathology to stuttered speech. *International Journal of Language & Communication Disorders, 47*, 603–608.

Hahn, H. (1997). Advertising the acceptably employable image: Disability and capitalism. In L. J. Davis (Ed.), *The disability studies reader* (pp. 172–186). New York, NY: Routledge.

Ham, R. E. (1990). What is stuttering: Variations and stereotypes. *Journal of Fluency Disorders, 15*, 259–273.

Hartford, E., & Leahy, M. M. (2007). The perceptions of primary school children of a person who stutters. In J. Au-Yeung & M. M. Leahy (Eds.), *Research, treatment, and self-help in fluency disorders: New Horizons. Proceedings of the Fifth World Congress on Fluency Disorders* (pp. 223–229). Dublin: International Fluency Association.

Hauser, R. M., & Warren, J. R. (1997). Socioeconomic indexes for occupations: A review, update, and critique. *Sociological Methodology, 27*, 177–298.

Healey, E. C., Gabel, R. M., Daniels, D. E., & Kawai, N. (2007). The effects of self-disclosure and non self-disclosure of stuttering on listeners' perceptions of a person who stutters. *Journal of Fluency Disorders, 32*, 51–69.

Hearne, A., Packman, A., Onslow, M., & Quine, S. (2008). Stuttering and its treatment in adolescence: The perceptions of people who stutter. *Journal of Fluency Disorders, 33*, 81–98.

Heite, L. B. (2000, October). *Icelandic teachers' attitudes toward stuttering and classroom decision making.* Paper presented at the International Stuttering Awareness Day (ISAD) online conference. Retrieved from www.mnsu.edu/comdis/ISAD3/papers/heite/heite3.html

Herek, G. M. (2007). Confronting sexual stigma and prejudice: Theory and practice. *Journal of Social Issues, 63*, 905–925.

Herring, R. D. (1994). The clown or contrary figure as a counseling intervention strategy with Native American Indian clients. *Journal of Multicultural Counseling and Development, 22*, 153–164.

Herzig, B. A., Roysircar, G., Kosyluk, K. A., & Corrigan, P. W. (2013). American Muslim college students: The impact of religiousness and stigma on active coping. *Journal of Muslim Mental Health, 7*, 33–42.

Hinson, J. A., & Swanson, J. L. (1993). Willingness to seek help as a function of self-disclosure and problem severity. *Journal of Counseling and Development, 71*, 465–470.

Hodges, E. V. E., Boivin, M., Vitaro, F., & Bukowski, W. M. (1999). The power of friendship:

Protection against an escalating cycle of peer victimization. *Developmental Psychology, 35,* 94–101.

Hodgkinson, H. L. (1990). *The demographics of American Indians: One percent of the people; fifty percent of the diversity.* Washington, DC: Institute of Educational Leadership.

Holcombe, K., & Eisert, S. (2012). *Understanding the impediment: Investigating the nature of people's attitudes toward stutterers.* Unpublished undergraduate capstone project, Pacific Lutheran University, Tacoma WA.

Horsley, I. A., & FitzGibbon, C. T. (1987). Stuttering children: Investigation of a stereotype. *British Journal of Disorders of Communication, 22,* 19–35.

Howell, P. (2010). Behavioral effects arising from the neural substrates for atypical planning and execution of word production in stuttering. *Experimental Neurology, 225,* 55–59.

Hugh-Jones, S., & Smith, P. K. (1999). Self-reports of short- and long-term effects of bullying on children who stammer. *British Journal of Educational Psychology, 69,* 141–158.

Hughes, S. (2008). *Exploring attitudes toward people who stutter: A mixed model approach.* Unpublished dissertation, Bowling Green State University, Bowling Green, OH.

Hughes, S., Gabel, R., Irani, F., & Schlagheck, A. (2010a). University students' explanations for their descriptions of people who stutter: An exploratory mixed model study. *Journal of Fluency Disorders, 35,* 280–298.

Hughes, S., Gabel, R., Irani, F., & Schlagheck, A. (2010b). University students' perceptions of the life effects of stuttering. *Journal of Communication Disorders, 43,* 45–60.

Hughes, C., Gabel, R., & Palasik, S. (2011). Talking about stuttering with a known person who stutters: Impact on perceptions towards stuttering. *Perspectives on Fluency and Fluency Disorders, 21,* 50–58.

Hulit, L. M., & Wirtz, L. (1994). The association of attitudes toward stuttering with selected variables. *Journal of Fluency Disorders, 19,* 247–267.

Hurst, M. A., & Cooper, E. B. (1983a). Employer attitudes toward stuttering. *Journal of Fluency Disorders, 8,* 1–12.

Hurst, M. A., & Cooper, E. B. (1983b). Vocational rehabilitation counselors' attitudes toward stuttering. *Journal of Fluency Disorders, 8,* 13–27.

Inbau, F. E., Reid, J. E., Buckley, J. B., & Jayne, B. P. (2001). *Criminal interrogation and confessions.* Baltimore, MD: Williams & Wilkins.

Ingham, R. J. (1979). Comment on "Stuttering therapy: The relation between attitude change and long-term outcome." *Journal of Speech and Hearing Disorders, 44,* 397–400.

Ingham, R. J. (2012). Comments on recent developments in stuttering treatment maintenance research using the Camperdown Program. *Journal of Speech, Language, and Hearing Research, 55,* 306–309.

International Stuttering Association. (2014, September). *Constitution.* Retrieved from http://www.isastutter.org/who-we-are/constitution

Ip, M. L., St. Louis, K. O., Myers, F. L., & An Xue, S. (2012). Stuttering attitudes in Hong Kong and Mainland China. *International Journal of Speech-Language Pathology, 14,* 543–556.

Iran Human Rights Documentation Center (IHRD). (2014, September). *Gender inequality and discrimination: The case of Iranian women.* Retrieved from http://www.iranhrdc. org/english/publications/legal-commentary/1000000261-gender-inequality-and-discrimination-the-case-of-iranian-women.html#ftn11

Irani, F., & Gabel, R. M. (2008). Schoolteachers' attitudes towards people who stutter: Results of a mail survey. *Canadian Journal of Speech-Language Pathology and Audiology, 32,* 129–134.

Irani, F., Gabel, R. M., Daniels, D., & Hughes, S. (2012). The long-term effectiveness of intensive stuttering therapy: A mixed methods study. *Journal of Fluency Disorders, 37,* 164–178.

Irani, F., Gabel, R., Hughes, S., Swartz, E. R., & Palasik, S. T. (2009). Role entrapment of people who stutter reported by K-12 teachers. *Contemporary Issues in Communication Science and Disorders, 36,* 45–54.

Iverach, L., Jones, M., O'Brian, S., Block, S., Lincoln, M., Harrison, E., Hewat, S., Menzies, R. G., Packman, A., & Onslow, M. (2009). Screening for personality disorders among adults seeking speech treatment for stuttering. *Journal of Fluency Disorders, 34,* 173–186.

Iverach, L., O'Brian, S., Jones, M., Block, S., Lincoln, M., Harrison, E., Hewat, S., Menzies, R. G., Packman, A., & Onslow, M. (2009). Prevalence of anxiety disorders among adults seeking speech therapy for stuttering. *Journal of Anxiety Disorders, 23,* 928–934.

Iverach, L., O'Brian, S., Jones, M., Block, S., Lincoln, M., Harrison, E., Hewat, S., Menzies, R. G., Packman, A., Onslow, M. (2010). The five factor model of personality applied to adults who stutter. *Journal of Communication Disorders, 43,* 120–132.

Iverach, L., & Rapee, R. M. (2014). Social anxiety disorder and stuttering: Current status and future directions. *Journal of Fluency Disorders, 40,* 69–82.

Jacoby, A. (1994). Felt versus enacted stigma: A concept revisited. *Social Science & Medicine, 38,* 269–274.

Joe, J. R., & Miller, D. (1987). *American Indian cultural perspectives on disability.* Tucson, AZ: Native American Research and Training Center.

Johns, M., Chen, S.-L., & Hall, G. (Eds.). (2003). *Online social research: Methods, issues, and ethics.* New York, NY: Peter Lang.

Johnson, G. F. (1987). A clinical study of Porky Pig cartoons. *Journal of Fluency Disorders, 12,* 235–238.

Johnson, J. K. (2008). The visualization of the twisted tongue: Portrayals of stuttering in film, television, and comic books. *The Journal of Popular Culture, 41,* 245–261.

Johnson, R. R. (2006). Confounding influences on police detection of suspiciousness. *Journal of Criminal Justice, 34,* 435–442.

Johnson, W. (1961). *Stuttering and what you can do about it.* Danville, IL: Interstate.

Johnson, W. (1934). Stutterers' attitudes toward stuttering. *Journal of Abnormal and Social Psychology, 29,* 32–44.

Johnson, W. (1944). The Indians have no word for it. *Quarterly Journal of Speech, 30,* 330-337.

Jones, E. E., Farina, A., Hastorf, A. H., Markus, H., Miller, D., & Scott, R. A. (1984). *Social stigma: The psychology of marked relationships.* New York, NY: Freeman.

Juvoven, J., Graham, S., & Schuster, M. (2003). Bullying among young adolescents: The strong, the weak, and the troubled. *Pediatrics, 112,* 1231–1237.

Kahn, J. H., & Hessling, R. M. (2001). Measuring the tendency to conceal versus disclose psychological distress. *Journal of Social & Clinical Psychology, 20,* 41–65.

Kalinowski, J., Armson, J., Stuart, A., & Lerman, J. W. (1993). Speech clinicians' and the general public's perceptions of self and stutterers. *Journal of Speech-Language Pathology and Audiology, 17*, 79–85.

Kalinowski, J. S., Lerman, J. W., & Watt, J. (1987). A preliminary examination of the perceptions of self and others in stutterers and nonstutterers. *Journal of Fluency Disorders, 12*, 317–331.

Kalinowski, J., Stuart, A., & Armson, J. (1996). Perceptions of stutterers and nonstutterers during speaking and nonspeaking situations. *American Journal of Speech-Language Pathology, 5*, 61–67.

Kamhi, A. (2003). Two paradoxes in stuttering treatment. *Journal of Fluency Disorders, 13*, 11–25.

Kanaka, G., St. Louis, K. O., Usmani, T., & Rajashekhar, B. (2012). *Public opinion about stuttering using POSHA–S among H-SES and M-SES Hindi speakers.* Unpublished research, Manipal University, Manipal, India.

Katz, P. A. (2003). Racists or tolerant multiculturalists? How do they begin? *American Psychologist, 58*, 897–909.

Keeffe, J. (2005). Psychosocial impact of vision impairment. *International Congress Series, 1282*, 167–173.

Keith, A., & Kuhn, T. (1996). *Effects of altered auditory feedback on stuttering frequency at normal and fast speaking rates* [videotape]. Department of Communication Sciences and Disorders, East Carolina University, Greenville, NC.

Kellison, I., Bussing, R., Bell, L., & Garvan, C. (2010). Assessment of stigma associated with attention-deficit hyperactivity disorder: Psychometric evaluation of the ADHD Stigma Questionnaire. *Psychiatry Research, 178*, 363–369.

Kelly, S. (2010). Stigma and silence: Oral histories of tuberculosis. *Oral History, 39*, 79–90.

Keltner, B. R., Crowell, N. A., & Taylor, W. (2005). Attitudes about disabilities in a southeastern American Indian tribe. *American Indian Culture and Research Journal, 29*, 57–74.

Kestenbaum, J., & Khnonov, M. (2011). *Effects of* The King's Speech *on adults' stuttering attitudes in New York City.* Unpublished undergraduate research. Brooklyn College, Brooklyn, NY.

Klassen, T. R. (2001). Perceptions of people who stutter: Re-assessing the negative stereotype. *Perceptual and Motor Skills, 92*, 551–559.

Klassen, T. R. (2002). Social distance and the negative stereotype of people who stutter. *Journal of Speech-Language Pathology and Audiology, 26*, 97–99.

Klein, E. R., & Amster, B. J. (2010). Does a graduate course in fluency make a difference? *Perspectives on Fluency and Fluency Disorders, 20*, 10–14.

Klein, J. F., & Hood, S. B. (2004). The impact of stuttering on employment opportunities and job performance. *Journal of Fluency Disorders, 29*, 255–273.

Klompas, M., & Ross, E. (2004). Life experiences of people who stutter, and the perceived impact of stuttering on quality of life: Personal accounts of South African individuals. *Journal of Fluency Disorders, 29*, 275–305.

Knack, J. M., Jensen-Campbell, L. A., & Baum, A. (2011). Worse than sticks and stones? Bullying is associated with altered HPA axis functioning and poorer health. *Brain and Cognition, 77*, 183–190.

Knudsen, P. F., Kathard, H., St. Louis, K. O., & Shrestha, S. (2004, November). *Selected attitudes toward stuttering: Denmark, South Africa, and Nepal (English)*. Poster presented at the Annual Convention of the American Speech-Language-Hearing Association, Philadelphia, PA.

Kochenderfer-Ladd, B. J., & Wardrop, J. L. (2001). Chronicity and instability of children's peer victimization experiences as predictors of loneliness and social satisfaction trajectories. *Child Development, 72*, 134–151.

Koedoot, C., Bouwmans, C., Franken, M. C., & Stolk, E. (2011). Quality of life in adults who stutter. *Journal of Communication Disorders, 44*, 429–443.

Kramer, B. (1996). Dementia and American Indian populations. In G. Yao & D. Gallagher-Thompson (Eds.), *Ethnicity and the dementias* (pp. 175–203). Washington DC: Taylor & Francis.

Krannich, R. L., & Krannich, C. R. (1993). *The best jobs for the 1990s and into the 21st century*. Manassas Park, VA: Impact Publishing.

Krieger, N. (2000). Discrimination and health. In L. Berkman & I. Kawachi (Eds.), *Social epidemiology* (pp. 36–75). Oxford, UK: Oxford University Press.

Kreiger, N. (2003). Genders, sexes, and health: What are the connections—and why does it matter? *International Journal of Epidemiology, 32*, 652–657.

Kristensen, S. M., & Smith, P. K. (2003). The use of coping strategies by Danish children classed as bullies, victims, bully/victims, and not involved, in response to different (hypothetical) types of bullying. *Scandinavian Journal of Psychology, 44*, 479–488.

Kroeger, B. (2003). *Passing: When people can't be who they are*. New York, NY: PublicAffairs.

LaFromboise, T. D. (1998). American Indian mental health policy. *American Psychologist, 43*, 388–397.

Lakhani, M., & Taylor, R. (2003). Beliefs about the cues to deception in high- and low-stake situations. *Psychology, Crime, and Law, 9*, 357–369.

Lamb, R., Weinberger, L. E., & DeCuir, W. J. (2002). The police and mental health. *Psychiatric Services, 53*, 1266–1271.

Landau, A. R. (2011). *Experiences and expectations of children who stutter and their significant others*. Unpublished master's dissertation, University College London, London, UK.

Langevin, M. (2000). *Teasing and bullying: Unacceptable behaviour (TAB)*. Edmonton, AB: Institute for Stuttering Treatment & Research.

Langevin, M. (2009). The Peer Attitudes Toward Children who Stutter Scale: Reliability, known groups validity, and negativity of elementary school-age children's attitudes. *Journal of Fluency Disorders, 34*, 72–86.

Langevin, M., Bortnick, K., Hammer, T., & Wiebe, E. (1998). Teasing/bullying experienced by children who stutter: Toward development of a questionnaire. *Contemporary Issues in Communication Science and Disorders, 25*, 12–24.

Langevin, M., & Gervais, C. (2013, October). *Teasing and bullying experienced by children who stutter: An update and comparison to reported incidence of children with SLI, ADHD, and autism*. Poster presented at the Annual Conference of the Alberta College of Speech-Language Pathologists and Audiologists, Edmonton, AB.

Langevin, M., & Hagler, P. (2004). Development of a scale to measure peer attitudes toward children who stutter. In A. K. Bothe (Ed.), *Evidence-based treatment of stuttering:*

Empirical bases and clinical applications (pp. 139–171). Mahwah, NJ: Lawrence Erlbaum Associates.

Langevin, M., Kleitman, S., Packman, A., & Onslow, M. (2009). The Peer Attitudes Toward Children who Stutter (PATCS) Scale: An evaluation of validity, reliability, and the negativity of attitudes. *International Journal of Language & Communication Disorders, 44,* 352–368.

Langevin, M., Kully, D. A., & Ross-Harold, B. (2007). The comprehensive stuttering program for school-age children with strategies for managing teasing and bullying. In E. G. Conture & R. F. Curlee (Eds.), *Stuttering and related disorders of fluency* (3rd ed.) (pp. 131–149). New York, NY: Thieme.

Langevin, M., Packman, A., & Onslow, M. (2009). Peer responses to stuttering in the preschool setting. *American Journal of Speech-Language Pathology, 18,* 264–276.

Langevin, M., Packman, A., & Onslow, M. (2010). Parent perceptions of the impact of stuttering on their preschoolers and themselves. *Journal of Communication Disorders, 43,* 407–423.

Langevin, M., & Prasad, N. G. N. (2012). A stuttering education and bullying awareness and prevention resource: A feasibility study. *Language, Speech, & Hearing Services in Schools, 43,* 344–358.

Lass, N. J., Ruscello, D. M., Pannbacker, M. D., Schmitt, J. F., & Everly-Myers, D. S. (1989). Speech-language pathologists' perceptions of child and adult female and male stutterers. *Journal of Fluency Disorders, 14,* 127–134.

Lass, N. J., Ruscello, D. M., Pannbacker, M., Schmitt, J. F., Kiser, A. M., Mussa, A. M., & Lockhart, P. (1994). School administrators' perceptions of people who stutter. *Language, Speech, and Hearing Services in Schools, 25,* 90–93.

Lass, N. J., Ruscello, D. M., Schmitt, J. F., Pannbacker, M. D., Orlando, M. B., Dean, K. A., Ruziska, J. C., & Bradshaw, K. H. (1992). Teachers' perceptions of stutterers. *Language, Speech, and Hearing Services in Schools, 23,* 78–81.

Lawrence, M., & Barclay, D. M. (1998). Stuttering: A brief review. *American Family Physician, 57,* 2175–2178.

Leahy, M. M. (1994). Attempting to ameliorate student therapists' negative stereotype of the stutterer. *International Journal of Language & Communication Disorders, 29,* 39–49.

LeBel, T. P. (2008). Perceptions of and responses to stigma. *Sociology Compass, 2,* 409–432.

Lee, K., & Manning, W. H. (2010). Listener responses according to stuttering self-acknowledgment and modification. *Journal of Fluency Disorders, 35,* 110–122.

Lees, R., Stark, C., Baird, J., & Birse, S. (2000). Primary care professionals' knowledge and attitudes on speech disfluency in pre-school children. *Child Language, Teaching, and Therapy, 20,* 241–254.

Lees, R. M., & Stewart, T. (2001). Students' attitudes and beliefs about stuttering. In H. G. Bosshardt, J. S. Yaruss, & H. Peters (Eds.), *Proceedings of the Third World Congress of Fluency Disorders* (pp. 610–613). Nijmegen, The Netherlands: University of Nijmegen Press.

Lemert, E. M. (1953). Some Indians who stutter. *Journal of Speech and Hearing Disorders, 18,* 168–174.

Lester, L., Cross, D., Dooley, J., & Shaw, T. (2013). Developmental trajectories of adolescent victimization: Predictors and outcomes. *Social Influence, 8,* 107–130.

Lewis, H. (1990). *A question of values.* San Francisco, CA: Harper & Row.

Lincoln, Y. S., & Guba, E. G. (1985). *Naturalistic inquiry.* Beverly Hills, CA: Sage.

Link, B. G., & Phelan, J. C. (2006). Stigma and its public health implications. *The Lancet, 367,* 528–529.

Livingston, J. D., & Boyd, J. E. (2010). Correlates and consequences of internalized stigma for people living with mental illness: A systematic review and meta-analysis. *Social Science & Medicine, 71,* 2150–2161.

Livingston, J. D., Milne, T., Fang, M. L., & Amari, E. (2012). The effectiveness of interventions for reducing stigma related to substance use disorders: A systematic review. *Addiction, 107,* 39–50.

Livingston, J. D., Tugwell, A., Korf-Uzan, K., Cianfrone, M., & Coniglio, C. (2012). Evaluation of a campaign to improve awareness and attitudes of young people towards mental health issues. *Social Psychiatry and Psychiatric Epidemiology, 48,* 1–9.

Logan, K. J., Mullins, M. S., & Jones, K. M. (2008). The depiction of stuttering in contemporary juvenile fiction: Implications for clinical practice. *Psychology in the Schools, 45,* 609–626.

Logan, K. J., & O'Connor, E. M. (2012). Factors affecting occupational advice for speakers who do and do not stutter. *Journal of Fluency Disorders, 37,* 25–41.

Lomay, V. T., & Hinkebein, J. H. (2006). Cultural considerations when providing rehabilitation services to American Indians. *Rehabilitation Psychology, 51,* 36–42.

London, B., Downey, G., Romero-Canyas, R., Rattan, A., & Tyson, D. (2012). Gender-based rejection sensitivity and academic self-silencing in women. *Journal of Personality and Social Psychology, 102,* 961–979.

Lowe, R., Guastella, A. J., Chen, N. M., Menzies, R. G., Packman, A., O'Brian, S., & Onslow, M. (2012). Avoidance of eye gaze by adults who stutter. *Journal of Fluency Disorders, 37,* 263–274.

Mackelprang, R. W., & Salsgiver, R. (1999). *Disability: A diversity model approach in human service practice.* Belmont, CA: Brookes/Cole.

MacKinnon, S. P., Hall, S., & MacIntyre, P. D. (2007). Origins of the stuttering stereotype: Stereotype formation through anchoring-adjustment. *Journal of Fluency Disorders, 32,* 297–309.

Mahady Wilton, M. M., Craig, W. M., & Pepler, D. J. (2000). Emotional regulation and display in classroom victims of bullying: Characteristic expressions of affect, coping styles, and relevant contextual factors. *Social Development, 9,* 226–245.

Major, B., & O'Brien, L. T. (2005). The social psychology of stigma. *Annual Review of Psychology, 56,* 393–421.

Mak, W. W. S., Poon, C. Y. M., Pun, L. Y. K., & Cheung, S. F. (2007). Meta-analysis of stigma and mental health. *Social Science & Medicine, 65,* 245–261.

Manning, W. (2001). *Clinical decision making in fluency disorders* (2nd ed.). San Diego, CA: Singular.

Manning, W. (2010). *Clinical decision making in fluency disorders* (3rd ed.). Albany, NY: Delmar-Cengage Learning.

Manning, W., & Beck, J. (2013). Personality dysfunction in adults who stutter: Another look. *Journal of Fluency Disorders, 38,* 184–192.

Manning, W. H., Burlison, A. E., & Thaxton, D. (1999). Listener response to stuttering modification techniques. *Journal of Fluency Disorders, 24,* 267–280.

Marini, Z. A., & Dane, A. V. (2008). Matching interventions to bullying subtypes: Ensuring programs fit the multifaceted needs of children involved in bullying. In D. Pepler & W. Craig (Eds.), *Understanding and addressing bullying: An international perspective* (pp. 97–126). Bloomington, IN: AuthorHouse.

Maviş, İ., St. Louis, K. O., Özdemir, S., & Toğram, B. (2013). Attitudes of Turkish speech and language therapists toward stuttering. *Journal of Fluency Disorders, 38,* 157–170.

Mayo, R., Mayo, C., Gentry, A., & Hildebrandt, M. (2008, November). *Can listener's attitudes towards person who stutter be modified?* Paper presented at the Annual Convention of the American Speech-Language-Hearing Association, Chicago, IL.

McAllister, J., Collier, J., & Shepstone, L. (2012). The impact of adolescent stuttering on educational and employment outcomes: Evidence from a birth cohort study. *Journal of Fluency Disorders, 37,* 106–121.

McAllister, J., Collier, J., & Shepstone, L. (2013). The impact of adolescent stuttering and other speech problems on psychological well being in adulthood: Evidence from a birth cohort study. *International Journal of Language & Communication Disorders, 48,* 458–468.

McCullough, D. R. C. (2014, September). When police encounter persons who stutter. *Community Policing Dispatch, 6.* Retrieved from http://cops.usdoj.gov/html/dispatch/01 2013/police-and-people-who-stutter.asp

McDavid, J., & Harari, H. (1974). *Psychology and social behavior.* New York, NY: Harper & Row.

McDonald, E. T., & Frick, J. V. (1954). Store clerks' reactions to stuttering. *Journal of Speech and Hearing Disorders, 19,* 306–311.

McGee, L., Kalinowski, J., & Stuart, A. (1996). Effect of a videotape documentary on high school students' perceptions of a high school male who stutterers. *Canadian Journal of Speech-Language Pathology and Audiology, 20,* 240–246.

Menzies, R. G., O'Brian, S., Onslow, M., Packman, A., St. Clare, T., & Block, S. (2008). An experimental clinical trial of a cognitive-behavioral therapy package for chronic stuttering. *Journal of Speech, Language, and Hearing Research, 51,* 1451–1464.

Menzies, R. G., Onslow, M., Packman, A., & O'Brian, S. (2009). Cognitive behavior therapy for adults who stutter: A tutorial for speech-language pathologists. *Journal of Fluency Disorders, 34,* 187–200.

Miller, W. R. (1972). Newe Natakwiappe: Shoshoni stories and dictionary. *University of Utah Anthropological Papers, 94.*

Ministry of Education, Sri Lanka. (2014, September). *Publications.* Retrieved from www.education.gov.lk

Modell, S. (2003, October). *Dependent adults and law enforcement: When worlds collide.* Paper presented at the Beyond Awareness: Advanced Training in the Detection, Investigation & Prosecution of Crimes against Elders & Dependent Adults Conference, Kelseyville, CA.

Modell, S. J., & Copp, D. (2007). Police officers and disability: Perceptions and attitudes. *Intellectual and Developmental Disabilities, 45,* 60–63.

Murphy, S., & Kaffenberger, C. (2007). ASCA national model®: The foundation for supervision of practicum and internship students. *Professional School Counseling, 10*, 289–296.

Murphy, W., & Quesal, R. (2004). Best practices for preparing students to work with people who stutter. *Contemporary Issues in Communication Sciences and Disorders, 31*, 25–39.

Murphy, W. (B.), Quesal, R. W., & Gulker, H. (2007). Covert stuttering. *Perspectives on Fluency and Fluency Disorders, 17*, 4–9.

Murphy, W. P., Yaruss, J. S., & Quesal, R. W. (2007a). Enhancing treatment for school-age children who stutter: I. Reducing negative reactions through desensitization and cognitive restructuring. *Journal of Fluency Disorders, 32*, 121–138.

Murphy, W. P., Yaruss, J. S., & Quesal, R. W. (2007b). Enhancing treatment for school-age children who stutter: II. Reducing bullying through role-playing and self-disclosure. *Journal of Fluency Disorders, 32*, 139–162.

Murugami, M. W. (2009). Disability and identity. *Disabilities Studies Quarterly, 29*. Retrieved from http://dsq-sds.org/article/view/979/1173

Nansel, T. R., Overpeck, M., Pilla, R. S., Ruan, W., Simons-Morton, B., & Scheidt, P. (2001). Bullying behaviors among U.S. youth: Prevalence and association with psychosocial adjustment. *Journal of the American Medical Association, 285*, 2094–2100.

Nario-Redmond, M. R., Noel, J. G., & Fern, E. (2012). Redefining disability, re-imagining the self: Disability identification predicts self-esteem and strategic responses to stigma. *Self and Identity, 12*, 1–21.

National Council on Disability. (2003). *Understanding disabilities in American Indian and Alaska Native communities.* Retrieved from http://www.ncd.gov/publications/2003/Aug12003

National Stuttering Association. (2014a, September). Retrieved from http://www.westutter.org

National Stuttering Association. (2014b, September). *What is stuttering?* Retrieved from http://www.westutter.org/what-is-stuttering/stuttering-info

Nespor, J. (1987). The role of beliefs in the practice of teaching. *Journal of Curriculum Studies, 19*, 317–328.

Nisbett, R., & Ross, L. (1980). *Human inference: Strategies and shortcomings of social judgment.* Englewood Cliffs, NJ: Prentice-Hall.

O'Brian, S., Jones, M., Packman, A., Menzies, R., & Onslow, M. (2011). Stuttering severity and educational attainment. *Journal of Fluency Disorders, 36*, 86–92.

O'Connell, J. C. (1985). A family systems approach for serving rural reservation Native American communities. *Journal of American Indian Education, 24*, 1–6.

O'Connor, H., Madge, C., Shaw, R., & Wellens, J. (2008). Internet-based interviewing. In N. Fielding, R. Less, & G. Blank (Eds.), *The SAGE handbook of online research methods* (pp. 271–289). Thousand Oaks, CA: Sage Publications.

Olweus, D. (1993). *Bullying at school: What we know and what we can do.* Cambridge, UK: Blackwell.

Ostrov, J. M., & Godleski, S. A. (2007). Relational aggression, victimization, and language development: Implications for practice. *Topics in Language Disorders, 27*, 146–166.

Özdemir, R. S., St. Louis, K. O., & Topbaş, S. (2011a). Public attitudes toward stuttering in Turkey: Probability versus convenience sampling. *Journal of Fluency Disorders, 36*, 262–267.

Özdemir, R. S., St. Louis, K. O., & Topbaş, S. (2011b). Stuttering attitudes among Turkish family generations and neighbors from representative samples. *Journal of Fluency Disorders, 36*, 318–333.

Pachigar, V., Stansfield, J., & Goldbart, J. (2011). Beliefs and attitudes of primary school teachers in Mumbai, India towards children who stutter. *International Journal of Disability, Development, and Education, 58*, 287–302.

Palasik, S., Gabel, R., Hughes, C., & Rusnak, E. (2012). Perceptions about occupational experiences by people who stutter. *Perspectives on Fluency and Fluency Disorders, 22*, 21–33.

Panico, J., Healey, E. C., Brouwer, K., & Susca, M. (2005). Listener perceptions of stuttering across two presentation modes: A quantitative and qualitative approach. *Journal of Fluency Disorders, 30*, 65–85.

Patterson, J. J., & Pring, T. T. (1991). Listeners' attitudes to stuttering speakers: No evidence for a gender difference. *Journal of Fluency Disorders, 16*, 201–205.

Pengra, L. M., & Godfrey, J. G. (2001). Different boundaries, different barriers: Disability studies and the Lakota culture. *Disability Studies Quarterly, 21*, 36–51.

Perkins, W. H. (1990). What is stuttering? *Journal of Speech and Hearing Disorders, 55*, 370–382.

Perren, S., & Alsaker, F. D. (2006). Social behaviour and peer relationships of victims, bully-victims, and bullies in kindergarten. *Journal of Child Psychology and Psychiatry, 45*, 45–57.

Petrunik, M., & Shearing, C. (1983). Fragile facades: Stuttering and the strategic manipulation of awareness. *Social Problems, 31*, 125–138.

Pewewardy, C. (2002). Learning styles of American Indian/Alaska Native students: A review of the literature and implications for practice. *Journal of American Indian Education, 41*. Retrieved from http://jaie.asu.edu/v41/V41I3A2.pdf

Phillips, K. W., Rothbard, N. P., & Dumas, T. L. (2009). To disclose or not to disclose? Status distance and self-disclosure in diverse environments. *Academy of Management Review, 34*, 710–732.

Plexico, L., Manning, W. H., & DiLollo, A. (2005). A phenomenological understanding of successful stuttering management. *Journal of Fluency Disorders, 30*, 1–22.

Plexico, L., Manning, W. H., & DiLollo, A. (2010). Client perceptions of effective and ineffective therapeutic alliances during treatment for stuttering. *Journal of Fluency Disorders, 35*, 333–354.

Plexico, L. W., Manning, W. H., & Levitt, H. (2009a). Coping responses by adults who stutter: Part I. Protecting the self and others. *Journal of Fluency Disorders, 34*, 87–107.

Plexico, L., Manning, W. H., & Levitt, H. (2009b). Coping responses by adults who stutter: Part II. Approaching the problem and achieving agency. *Journal of Fluency Disorders, 34*, 108–126.

Plexico, L. W., Plumb, A. M., & Beacham, J. (2013). Teacher knowledge and perceptions of stuttering and bullying in school-age children. *Perspectives on Fluency and Fluency Disorders, 23*, 39–53.

Porter, S., Woodworth, M., & Birt, A. (2000). Truth, lies, and videotape: An investigation of the ability of federal parole officers to detect deception. *Law and Human Behavior, 24*, 643–658.

Prausse, J. E., & Kikano, G. E. (2008). Stuttering: An overview. *American Family Physician, 77*, 1271–1276.

Preston, D. B., D'augelli, A. R., Kassab, C. D., & Starks, M. T. (2007). The relationship of stigma to the sexual risk behavior of rural men who have sex with men. *AIDS Education & Prevention, 19*, 218–230.

Przepiórka, A., Błachnio, A., St. Louis, K. O., & Wozniak, T. (2013). Public attitudes toward stuttering in Poland. *International Journal of Language and Communication Disorders, 48*, 703–714.

Puglik, I. (2010). *Effects of brief brochures on stuttering versus dysarthria on adults' stuttering attitudes in New York City.* Unpublished undergraduate research, Brooklyn College, Brooklyn, NY.

Quesal, R. W. (2010). Empathy: Perhaps the most important *E* in EBP. *Seminars in Speech and Language, 31*, 217–226.

Quinn, D. M., & Chaudoir, S. R. (2009). Living with a concealable stigmatized identity: The impact of anticipated stigma, centrality, salience, and cultural stigma on psychological distress and health. *Journal of Personality and Social Psychology, 97*, 634–651.

Rafuse, J. (1994). Early intervention, intensive therapy can help people who stutter. *Canadian Medical Association Journal, 150*, 754–755.

Ragins, B. R. (2008). Disclosure disconnects: Antecedents and consequences of disclosing invisible stigmas across life domains. *Academy of Management Review, 33*, 194–215.

Ragsdale, J. D., & Ashby, J. K. (1982). Speech and language pathologist's connotations of stuttering. *Journal of Speech and Hearing Research, 25*, 75–80.

Ramig, P. R. (1993). The impact of self-help groups on persons who stutter: A call for research. *Journal of Fluency Disorders, 18*, 351–361.

Raskauskas, J., & Stoltz, A. D. (2007). Involvement in traditional and electronic bullying among adolescents. *Developmental Psychology, 43*, 564–575.

Reed, P., & Wu, Y. (2013). Logistic regression of risk factor modelling in stuttering research. *Journal of Fluency Disorders, 38*, 88–101.

Reese, S., Hoffmann, S., & Li, S. L. (1999, October). *The state of stuttering in China.* Paper presented at the 1999 International Stuttering Awareness Day Online Conference. Retrieved from http://www.mnsu.edu/comdis/isad2/papers/reese.html

Reeves, L. (2006). The role of self-help/mutual aid in addressing the needs of individuals who stutter. In N. Bernstein Ratner & J. Tetnowski (Eds.), *Current issues in stuttering research and practice* (pp. 255–278). Mahwah, NJ: Lawrence Erlbaum Associates.

Reeves, L. (2007). Are self-help/mutual aid groups and professional intervention mutually exclusive concepts for helping those affected by stuttering? *Perspectives on Fluency and Fluency Disorders, 17*, 4–8.

Reichel, I., & St. Louis, K. O. (2004). Effects of emotional intelligence training in graduate fluency disorders courses. In A. Packman, A. Meltzer, & H. F. M. Peters (Eds.), *Proceedings of the 4th World Congress on Fluency Disorders* (pp. 474–481). Nijmegen, The Netherlands: Nijmegen University Press.

Reichel, I., & St. Louis, K. O. (2007). Mitigating negative stereotyping of stuttering in a fluency disorders class. In J. Au-Yeung & M. M. Leahy (Eds.), *Research, treatment, and self-help in fluency disorders: New Horizons. Proceedings of the Fifth World Congress on Fluency Disorders* (pp. 236–243). Dublin: International Fluency Association.

Reichel, I. K., & St. Louis, K. O. (2011, November). *Effects of multidisciplinary curricula in graduate fluency disorders courses.* Seminar presented at the Annual Convention of the American Speech-Language-Hearing Association, San Diego, CA.

Remsberg, C. (1997). *Tactics for criminal patrol: Vehicle stops, drug discovery, and officer survival.* Northbrook, IL: Calibre Press.

Rex-Lear, M., Knack, J. M., & Jensen-Campbell, L. A. (2012). Beyond the playground: Bullying in the workplace and its relation to mental and physical health outcomes. In R. J. Gatchel & I. Z. Schultz (Eds.), *Handbook of occupational health and wellness* (pp. 219–240). New York, NY: Springer Science & Business Media.

Reynolds, W. M. (2003). *Reynolds Bully–Victimization Scales for Schools.* San Antonio, TX: The Psychological Corp.

Rice, M., & Kroll, R. (1994). A survey of stutterers' perceptions of challenges and discrimination in the workplace. In C. W. Starkweather & H. F. M. Peters (Eds.), *Stuttering: Proceedings of the First World Congress on Fluency Disorders* (pp. 559–562). International Fluency Association. Nijmegen, The Netherlands: University Press Nijmegen.

Rice, M., & Kroll, R. (1997). Workplace experiences of people who stutter. *Journal of Fluency Disorders, 22,* 61–62.

Richwood, D. J., & Braithwaite, V. A. (1994). Social-psychological factors affecting help seeking for emotional problems. *Social Science & Medicine, 39,* 563–572.

Rigby, K. (2003). Consequences of bullying in schools. *Canadian Journal of Psychiatry, 48,* 583–590.

Rigby, K., & Slee, P. T. (1991). Bullying among Australian school children: Reported behavior and attitudes toward victims. *The Journal of Social Psychology, 13,* 615–627.

Rigby, K., & Slee, P. T. (1993). *The Peer Relations Questionnaire.* Adelaide, Australia: Institute of Social Research, University of South Australia.

Riley, G. D., (2009). *Stuttering Severity Instrument* (4th ed.). Austin, TX: Pro-Ed.

Robinson, T., & Crowe, T. (2002). Fluency disorders. In D. E. Battle (Ed.), *Communication disorders in multicultural populations* (pp. 267–298). Boston: Butterworth-Heinemann.

Rosenfield, D. (1981). Response of physicians to a mailing about stuttering. *Journal of Fluency Disorders, 6,* 187–188.

Runyan, C. M., & Runyan, S. E. (2007). The fluency rules program for school-age children who stutter. In E. G. Conture & R. F. Curlee (Eds.), *Stuttering and related disorders of fluency* (pp. 100–114). New York, NY: Thieme.

Ruscello, D. M., Lass, N. J., & Brown, J. (1988). College students' perceptions of stutterers. *National Student Speech Language Hearing Association Journal, 16,* 115–120.

Ruscello, D. M., Lass, N. J., Schmitt, J. F., & Pannbacker, M. D. (1994). Special educators' perceptions of stutterers. *Journal of Fluency Disorders, 19,* 125–132.

Ruscello, D. M., Lass, N. J., Schmitt, J. F., Pannbacker, M. D., Hoffman, F. M., Miley, M. A., & Robison, K. L. (1990). Professors' perceptions of stutterers. *National Student Speech Language Hearing Association Journal, 18,* 142–145.

Ryan, B. P. (2001). *Programmed therapy for stuttering in children and adults* (2nd ed.). Springfield, IL: Charles C. Thomas.

Salmivalli, C. (2010). Bullying and the peer group: A review. *Aggression and Violent Behavior, 15*, 112–120.

Salmivalli, C., Karhunen, J., & Lagerspetz, K. M. J. (1996). How do the victims respond to bullying? *Aggressive Behavior, 22*, 99–109.

Salmivalli, C., Lagerspetz, K., Björkqvist, K., Österman, K., & Kaukiainen, A. (1996). Bullying as a group process: Participant roles and their relations to social status within the group. *Aggressive Behavior, 22*, 1–15.

Salmivalli, C., & Peets, K. (2009). Bullies, victims, and bully-victim relationships in middle childhood and early adolescence. In K. H. Rubin, W. M. Bukowski, & B. Laursen (Eds.), *Handbook of peer interactions, relationships, and groups* (pp. 322–340). New York, NY: The Guildford Press.

Salmon, G., James, A., & Smith, D .M. (1998). Bullying in schools: Self-reported anxiety, depression, and self-esteem in secondary school children. *British Medical Journal, 317*, 924–925.

Sanchez, D. T., & Garcia, J. A. (2009). When race matters: Racially stigmatized others and perceiving race as a biological construction affect biracial people's daily well-being. *Personality and Social Psychology Bulletin, 35*, 1154–1164.

Schlagheck, A., Gabel, R., & Hughes, S. (2009). A mixed method study of stereotypes of people who stutter. *Contemporary Issues in Communication Science and Disorders, 36*, 108–117.

Schmader, T., Croft, A., Whitehead, J., & Stone, J. (2013). A peek inside the targets' toolbox: How stigmatized targets deflect discrimination by invoking a common identity. *Basic and Applied Social Psychology, 35*, 141–149.

Schneider, J. (2007). *True life: I stutter* [Television series episode]. New York, NY: MTV.

Schneider, J. W., & Conrad, P. (1980). In the closet with illness: Epilepsy, stigma potential, and information control. *Social Problems, 28*, 32–44.

Schutte, N., & Malouff, J. (1999). *Measuring emotional intelligence and related constructs.* Lewiston, NY: Edwin Mellen Press.

Schwartz, D., Gorman, A. H., Nakamoto, J., & Toblin, R. L. (2005). Victimization in the peer group and children's academic functioning. *Journal of Educational Psychology, 97*, 425–435.

Schwartz, D., Proctor, L. J., & Chien, D. H. (2001). The aggressive victim of bullying: Emotional and behavioural dysregulation as a pathway to victimization by peers. In J. Juvonen & S. Graham (Eds.), *Peer harassment in school: The plight of the vulnerable and the victimized* (pp. 147–174). New York, NY: The Guilford Press.

Schwarz, N. (2007). Attitude construction: Evaluation in context. *Social Cognition, 25*, 638–656.

Selig, R. (1998). Investigating the origins, nature, and cultures of humankind. In R. Selig & M. London (Eds.), *Anthropology explored* (pp. 1–10). Washington, DC: Smithsonian Institution Press.

Sengupta, S., Banks, B., Jonas, D., Miles, M. S., & Smith, G. C. (2011). HIV interventions to reduce HIV/AIDS stigma: A systematic review. *AIDS and Behavior, 15*, 1075–1087.

Shapiro, D. A. (1999). *Stuttering intervention: A collaborative journey to fluency freedom.* Austin, TX: Pro-Ed.

Shapiro, D. A. (2011). *Stuttering intervention: A collaborative journey to fluency freedom* (2nd ed.). Austin, TX: Pro-Ed.

Sheehan, J. G. (1970). *Stuttering: Research and therapy.* New York, NY: Harper & Row.

Sheehan, J. G. (1975). Conflict theory and avoidance-reduction therapy. In J. Eisenson (Ed.), *Stuttering: A second symposium* (pp. 97–198). New York, NY: Harper & Row.

Shelton, J., Alegre, J., & Son, D. (2010). Social stigma and disadvantage: Current themes and future prospects. *Journal of Social Issues, 66,* 618–633.

Siegel, S. (1956). *Nonparametric statistics for the behavioral sciences.* New York, NY: McGraw-Hill.

Silverman, E.-M. (1982). Speech-language clinicians' and university students' impressions of women and girls who stutter. *Journal of Fluency Disorders, 7,* 469–478.

Silverman, E.-M. (2012). *Mindfulness and stuttering: Using eastern strategies to speak with greater ease.* North Charleston, SC: CreateSpace.

Silverman, E.-M., & Zimmer, C. H. (1979). Women who stutter: Personality and speech characteristics. *Journal of Speech and Hearing Research, 22,* 553–564.

Silverman, E.-M., & Zimmer, C. H. (1982). Demographic characteristics and treatment experiences of women and men who stutter. *Journal of Fluency Disorders, 7,* 273–285.

Silverman, F. H. (1985). *Research design and evaluation in speech-language pathology and audiology* (2nd ed.). Englewood Cliffs, NJ: Prentice Hall.

Silverman, F. H. (1988). Impact of a T-shirt message on stutterer stereotypes. *Journal of Fluency Disorders, 13,* 279–281.

Silverman, F. H., & Bongey, T. A. (1997). Nurses' attitudes toward physicians who stutter. *Journal of Fluency Disorders, 22,* 61–62.

Silverman, F. H., & Paynter, K. K. (1990). Impact of stuttering on perception of occupational competence. *Journal of Fluency Disorders, 15,* 87–91.

Silvers, A. (1998). Formal justice. In A. Silvers, D. Wasserman, & M. B. Mahowald (Eds.), *Disability, difference, discrimination: Perspectives on justice in public policy* (pp. 13–145). Lanham, MD: Rowman and Littlefield.

Sirey, J. A., Bruce, M. L., Alexopoulos, G. S., Perlick, D. A., Friedman, S. J., & Meyers, B. S. (2001). Perceived stigma and patient-rated severity of illness as predictors of antidepressant drug adherence. *Psychiatric Services, 52,* 1615–1620.

Siyahhan, S., Aricak, O. T., & Cayirdag-Acar, N. (2012). The relation between bullying, victimization, and adolescents' level of hopelessness. *Journal of Adolescence, 35,* 1053–1059.

Smart, J. (2001). *Disability, society, and the individual.* Austin, TX: Pro-Ed.

Smith, J. A., & Osborn, M. (2003). Interpretive phenomenology analysis. In J. A. Smith (Ed.), *Qualitative psychology* (pp. 51–80). Thousand Oaks, CA: Sage Publications.

Smith, P. K., Shu, S., & Madsen, K. (2001). Characteristics of victims of school bullying: Developmental changes in coping strategies and skills. In J. Juvonen & S. Graham (Eds.), *Peer harassment in school* (pp. 332–351). New York, NY: The Guilford Press.

Smith, P. K., Talamelli, L., Cowie, H., Naylor, P., & Chauhan, P. (2004). Profiles of non-victims, escaped victims, continuing victims, and new victims of school bullying. *British Journal of Educational Psychology, 74,* 565–581.

Snidecor, J. (1947). Why the Indian does not stutter. *Quarterly Journal of Speech, 33,* 493–495.

Snyder, G. J. (2001). Exploratory research in the measurement and modification of attitudes toward stuttering. *Journal of Fluency Disorders, 26,* 149–160.

Soderberg, G. A. (1962). What is "average" stuttering? *Journal of Speech and Hearing Disorders, 27,* 85–86.

Spradley, J. P. (1979). *The ethnographic interview.* New York, NY: Holt, Rinehart, & Winston.

St. Louis, K. O. (1994). Speaking of courage and voices to remember [Review of videos]. *Journal of Fluency Disorders, 19,* 289–293.

St. Louis, K. O. (1999). Person-first labeling and stuttering. *Journal of Fluency Disorders, 24,* 1–24.

St. Louis, K. O. (2001). *Living with stuttering: Stories, basics, resources, and hope.* Morgantown, WV: Populore.

St. Louis, K. O. (2005). A global project to measure public attitudes of stuttering. *The Asha Leader, 10,* 12–13, 22.

St. Louis, K. O. (2006). Measurement issues in fluency disorders. In N. Bernstein Ratner & J. Tetnowski (Eds.), *Current issues in stuttering research and practice* (pp. 61–86). Mahwah, NJ: Lawrence Erlbaum.

St. Louis, K. O. (2008, November). *Surveying public attitudes toward stuttering: Considerations of sample size.* Technical paper presented at the Annual Convention of the Speech-Language-Hearing Association, Chicago, IL.

St. Louis, K. O. (2010, April). *Progress, benefits, and challenges in measuring public opinions about stuttering worldwide.* Invited keynote address at the European Symposium on Fluency Disorders, Antwerp, Belguim.

St. Louis, K. O. (2011a). The Public Opinion Survey of Human Attributes–Stuttering (POSHA–S): Summary framework and empirical comparisons. *Journal of Fluency Disorders, 36,* 256–261.

St. Louis, K. O. (2011b). *User's Guide: Public Opinion Survey of Human Attributes–Stuttering (POSHA–S): Measuring public attitudes toward stuttering.* Morgantown, WV: Populore.

St. Louis, K. O. (2012a). Male versus female attitudes toward stuttering. *Journal of Communication Disorders, 45,* 246–253.

St. Louis, K. O. (2012b). POSHA–S public attitudes toward stuttering: Online versus paper surveys. *Canadian Journal of Speech-Language Pathology and Audiology, 36,* 116–122.

St. Louis, K. O. (2012c). Research and development for a public attitude instrument for stuttering. *Journal of Communication Disorders, 45,* 129–146.

St. Louis, K. O. (2014, September). *International project on attitudes toward human attributes (IPATHA).* Morgantown, WV: Populore. Retrieved from http://www.stutteringattitudes.com

St. Louis, K. O., Andrade, C. R. F., Georgieva, D., & Troudt, F. O. (2005). Experience and personal report about an international cooperation research—Brazil, Bulgaria, and Turkey—attitudes toward stuttering. *Pró-Fono Revista de Atualização Científica, 17,* 413–416.

St. Louis, K. O., & Durrenberger, C. H. (1993, December). What communication disorders do experienced clinicians prefer to manage? *American Speech and Hearing Association, 35,* 23–30.

St. Louis, K. O., Filatova, Y., Coşkun, M., Topbaş, S., Özdemir, S., Georgieva, D., McCaffrey, E., & George, R. D. (2011). Public attitudes toward cluttering and stuttering in four countries.

In E. L. Simon (Ed.), *Psychology of stereotypes* (pp. 81–113). Hauppauge, NY: Nova Science. (Also available online.) Retrieved from https://www.novapublishers.com/catalog/product_info.php?products_id=23253

St. Louis, K. O., & George, R. D. (2008, November). *Attitudes toward stuttering: In search of a gold standard.* Poster presented at the Annual Convention of the Speech-Language-Hearing Association, Chicago, IL.

St. Louis, K. O., & Lass, N. J. (1981). A survey of communicative disorders students' attitudes toward stuttering. *Journal of Fluency Disorders, 6*, 49–79.

St. Louis, K. O., Lubker, B. B., Yaruss, J. S., Adkins, T. A., & Pill, J. C. (2008). Development of a prototype questionnaire to survey public attitudes toward stuttering: Principles and methodologies in the first prototype. *The Internet Journal of Epidemiology, 5.* Retrieved from http://www.ispub.com/journal/the-internet-journal-of-epidemiology/volume-5-number-2/development-of-a-prototype-questionnaire-to-survey-public-attitudes-toward-stuttering-principles-and-methodologies-in-the-first-prototype.html

St. Louis, K. O., Lubker, B. B., Yaruss, J. S., & Aliveto, E. F. (2009). Development of a prototype questionnaire to survey public attitudes toward stuttering: Reliability of the second prototype. *Contemporary Issues in Communication Sciences and Disorders, 36*, 101–107.

St. Louis, K. O., Przepiórka, A. M., Beste-Guldborg, A., Williams, M. J., Błachnio, A., Guendouzi, J., Reichel, I. K., & Ware, M. B. (2014). Stuttering attitudes of students: Professional, intracultural, and international comparisons. *Journal of Fluency Disorders, 39*, 34–50.

St. Louis, K. O., Reichel, I., Yaruss, J. S., & Lubker, B. B. (2009). Construct and concurrent validity of a prototype questionnaire to survey public attitudes toward stuttering. *Journal of Fluency Disorders, 34*, 11–28.

St. Louis, K. O., & Roberts, P. M. (2010). Measuring attitudes toward stuttering: English-to-French translations in Canada and Cameroon. *Journal of Communication Disorders. 43*, 361-377.

St. Louis, K. O., & Roberts, P. M. (2013). Public attitudes toward mental illness in Africa and North America. *African Journal of Psychiatry, 16*, 123–133.

St. Louis, K. O., & Rogers, A. L. (2011a, November). *Predicting stuttering attitudes: Familiarity with stuttering, mental illness, and obesity.* Poster presented at the Annual Convention of the American Speech-Language-Hearing Association, San Diego, CA.

St. Louis, K. O., & Rogers, A. L. (2011b, November). *Predicting stuttering attitudes from socioeconomic indicators: Education, occupation, and income.* Poster presented at the Annual Convention of the American Speech-Language-Hearing Association, San Diego, CA.

St. Louis, K. O., & Schulte, K. (2011). Defining cluttering: The lowest common denominator. In D. Ward & K. Scaler Scott (Eds.), *Cluttering: Research, intervention, and education* (pp. 233–253). East Sussex, UK: Psychology Press.

St. Louis, K. O., Sønsterud, H., Carlo, E. J., Heitmann, R. R., & Kvenseth, H. (2014). Cluttering versus stuttering attitudes in Norway and Puerto Rico. *Journal of Fluency Disorders, 42*, 21–34.

St. Louis, K. O., Tellis, G., Tuanquin, T. C., Wolfenden, R. P., & Nicholson, R. M. (2004, November). *Selected attitudes toward stuttering: SLP fluency specialists, generalists, and students.* Poster presented at the Annual Convention of the American Speech-Language-Hearing Association, Philadelphia, PA.

St. Louis, K. O., Weidner, M. E., Gabel, R., Hughes, S., & Coleman, C. (2014). Stuttering Attitudes Research Symposium: Reflecting on a landmark event. *Perspectives on Fluency and Fluency Disorders, 24*, 5–7.

St. Louis, K. O., Williams, M. J., Ware, M. B., Guendouzi, J., & Reichel, I. (2014). The Public Opinion Survey of Human Attributes–Stuttering (POSHA–S) and Bipolar Adjective Scale (BAS): Aspects of validity. *Journal of Communication Disorders, 50*, 36–50.

Steele, C. M. (1997). A threat in the air: How stereotypes shape intellectual identity and performance. *American Psychologist, 52*, 613–629.

Stewart, J. L. (1960). The problem of stuttering in certain North American Indian societies. *Journal of Speech and Hearing Disorders, Monograph Supplement 6,* 22.

Stonehouse, J. M., & Forrester, G. J. (1998). Robustness and the *t* and *U* tests under combined assumption violations. *Journal of Applied Statistics, 25*, 63–74.

Stromwall, L., & Granhag, P. (2003). How to detect deception? Arresting the beliefs of police officers, prosecutors, and judges. *Psychology, Crime, and Law, 9*, 19–36.

Sugarman, M. (1980). It's OK to stutter: A personal account. *Journal of Fluency Disorders, 5*, 149–157.

Sugden, K., Arseneault, L., Harrington, H., Moffitt, T. E., Williams, B., & Caspi, A. (2010). The serotonin transporter gene moderates the development of emotional problems among children following bullying victimization. *Journal of the American Academy of Child & Adolescent Psychiatry, 49*, 830–840.

Susca, M., & Healey, E. C. (2001). Perceptions of simulated stuttering and fluency. *Journal of Speech, Language, and Hearing Research, 44*, 61–72.

Susca, M., & Healey, E. C. (2002). Listener perceptions along a fluency-disfluency continuum: A phenomonological analysis. *Journal of Fluency Disorders, 27*, 135–161.

Swartz, E., Gabel, R., Hughes, S., & Irani, F. (2009). Speech–language pathologists' responses on surveys on vocational stereotyping (role entrapment) regarding people who stutter. *Contemporary Issues in Communication Sciences and Disorders, 36*, 157–165.

Swartz, E., Gabel, R., & Irani, F. (2009). Speech-language pathologists' attitudes towards people who stutter. *Canadian Journal of Speech-Language Pathology and Audiology, 33*, 99–105.

Swearer, S. M. (2011). *Risk factors for and outcomes of bullying and victimization.* White paper prepared for the United States White House conference on bullying prevention. Retrieved from http://digitalcommons.unl.edu/edpsychpapers/132/

Swim, J. K., Hyers, L. L., Cohen, L. L., & Ferguson, M. J. (2001). Everyday sexism: Evidence for its incidence, nature, and psychological impact from three daily diary studies. *Journal of Social Issues, 57*, 31–53.

Swim, J. K., Mallett, R. K., & Stangor, C. (2004). Understanding subtle sexism: Detection and use of sexist language. *Sex Roles, 51*, 117–128.

Tarkowski, Z. (2005). The social and professional image of a speech-language therapist. In M. Młynarska, T. Smereka (Eds.), *Speech pathology: Theory and practice* (pp. 395–405). Wrocław: Agencja Wydawnicza A linea.

Tatchell, R. H., van den Berg, S., & Lerman, J. W. (1983). Fluency and eye contact as factors influencing observers' perceptions of stutterers. *Journal of Fluency Disorders, 8*, 221–231.

Tellis, G. M., Blood, G. W., Blood, I. M., Lubker, B. B., St. Louis, K. O., Yaruss, J. S., Pill, J., et al. (2000, November). *Multicultural perspectives of stuttering and people who stutter.* Mini-seminar presented at the Annual Convention of the American Speech-Language-Hearing Association, Washington, DC.

Tellis, G., Bressler, L., & Emerick, K. (2008). An exploration of clinician views about assessment and treatment of stuttering. *Perspectives on Fluency and Fluency Disorders, 18*, 16–23.

Tetnowski, J. A., & Damico, J. S. (2001). A demonstration of the advantages of qualitative methodologies in stuttering research. *Journal of Fluency Disorders, 26*, 17–42.

The Stuttering Foundation. (2014a, September). Retrieved from http://www.stutteringhelp.org

The Stuttering Foundation. (2014b, September). *Brief history.* Retrieved from http://www.stutteringhelp.org/brief-history

Tomaiuoli, D., Del Gado, F., Capparelli, E., & St. Louis, K. O. (2013, August). *Stuttering attitudes in Italy.* Paper presented at the 29th World Congress of the International Association of Logopedics and Phoniatrics, Turin, Italy.

Tops, M., Riese, H., Oldehinkel, A. J., Rijsdijke, F. V., & Ormel, J. (2008). Rejection sensitivity relates to hypocortisolism and depressed mood state in young women. *Psychoneuroendocrinology, 33*, 551–559.

Tran, Y., Blumgart, E., & Craig, A. (2011). Subjective distress associated with chronic stuttering. *Journal of Fluency Disorders, 36*, 17–26.

Treasa, J., & Kanaka, G. (2013). *Measuring the teachers' knowledge and attitude towards stuttering using POSHA–S in Udupi district.* Unpublished dissertation, Manipal University, Manipal, India.

Trichon, M. (2007). Getting the maximum benefits from support groups: Perspectives of members and group leaders. *Perspectives on Fluency and Fluency Disorders, 17*, 10–13.

Trichon, M., & Tetnowski, J. (2011). Self-help conferences for people who stutter: A qualitative investigation. *Journal of Fluency Disorders, 36*, 290–295.

Tudor, H., Davis, S., Brewin, C. R., & Howell, P. (2013). Recurrent involuntary imagery in people who stutter and people who do not stutter. *Journal of Fluency Disorders, 38*, 247–259.

Turnbaugh, K. R., Guitar, B. E., & Hoffman, P. R. (1979). Speech clinicians' attribution of personality traits as a function of stuttering severity. *Journal of Speech and Hearing Research, 22*, 37–45.

Turnbaugh, K., Guitar, B., & Hoffman, P. (1981). The attribution of personality traits: The stutterer and nonstutterer. *Journal of Speech and Hearing Research, 24*, 288–291.

Turnbull, A. P., Brotherson, M. J., & Summers, J. A. (1985). The impact of deinstitutionalization of families. In R. Bruininks & K. Lakin (Eds.), *Living and learning in the least restrictive environment* (pp, 115–152). Baltimore, MD: Paul H. Brookes.

Turnbull, J. (2006). Promoting greater understanding in peers of children who stammer. *Emotional & Behavioural Difficulties, 11*, 237–247.

Turner, J. S., & Helms, D. B. (1995). *Lifespan development.* Fort Worth, TX: Harcourt Brace College.

Ulliana, L., & Ingham, R. J. (1984). Behavioral and nonbehavioral variables in the measurement of stutterers' communication attitudes. *Journal of Speech and Hearing Disorders, 49,* 83–93.

U.S. Department of Health and Human Services, Centers for Disease Control and Prevention. (2014a, September). *Vital and health statistics: Summary Health Statistics for U.S. Adults: National Health Interview Survey, 2012* (DHHS Publication no. 260). Retrieved from http://www.cdc.gov/nchs/data/series/sr_10/sr10_260.pdf

U.S. Department of Health and Human Services, Centers for Disease Control and Prevention. (2014b, September). *Vital and health statistics: Summary Health Statistics for U.S. Children: National Health Interview Survey, 2012* (DHHS Publication no. 258). Retrieved from http://www.cdc.gov/nchs/data/series/sr_10/sr10_258.pdf

Usmani, T., Kanaka, G., & Rajashekhar, B. (2012). *Measurement of public attitude towards stuttering in Hindi speaking population.* Unpublished undergraduate dissertation, Manipal University, Manipal, India.

Vaillancourt, T., Clinton, J., McDougall, P., Schmidt, L. A., & Hymel, S. (2010). The neurobiology of peer victimization and rejection. In S. R. Jimerson, S. M. Swearer, & D. L. Espelage (Eds.), *Handbook of bullying in schools: An international perspective* (pp. 293–304). New York, NY: Routledge.

Vaillancourt, T., Duku, E., Becker, S., Schmidt, L. A., Nicol, J., Muir, C., & MacMillan, H. (2011). Peer victimization, depressive symptoms, and high salivary cortisol predict poorer memory in children. *Brain and Cognition, 77,* 191–199.

Valente, A. R. S., Jesus, L. M. T., Leahy, M., & St. Louis, K. O. (2014, March). *Attitudes and knowledge of the Portuguese population about stuttering.* Paper presented at the European Symposium on Fluency Disorders, Antwerp, Belgium.

Van Borsel, J., Brepoels, M., & De Coene, J. (2011). Stuttering, attractiveness, and romantic relationships: The perception of adolescents and young adults. *Journal of Fluency Disorders, 36,* 41–50.

Van Borsel, J., Verniers, I., & Bouvry, S. (1999). Public awareness of stuttering. *Folia Phoniatrica Logopaedica, 51,* 124–132.

Van Riper, C. (1971). *The nature of stuttering.* Englewood Cliffs, NJ: Prentice-Hall.

Van Riper, C. (1973). *The treatment of stuttering.* Englewood Cliffs, NJ: Prentice-Hall.

Van Riper, C. (1982). *The nature of stuttering* (2nd ed.). Englewood Cliffs, NJ: Prentice Hall.

Vescio, T. K., Gervais, S. J., Heiphetz, L., & Bloodhart, B. (2009). The stereotypic behaviors of the powerful and their effect on the relatively powerless. In T. D. Nelson (Ed.), *The handbook of prejudice, stereotyping, and discrimination* (pp. 247–265). New York, NY: Psychology Press.

Von Tiling, J. (2011). Listener perceptions of stuttering, prolonged speech, and verbal avoidance behaviors. *Journal of Communication Disorders, 44,* 161–172.

Vrij, A., & Semin, G. (1996). Lie experts' beliefs about nonverbal indicators of deception. *Journal of Nonverbal Behavior, 20,* 65–80.

Wang, J., Iannotti, R. J., & Nansel, T. R. (2009). School bullying among adolescents in the

United States: Physical, verbal, relational, and cyber. *Journal of Adolescent Health, 45,* 368–375.

Watson, A. C., Corrigan, P. W., Ottati, V. (2004). Police officers' attitudes toward and decisions about persons with mental illness. *Psychiatric Services, 55,* 49–53.

Webster, R. L. (1977). A few observations on the manipulation of speech response characteristics in stutterers. *Journal of Communication Disorders, 10,* 73–76.

Weisel, A., & Spektor, G. (1998). Attitudes toward own communication and toward stuttering. *Journal of Fluency Disorders, 23,* 157–172.

Weiss, M. G., Ramakrishna, J., & Somma, D. (2006). Health-related stigma: Rethinking concepts and interventions. *Psychology, Health, & Medicine, 11,* 277–287.

Węsierska, K. (2012). Speech-language therapists' attitudes towards diagnosis and therapy of early stuttering. In A. Podstolec & K. Węsierska (Eds.), *In the world of speech pathology: Academic resources,* vol. 1 (pp. 211–236). Katowice: Wydawnictwo Uniwersytetu Śląskiego—Agencja Artystyczna PARA.

Węsierska, M., & St. Louis, K. O. (2014). Comparison of attitudes towards stuttering among Polish and English university students. *Chowanna, 42,* 263–284.

Westby, C. (1990). Ethnographic interviewing: Asking the right questions to the right people in the right ways. *Communication Disorders Quarterly, 13,* 101–111.

Whaley, B. B., & Parker, R. G. (2000). Expressing the experience of communicative disability: Metaphors of persons who stutter. *Communication Reports, 13,* 115–125.

White, P. A., & Collins, S. R. (1984). Stereotype formation by inference: A possible explanation for the "stutterer" stereotype. *Journal of Speech and Hearing Research, 27,* 567–570.

Wingate, V. S., Minney, J. A., & Guadagno, R. E. (2013). Sticks and stones may break your bones, but words will always hurt you: A review of cyberbullying. *Social Influence, 8,* 87–106.

Woods, C. L., & Williams, D. E. (1971). Speech clinicians' conceptions of boys and men who stutter. *Journal of Speech and Hearing Disorders, 36,* 225–234.

Woods, C. L., & Williams, D. E. (1976). Traits attributed to stuttering and normally fluent males. *Journal of Speech and Hearing Research, 19,* 267–278.

Woolf, G. (1967). The assessment of stuttering as struggle, avoidance, and expectancy. *British Journal of Disorders of Communication, 2,* 158–171.

World Health Organization. (2001). *The International Classification of Functioning, Disability, and Health: A new tool for understanding disability and health.* Geneva, Switzerland: Author.

World Health Organization. (2012). *Sudan launches Arabic version of the world report on disability.* Retrieved from http://www.emro.who.int/sdn/sudan-events/disability-arabicreport-launch.html

Wright, B. A. (1983). *Physical disability: A psychosocial approach.* New York, NY: Harper & Row.

Xing Ming, J., Jing, Z., Yi Wen, Z., & Van Borsel, J. (2001). Public awareness of stuttering in Shanghai, China. *Logopedics Phoniatrics Vocology, 26,* 145–150.

Yairi, E., & Carrico, D. M. (1992). Early childhood stuttering: Pediatricians' attitudes and practices. *American Journal of Speech-Language Pathology, 1,* 54–62.

Yairi, E., & Seery, C. H. (2011). *Stuttering: Foundations and clinical applications.* Upper Saddle River, NJ: Pearson Higher Education.

Yairi, E., & Williams, D. E. (1970). Speech clinicians' stereotypes of elementary-school boys who stutter. *Journal of Communication Disorders, 3,* 161–170.

Yaruss, J. S. (1998). Describing the consequences of disorders: Stuttering and the International Classification of Impairments, Disabilities, and Handicaps. *Journal of Speech, Language, and Hearing Research, 41,* 249–257.

Yaruss, J. S. (2001). Evaluating treatment outcomes for adults who stutter. *Journal of Communication Disorders, 34,* 163–182.

Yaruss, J. S. (2010). Assessing quality of life in stuttering treatment outcomes research. *Journal of Fluency Disorders, 35,* 190–202.

Yaruss, J. S., & Quesal, R. W. (2002). Academic and clinical education in fluency disorders: An update. *Journal of Fluency Disorders, 27,* 43–63.

Yaruss, J. S., & Quesal, R. W. (2004a). Describing the consequences of disorders: Stuttering and the International Classification of Impairments, Disabilities, and Handicaps. *Journal of Communication Disorders, 37,* 35–52.

Yaruss, J. S., & Quesal, R.W. (2004b). Stuttering and the International Classification of Functioning, Disability, and Health (ICF): An update. *Journal of Communication Disorders, 37,* 35–52.

Yaruss, J. S., & Quesal, R. W. (2008). *Overall Assessment of the Speaker's Experience of Stuttering (OASES).* Bloomington, MN: Pearson Assessments.

Yaruss, J. S., Quesal, R. W., & Coleman, C. (2010). *Overall Assessment of the Speaker's Experience of Stuttering: Ages 13–17 (OASES-T) Response form.* Bloomington, MN: Pearson Assessments.

Yaruss, J. S., Quesal, R. W., & Murphy, B. (2002). National stuttering association members' opinions about stuttering treatment. *Journal of Fluency Disorders, 27,* 227–242.

Yaruss, J. S., Quesal, R. W., Reeves, L., Molt, L. F., Kluetz, B., Caruso, A. J., & Lewis, F. (2002). Speech treatment and support group experiences of people who participate in the National Stuttering Association. *Journal of Fluency Disorders, 27,* 115–134.

Yeakle, M. K., & Cooper, E. B. (1986). Teacher perceptions of stuttering. *Journal of Fluency Disorders, 11,* 345–359.

Yen, C. F., Chen, C. C., Lee, Y., Tang, T. C., Yen, J. Y., & Ko, C. H. (2005). Self-stigma and its correlates among outpatients with depressive disorders. *Psychiatric Services, 56,* 599–601.

Zimmerman, G., Liljeblad, S., Frank, A., & Cleeland, C. (1983). The Indians have many terms for it. *Journal of Speech and Hearing Research, 26,* 315–331.

About the Authors

Fauzia Abdalla, PhD, CCC-SLP, earned her doctoral degree in speech-language pathology from McGill University, Montreal, Canada. She is currently an Associate Professor in the Department of Communication Disorders at Kuwait University. Dr. Abdalla's research has focused on morpho-syntax and gestures in developmental language disorders and psychosocial aspects of communication disorders and stuttering. Her studies of Arab attitudes toward stuttering and controlled procedures for changing public attitudes toward stuttering were recognized with research awards from the University of Kuwait.

Julie Atwood, MEd, is Professor Emerita in the Communication Sciences and Disorders Department at the Massachusetts General Hospital Institute of Health Professions, Boston, MA. While Director of the MGH's Speech-Language Pathology and Swallowing Department, she was the primary developer of the MGH Institute's Communication Sciences and Disorders degree granting program and the first graduate program's Director. The highest honor awarded to a graduating speech-language pathology student each year is the Julie Atwood Award for Excellence in CSD. Professor Atwood is an ASHA Fellow and recipient of the MA Speech-Language Hearing Association's Distinguished Service Award.

Ann Beste-Guldborg, PhD, is an Assistant Professor of Communication Disorders at Minot State University. She has been a practicing speech-language pathologist, teacher, administrator, and mentor for 29 years. Dr. Guldborg's research passion involves exploring and understanding attitudes and attitudinal change surrounding communication disorders. She has presented her research widely in various professional realms.

Gordon W. Blood, PhD, CCC-SLP, is currently Professor and Department Head in the Department of Communication Sciences and Disorders at The Pennsylvania State University, where he also teaches graduate courses in fluency disorders. He has published extensively and shared the results of his funded research and specific treatment ideas at state, national, and international conferences. He specializes in the treatment of children, adolescents, and adults who stutter. His core research interests encompass the psychosocial aspects of stuttering, including the negative influences of anxiety, communication apprehension, physiological and psychological stress, and bullying. Additionally, he studies effective ways of dealing and coping with these adverse factors to improve the quality of life for individuals who stutter. Other research has addressed auditory and brain processing in people who stutter.

Dinamichele Boyer pursued her master's studies at Misericordia University in speech-language pathology. She has an interest in the identification and analysis of stuttering attitudes and experiences among people who stutter.

Michael P. Boyle, PhD, CCC-SLP, received his doctorate in Communication Sciences and Disorders from The Pennsylvania State University in 2012. He is an Assistant Professor of Communication Sciences and Disorders at Oklahoma State University, where he teaches graduate courses in fluency disorders and research methods. His research focuses on psychosocial aspects of stuttering, including stigma and well-being.

Megan Burgess, MS, earned her bachelor's and master's degrees from West Virginia University in Communication Sciences and Disorders. She was involved in independent research that focused on measuring stuttering attitudes in both children and adults. Her research has been presented at state and national conventions.

Nichole Campanele, MS, completed her undergraduate studies in Communications at Temple University and graduate studies in Speech-Language Pathology from Minot State University. While pursuing her degree at Minot University, Nichole worked as a graduate research assistant and was involved in research examining perceptions, attitudes, and beliefs of Eastern American Indians. She has presented her research at various conventions and symposiums.

Susanne Cook, PhD, is a speech-language pathologist and stuttering specialist from Germany. She completed her doctorate in Developmental Science at University College London in 2011. She has been running an intensive therapy summer program for stuttering children and adolescents for 10 years wherein she has developed a multifactor model to predict therapy outcomes for children who stutter. Her research interests include therapy outcomes for children who stutter, orofacial training for people who stutter, the psychosocial impact of stuttering on a person's life, and bullying related to stuttering.

Derek E. Daniels, PhD, CCC-SLP, earned his doctorate from Bowling Green State University in 2007. He is a speech-language pathologist and Associate Professor of Communication Sciences and Disorders at Wayne State University in Detroit, MI. There, Derek is Director of the Stuttering Clinic, teaches courses in the area of stuttering, and has published and presented on stuttering as it relates to identity development, school experiences, psychosocial experiences, and treatment outcomes.

Jill Douglass, PhD, CCC-SLP, is a speech-language pathologist and Associate Professor at Sacred Heart University in Fairfield, Connecticut. As a result of her involvement in local and national self-help groups for people who stutter, she has dedicated her career to advocating and giving a voice to people who stutter and to educating future clinicians.

Yomna Elsiddig, MS, CCC-SLP, received her bachelor's degree from Northwestern University and her master's degree in Speech-Language Pathology from MGH Institute of Health Professions. Her interests and experiences include children and adults with developmental delays, hearing impairment, fluency disorders, and aphasia. As a bilingual SLP in English and Arabic, she has a special interest in working with culturally and linguistically diverse populations.

Rodney Gabel, PhD, CCC-SLP, BCS-F, is an Associate Professor at the University of Toledo. He teaches courses in stuttering and directs the Northwest Ohio Intensive Stuttering Clinics, which serves children, adolescents, and adults who stutter and their families. Dr. Gabel has published more than 50 articles and presented nearly 100 papers and posters at international, national, and state conventions. He continues to conduct research that explores outcomes of stuttering therapy and psychosocial impact of stuttering.

Charles Haynes, EdD, CCC-SLP, is a Professor in the Communication Sciences and Disorders Department at the MGH Institute of Health Professions in Boston. A practicing speech-language pathologist, he received his doctorate in reading, language and learning disabilities at the Harvard Graduate School of Education. Dr. Haynes has been principal or coprincipal investigator on many externally funded studies in the United States and the Middle East, and is currently collaborating with researchers from Tunisia, Egypt, and Saudi Arabia to develop diagnostic and intervention tools for spoken and written Arabic.

Peter Howell, PhD, has worked at University College London since 1972. He is Professor of Experimental Psychology and codirector of the Centre for Human Communications. His work spans music perception, auditory perception, and speech perception and production. His interest in the field of stuttering stems from his early research into the relationship between speech perception and production. He has worked in the area of stuttering for about 25 years.

Stephanie Hughes, PhD, CCC-SLP is on the faculty at the University of Toledo, where she is also the Assistant Director of the Northwest Ohio Stuttering Clinics. Stephanie's research has investigated fluent speakers' perceptions of people who stutter, as well as other psychosocial issues, such as childhood bullying and quality of life for people with communication disorders.

Chantha K. Jayawardena, received her Bachelor of Dental Surgery at University of Peradeniya, Sri Lanka, and completed her doctoral studies at Tokyo Medical and Dental University, Japan. She is a Senior Lecturer in the Department of Basic Sciences, Faculty of Dental Science at the University of Peradeniya, Sri Lanka. She teaches anatomy and carries out research in the fields of craniofacial development and adult education.

Lejla Junuzović-Žunić, PhD, is an Associate Professor and Department Chair of Speech and Language Pathology in the Faculty of Education and Rehabilitation at University of Tuzla, Bosnia and Herzegovina. She teaches courses and carries out research in the field of fluency disorders, as well as in articulation and phonological disorders.

Chelsea Kuhn, MS, earned her bachelor's and master's degrees from West Virginia University in Communication Sciences and Disorders. Having a strong interest in stuttering, she was involved in independent research with focus on measuring stuttering attitudes in children and adults that was presented at state and national conventions. Her master's studies also involved examining attitude change in middle school students.

K. A. S. Saminda Kuruppu, BSc, received her degree in Speech & Language Therapy from the University of Kelaniya, Sri Lanka, and her diploma in

Special Education from the National Institute of Education, Sri Lanka. She is a speech-language pathologist in the Lyceum International School, Colombo, Sri Lanka, and resource person for Diploma in Special Education in National Institute of Education. Her research interests focus on fluency disorders.

Marilyn Langevin, PhD, is the Director of Research at the Institute for Stuttering Treatment and Research and Associate Professor of Communication Sciences and Disorders in the Faculty of Rehabilitation Medicine, University of Alberta. Dr. Langevin's research interests include the social impact of stuttering on children, evidence-based treatment and clinical training practices, and neural function associated with stuttering. She developed *Teasing and Bullying: Unacceptable Behaviour* (*TAB*), a resource that aims to prevent bullying in schools and educate students about stuttering.

Staci LeMasters, MS, earned her bachelor's and master's degrees from West Virginia University in Communication Sciences and Disorders. She was involved in independent research projects examining public attitudes toward stuttering, both in children and adults. Her undergraduate research was recognized by an award by the College of Education and Human Services.

Lindsey Lytwak, MS, CCC-SLP, received her master's degree in speech-language pathology from West Virginia University. Lindsey was involved in stuttering research focusing on developing a new clinical instrument to measure attitudes among the family and friends of people who stutter. She currently works clinically as a speech-language pathologist in acute care.

Ahmad Poormohammad, MSC, is a speech-language pathologist and part-time lecturer at the Mashhad University of Medical Sciences in Iran. He is employed at the Ebnesina Mental Hospital of Mashhad, where he is involved in the evaluation and treatment of adolescents who stutter. He formerly worked for six years at primary exceptional schools with mentally deficient students.

Isabella K. Reichel, EdD, CCC-SLP/A, is an Associate Professor at Touro College, New York. She has integrated additional curricula into fluency disorders courses to investigate and mitigate negative stereotyping toward stuttering. She serves as Chair of the International Representatives Committee of the International Cluttering Association. Her papers on cluttering in collaboration with colleagues from around the world are published and presented nationally and internationally.

Christopher P. Roseman, PhD, is an Associate Professor in the Counselor Education Program at The University of Toledo. He is licensed as a Professional Counselor-Clinical Resident (PC-CR) in Ohio and an instructor in Non-violent Crisis Intervention for the Crisis Prevention Institute. Dr. Roseman has authored refereed articles and book chapters in the areas of substance abuse, sexual offending/victimization, and empathic accuracy.

Kathleen Scaler Scott, PhD, is a Board Certified Specialist in Fluency Disorders, practicing clinician, and Assistant Professor of Speech-Language Pathology at Misericordia University. Her research interests are largely in cluttering and atypical disfluencies. Dr. Scaler Scott is the author of numerous publications and has spoken nationally and internationally on the topics of fluency, learning differences, and social pragmatic disorders.

Kenneth O. St. Louis, PhD, is a Professor in the Department of Communication Sciences & Disorders at West Virginia University. For 40 years, he has taught and treated fluency disorders; presented papers at state, national, and international venues; and published numerous articles, chapters, and books. He is an ASHA Fellow, was a cofounder of the International Fluency Association and the International Cluttering Association, and is a recipient of the Deso Weiss Award for Excellence in cluttering. In 1999, he founded the International Project of Attitudes Toward Human Attributes and has collaborated with numerous colleagues internationally on measuring public attitudes toward stuttering. Other current research interests include the definition and symptoms of cluttering and stories of stuttering.

Edward Strugalla, MHS, is a speech-language pathologist with a Master of Health Science in Communication Disorders from Governors State University. He provides speech-language services in the Illinois Early Intervention program and Illinois public schools through his employment at Therapy Care, Ltd. He has presented clinical research at state and national conventions and also conducted presentations on student-initiated research and clinical applications.

Glen Tellis, PhD, is a Board-Certified Fluency Specialist and is Professor and Chair of the Speech-Language Pathology Department at Misericordia University in Dallas, Pennsylvania. He completed his doctorate at The Pennsylvania State University. His research interests include fluency disorders, multicultural issues, research designs, treatment efficacy research, advanced digital technology, and clinical outcomes. He has regularly presented papers at national and international conferences and has published articles that pertain to stuttering and other fluency disorders, as well as articles addressing culturally and linguistically diverse populations.

John A. Tetnowski, PhD, is the Ben Blanco Endowed Professor of Communicative Disorders at the University of Louisiana–Lafayette, where he is also the Coordinator of the Graduate Program in Communicative Disorders and the PhD Program in Applied Language and Speech Sciences. He is a Board-Certified Specialist in Fluency Disorders and has treated people who stutter for over 25 years. In addition, he has published over 60 manuscripts in journals, textbooks, and other outlets in the areas of stuttering, cluttering, and research design. He is a Fellow of the American Speech-Language-Hearing Association, and is a past winner of the National Stuttering Association's Speech-Language Pathologist of the Year.

Mercedes Ware, MS, received her bachelor's degree from West Virginia University and master's degree from Ohio University in speech-language pathology. She has been involved in numerous studies pertaining to students' attitudes toward stuttering, presented at national conventions and published in peer-reviewed journals. She is currently a clinical speech-language pathologist in a residential health care facility.

Mary Weidner, MS, is a doctoral student in Communication Sciences and Disorders at West Virginia University. She received her bachelor's and master's degrees from Indiana University of Pennsylvania and worked clinically at Children's Hospital of Pittsburgh. Her research interests include measuring and improving attitudes of young children toward peers who stutter. She also is codirector of Stuttering U., a camp for children who stutter and their families.

Katarzyna Węsierska, PhD, is a Professor in the Department of Sociolinguistics and Social Communication Practices at the University of Silesia, Poland. She is the founder and speech-language pathologist at the Logopedic Centre in Katowice, Poland. She was the first Polish recipient of the European Clinical Specialization in Fluency Disorders. Her research and clinical interests focus mainly on fluency disorders.

Marta Węsierska is a doctoral student at the University of York, UK. She completed her master's degree in Developmental Psychology at the University of

York, and bachelor's degree in Psychology from the University of Warwick, UK. Her research interests include language development in bilingual Polish–English children, speech and fluency disorders, and public attitudes toward people with communication disorders.

Author Index

Authors are listed alphabetically and followed by the chapter number(s) in which they are cited. A single citation of an author of one reference is listed only by the chapter number; two or more different citations of the author are listed by chapter numbers followed, in parentheses, by the number of different citations.

Abdalla, F. 1, 2(2), 5(4), 6, 7, 8, 9(2), 11, 12(2), 13, 14(2), 16, 21
Action for Stammering Children 5
Adkins, T. 1, 6, 16
Akehurst, L. 11
Al-Khaledi, M. 1, 6, 7, 9
Al-Saddah, A. 5
Alegre, J. 2
Alexopoulos, G. 2
Alghazo, E. 13
Aliveto, E. 1, 13, 14
Allard, E. 6, 11
Allport, G. 4
Alsaker, F. 3
Alshatti, T. 1, 6, 7, 9
Altholz, S. 11(2)
Althouse, M. 2, 4(2), 5, 9, 10, 11, 21(2)
Amari, E. 2
Amatya, K. 3, 20
American Psychiatric Association 19
American Speech-Language-Hearing Association 2, 6
Amster, B. 14
An Xue , S. 1, 2, 5, 6, 8, 9, 13, 14, 16, 21
Andel, S. 2
Andrade, C. 1, 5
Andreou, E. 3
Andrews, G. 11, 13
Areseneault, L. 3(2)

Aricak , O. 3
Armson, J. 2(2), 5, 6, 7, 21(3)
Arnold, H. 1(2), 2, 4, 12
Arora, C. 3
Arthur, B. 6, 7, 21
Ashby, J. 4, 11, 13, 21
Ashurst, J. 11
Atadzhanov, M. 2
Baird, J. 11
Baker, J. 5
Baldry, A. 3
Ball 3
Baly, M. 3
Bandura, A. 2
Bandyopadhyay, S. 3
Banerjee, S. 2
Banks, B. 2
Bar, A. 21
Barclay, D. 21
Barney, E. 5
Barr, L. 2
Barreto, M. 2
Bass, C. 13
Baum, A. 3
Bauman, A. 15
Beacham, J. 11
Beals, K. 2
Beatty, J. 2
Bebout, L. 6, 7, 21

www.ingramcontent.com/pod-product-compliance
Lightning Source LLC
Chambersburg PA
CBHW072059040426
42334CB00041B/1360